Controversies in Acute Trauma and Reconstruction

Editors

JORGE FILIPPI
GERMAN JOANNAS

FOOT AND ANKLE CLINICS

www.foot.theclinics.com

Consulting Editor
MARK S. MYERSON

December 2020 • Volume 25 • Number 4

ELSEVIER

1600 John F. Kennedy Boulevard • Suite 1800 • Philadelphia, Pennsylvania, 19103-2899

http://www.theclinics.com

FOOT AND ANKLE CLINICS Volume 25, Number 4
December 2020 ISSN 1083-7515, ISBN-978-0-323-77542-7

Editor: Lauren Boyle
Developmental Editor: Nicole Congleton

Foot and Ankle Clinics (ISSN 1083-7515) is published quarterly by Elsevier, Inc., 360 Park Avenue South, New York, NY 10010-1710. Months of issue are March, June, September, and December. Periodicals postage paid at New York, NY, and additional mailing offices. Subscription price per year is $340.00 (US individuals), $582.00 (US institutions), $100.00 (US students), $371.00 (Canadian individuals), $669.00 (Canadian institutions), $100.00 (Canadian students), $470.00 (international individuals), $669.00 (international institutions), and $215.00 (international students). To receive student/resident rate, orders must be accompanied by name of affiliated institution, date of term, and the *signature* of program/residency coordinator on institution letterhead. Orders will be billed at individual rate until proof of status is received. Foreign air speed delivery is included in all *Clinics* subscription prices. All prices are subject to change without notice. **POSTMASTER:** Send address changes to *Foot and Ankle Clinics*, Elsevier Health Sciences Division, Subscription Customer Service, 3251 Riverport Lane, Maryland Heights, MO 63043. **Customer Service: 1-800-654-2452 (US and Canada). From outside of the United States and Canada, call 314-447-8871. Fax: 314-447-8029. E-mail: JournalsCustomerService-usa@ elsevier.com (for print support); JournalsOnlineSupport-usa@elsevier.com (for online support).**

Reprints. For copies of 100 or more, of articles in this publication, please contact the Commercial Reprints Department, Elsevier Inc., 360 Park Avenue South, New York, NY 10010-1710. Tel.: 212-633-3874; Fax: 212-633-3820; E-mail: reprints@elsevier.com.

Contributors

CONSULTING EDITOR

MARK S. MYERSON, MD
Professor of Orthopedic Surgery, University of Colorado, Past President American Orthopedic Foot and Ankle Society, Editor in Chief, Foot and Ankle Clinics of North America, Executive Director and Founder, Steps2Walk, Denver, Colorado, USA

EDITORS

JORGE FILIPPI, MD, MBA
Department of Orthopedic Surgery, Foot and Ankle Unit, Clinica Las Condes, Las Condes, Santiago, Chile; Department of Orthopedic Surgery, Foot and Ankle Unit, Hospital del Trabajador, Providencia, Santiago, Chile

GERMAN JOANNAS, MD
Foot and Ankle Division "CEPP," Instituto Dupuytren, Foot and Ankle Division, Orthopaedics Department, Centro Artroscopico Jorge, Batista SA, Ciudad Autonoma de Buenos Aires, Argentina; Instituto Barrancas Buenos Aires, Argentina

AUTHORS

PAUL ANDRZEJOWSKI, BMedSci(Hons), BMBS, MRCS
Clinical Research Fellow (Registrar), Academic Department of Trauma and Orthopaedics, School of Medicine, University of Leeds, Leeds General Infirmary, Leeds, United Kingdom

GUILLERMO MARTIN ARRONDO, MD
Foot and Ankle Division "CEPP," Instituto Dupuytren, Ciudad Autónoma de Buenos Aires, Argentina

CHRISTIAN BASTIAS, MD
Foot and Ankle Surgeon, Chief, Foot and Ankle Unit, Hospital Mutual de Seguridad, Chief, Foot and Ankle Unit, Clínica Santa María, Santiago,Chile

GONZALO F. BASTIAS, MD
Department of Orthopedic Surgery, Foot and Ankle Unit, Clinica Las Condes, Department of Orthopedic Surgery, Foot and Ankle Unit, Hospital del Trabajador, Department of Orthopedic Surgery, Universidad de Chile, Complejo Hospitalario San Jose, Santiago, Chile

ANDRZEJ BOSZCZYK, MD, PhD
Department of Traumatology and Orthopaedics, Centre of Postgraduate Medical Education, Professor, Adam Gruca Clinical Hospital, Otwock, Poland

JORGE BRICENO, MD
Assistant Professor, Department of Orthopaedic Surgery, Pontificia Universidad Catolica de Chile, Santiago, Chile

MICHELLE M. COLEMAN, MD, PhD
Foot and Ankle Fellow, Department of Orthopaedic Surgery, MedStar Union Memorial Hospital, Baltimore, Maryland, USA

CESAR DE CESAR NETTO, MD, PhD
Professor, Department of Orthopedics and Rehabilitation, University of Iowa, Iowa City, Iowa, USA

SANTIAGO ESLAVA, MD
Foot and Ankle Division, Instituto Dupuytren, Ciudad Autónoma de Buenos Aires, Argentina

JORGE FILIPPI, MD, MBA
Department of Orthopedic Surgery, Foot and Ankle Unit, Clinica Las Condes, Las Condes, Santiago, Chile; Department of Orthopedic Surgery, Foot and Ankle Unit, Hospital del Trabajador, Providencia, Santiago, Chile

PETER V. GIANNOUDIS, MD, FACS, FRCS
Professor, Academic Department of Trauma and Orthopaedics, School of Medicine, University of Leeds, Leeds General Infirmary, Leeds, United Kingdom

ALEXANDRE LEME GODOY-SANTOS, MD, PhD
Professor, Department of Orthopedic Surgery, Faculdade de Medicina, Universidade de São Paulo, Foot and Ankle Surgeon, Hospital Israelita Albert Einstein, São Paulo, São Paulo, Brazil

GREGORY P. GUYTON, MD
Attending and Foot and Ankle Fellowship Director, Department of Orthopaedic Surgery, MedStar Union Memorial Hospital, Baltimore, Maryland, USA

GERMAN JOANNAS, MD
Foot and Ankle Division "CEPP," Instituto Dupuytren, Foot and Ankle Division, Orthopaedics Department, Centro Artroscopico Jorge, Batista SA, Ciudad Autonoma de Buenos Aires, Argentina; Instituto Barrancas Buenos Aires, Argentina

GABRIEL KHAZEN, MD
Hospital de Clinicas Caracas, San Bernardino, Caracas, Venezuela

JOHN Y. KWON, MD
Chief, Orthopaedic Foot and Ankle Service, Associate Professor, Department of Orthopaedic Surgery, Harvard Medical School, Beth Israel Deaconess Medical Center, Boston, Massachusetts, USA

LEONARDO LAGOS, MD
Foot and Ankle Surgeon, Foot and Ankle Unit, Hospital Mutual de Seguridad, Foot and Ankle Unit, Clínica Santa María, Santiago, Chile

ANNA-KATHRIN LEUCHT, MD
Department of Orthopaedic Surgery and Traumatology, Cantonal Hospital of Winterthur, Switzerland

ALAIN MASQUELET, MD
Professor, Department of Orthopaedic Surgery, Avicenne Hospital AP–HP, Bobiny, France

STEFAN RAMMELT, MD, PhD
Professor, Head of the Foot and Ankle Center, University Center for Orthopaedics, Trauma and Plastic Surgery, University Hospital Carl Gustav Carus at the TU Dresden, Dresden, Germany

CESAR KHAZEN RASSI, MD
Hospital de Clinicas Caracas, San Bernardino, Caracas, Venezuela

TIM SCHEPERS, MD, PhD
Traumasurgeon, Trauma Unit, Amsterdam UMC location AMC, Amsterdam, The Netherlands

FLORENCIO PABLO SEGURA, MD
Department of Orthopaedics, Faculty of Medicine, Universidad Nacional de Córdoba, Nuevo Hospital San Roque; Centro Privado de Ortopedia y Traumatología, Ciudad de Córdoba, Argentina

DEREK S. STENQUIST, MD
Harvard Combined Orthopaedic Residency Program, Massachusetts General Hospital, Boston, Massachusetts, USA

MICHAEL P. SWORDS, DO
Michigan Orthopedic Center, Chair, Department of Orthopedic Surgery, Director of Orthopedic Trauma, Sparrow Hospital, Lansing, Michigan, USA

ANDREA VELJKOVIC, MD, BComm, MPH, FRCSC
Associate Clinical Professor, University of British Columbia, Department of Orthopedics, St. Paul's Hospital, Footbridge Centre for Integrated Orthopaedic Care, Footbridge Clinic, Vancouver, Canada

BRIAN WEATHERFORD, MD
Orthopaedic Trauma, Reconstructive Foot and Ankle Surgery, Illinois Bone and Joint Institute, Glenview, Illinois, USA; Clinical Assistant Professor of Orthopaedics, University of Chicago Pritzker School of Medicine, Chicago, Illinois, USA

ALASTAIR YOUNGER, MB, ChB, MSc, ChM, FRCSC
Professor Head of Distal Extremities, University of British Columbia, Department of Orthopaedics, St. Paul's Hospital, Footbridge Centre for Integrated Orthopaedic Care, Footbridge Clinic, Vancouver, British Columbia, Canada

Editorial Advisory Board

Contents

> The tibial pilon fracture is a complex lesion, which requires experienced clinical judgment and adequate planning to achieve good results. Treatment concepts enunciated by Rüedi and Allgöwer remain valid but have undergone modifications. The reconstitution of the fibular length is not always the first step to be performed. In the reconstruction of the articular surface, the prognosis is already sealed by the initial cartilage damage, and it is better to achieve stability and alignment. The stabilization of the medial column is essential, but it must be associated with the stabilization of at least one other column in complex fractures.

> External fixation is an essential tool in the management of high-energy pilon fractures. Reduction techniques using the external fixator and fixation constructs for use with external fixation as a part of stage management are reviewed. The concepts of external fixation with limited articular fixation is discussed. The use of circular external fixation in both acute management of high-energy pilon fractures, as well as the indications and technique for acute ankle arthrodesis as part of primary treatment of pilon fractures are outlined.

> Bone defects to the distal tibia, foot, and ankle can be challenging to reconstruct. The induced membrane (Masquelet) technique has become an established method of repair for challenging areas of bone loss. It has been applied in acute open fractures, chronic nonunion, osteomyelitis, and gout erosion. This article presents a systematic review of distal tibia, foot, and ankle results using the Masquelet procedure, which should be considered in cases of challenging critical bone loss. Further work is needed to present large studies of the procedure on foot and ankle patients to consolidate current knowledge.

Anatomic reduction of the posterior malleolus is mandatory for a good functional outcome. Preoperative planning with a computed tomography scan's axial view helps to decide which approach and surgical position we should choose. Based on posterior malleolus fracture anatomy, a guideline is suggested to facilitate decision making on which approach seems to give the best exposure with minimum complications.

There is no consensus on whether the deltoid ligament must be repaired in ankle fractures. Recent studies have shown better early radiologic results when the deltoid ligament is repaired, but no differences in long term functional outcomes. However, there is evidence suggesting that patients with high fibular fractures or injuries with concomitant syndesmotic instability may benefit from repair. The authors recommend repairing the deltoid ligament complex in bimalleolar equivalent fractures associated with syndesmotic or gross multiligamentous instability as well as in heavier patients with greater mechanical requirements.

Nearly half of surgically treated ankle fractures may have associated syndesmotic disruption, and the quality of reduction has been shown to affect functional outcomes. Malreduction ranges from 15% to 50% in the literature, and achieving anatomic reduction remains a significant challenge, even for experienced surgeons. Keys to success include having a stepwise plan and an understanding of reliable fluoroscopic parameters to help achieve reduction in both the coronal and sagittal planes. This article summarizes the literature on syndesmotic reduction and provides the authors' preferred reduction technique using fluoroscopy.

Chronic syndesmotic injury covers a broad range of symptoms and pathologies. Anterolateral ankle impingement without instability is treated by arthroscopic debridement. Subacute, unstable, syndesmotic injuries are treated by arthroscopic or open debridement followed by secondary stabilization using suture button device or permanent screw placement. Chronic syndesmotic instability is treated by a near-anatomic ligamentoplasty supplemented by screw fixation. In case of poor bone stock, failed ligament reconstruction, or comorbidities, tibiofibular fusion with bone grafting is preferred. Malleolar malunions and particularly anterior or posterior syndesmotic avulsions must be corrected in order to achieve a stable and congruent ankle mortise.

Correct approach selection in talar neck injuries is crucial to obtain adequate access to the entire fracture site avoiding malreduction and angular deformity. The major concern about a single incision technique is lack of visualization. Combined lateral and medial approaches are strongly recommended in complex talar neck fractures providing better control of dorsal and varus displacement of the talar head.

Displaced intra-articular calcaneal fractures are among the most difficult articular fractures to treat, with a high rate of potential complications. Is important to restore calcaneus posterior facet anatomy as well as calcaneus width, length, and height. The extensile lateral approach provides excellent fracture visualization and allows reduction of the displaced fracture fragments, but high complication rate has been described with this approach, so many studies favor the sinus tarsi approach. Recent evidence favoring sinus tarsi rather than the extensile lateral approach has shifted opinion toward this less invasive approach, which can be considered the new gold standard.

The quest for the best treatment of displaced intraarticular calcaneal fractures continues. The open reduction and internal fixation of displaced intraarticular calcaneal fractures yields the best results if anatomic reduction is obtained and complications are avoided. The sinus tarsi approach is becoming the new gold standard. In cases with severe comminution or when anatomic reduction cannot be obtained, a primary subtalar arthrodesis is a valuable option, if the overall anatomy of the calcaneus is corrected first. This review discusses the open reduction and internal fixation of displaced intraarticular calcaneal fractures and the indications and technique of the primary arthrodesis.

Misdiagnosed Lisfranc injuries can be as high as 50%, leading to chronic pain, functional impairment, and posttraumatic arthritis. Subtle or incomplete lesions are the most problematic group for an adequate diagnosis. Conventional non–weight-bearing radiographs can overlook up to 30% of unstable cases. Abduction stress radiographs and anteroposterior monopodial comparative weight-bearing radiographic views are very useful to identify instability. Computed tomography gives detailed information about fracture patterns and comminution. MRI can predict instability but it is expensive and not readily available in the acute setting.

The management of Lisfranc injuries is challenging considering the broad spectrum of energy involved and highly variable clinical presentation. Despite the advances in surgical techniques, subtle Lisfranc injuries can lead to chronic pain and permanent disability. Surgical treatment is mandatory for all the unstable injuries; however, the best surgical technique remains controversial. The most predictive factor for a successful outcome is the maintenance of anatomic alignment; therefore, the selection of the appropriate surgical technique is of paramount importance. This article reviews the current treatment options and describes the selection of the surgical technique based on the different clinical presentations.

The reported incidence of Lisfranc injuries is 9.2/100.000 person-years; two-thirds of the injuries are nondisplaced. Tarsometatarsal injuries range from minor sprains and isolated ligamentous injuries to grossly unstable and multiligamentous lesions. High-energy injuries are usually linked with mechanical energy dissipation through the soft tissues. Operative treatment options include open reduction and internal fixation, open reduction with hybrid internal and external fixation, closed reduction with percutaneous internal or external fixation, and primary arthrodesis. Treatment goals are to obtain a painless, plantigrade, and stable foot. Anatomic reduction is a key factor for improved outcomes and decreased rates of post-traumatic arthritis.

Fractures of the proximal fifth metatarsal are common injuries with a unique history. Treatment of these fractures is controversial partly because of confusion regarding fracture subtype nomenclature. Today "Jones fracture" refers to proximal fifth metatarsal fracture in zones 2 or 3. Zone 2 fractures are acute injuries, and their optimal treatment is unclear. Zone 3 fractures commonly occur in the presence of a chronic stress reaction. Because of poor healing potential, zone 3 fractures typically require operative treatment. Zone 1 fractures have excellent healing potential and may be treated nonoperatively with a weightbearing as tolerated protocol.

FOOT AND ANKLE CLINICS

RELATED SERIES

Clinics in Sports Medicine
Orthopedic Clinics
Physical Medicine and Rehabilitation Clinics

THE CLINICS ARE NOW AVAILABLE ONLINE!
Access your subscription at:
www.theclinics.com

Preface

Controversies in Acute Trauma and Reconstruction

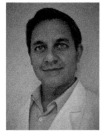　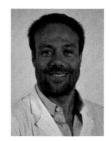

Jorge Filippi, MD, MBA　　German Joannas, MD
Editors

Foot and ankle trauma is a common problem for subspecialists and general orthopedic surgeons in the emergency department setting. This issue tries to give a practical approach for the most frequent clinical dilemmas in terms of diagnosis and treatment. In some articles, we asked the authors to defy some established knowledge or "gold standards"; in others, we asked the authors to organize and clarify classic contents, and in all of them, we asked the authors to share their experience and innovative vision on these problems.

Thanks to all our colleagues participating in this issue of *Foot and Ankle Clinics of North America*. Most of the work done for this issue was during the stressful COVID-19 pandemic. We are extremely grateful to the authors for sharing their time, knowledge, and experience. Their commitment and generosity are remarkable and were vital for achieving a good ending.

Our thanks to our teacher, leader, and friend, Mark Myerson, for the opportunity to organize this issue. Also, thanks for teaching us that the best way of learning is by sharing knowledge with friends. Thanks to all the staff in Elsevier for their kind support, especially to Nicole Congleton.

All this work is impossible without the help of our families and friends. Special thanks to Guillermo Arrondo for his mentoring, friendship, and support (G.J.); and Constanza, Anibal, and Adela for being the energy for life (J.F.).

Foot Ankle Clin N Am 25 (2020) xv–xvi
https://doi.org/10.1016/j.fcl.2020.09.001
1083-7515/20/© 2020 Published by Elsevier Inc.

We hope this *Foot and Ankle Clinics of North America* issue, "Controversies in Acute Trauma and Reconstruction," can be helpful for your clinical practice and could stimulate more research for our patients' benefit.

Jorge Filippi, MD, MBA
Estoril 450, Las Condes
Santiago 7591047, Chile

German Joannas, MD
Av. Belgrano 3402
Ciudad Autónoma de Buenos Aires CP 1078, Argentina

Instituto Barrancas
Hipolito Yrigoyen 902
Quilmes, CP 1878
Buenos Aires, Argentina

E-mail addresses:
jfilippi@clinicalascondes.cl; jlfilippi@gmail.com (J. Filippi)
germanjoannas@icloud.com; german_joannas@cepp.org.ar (G. Joannas)

New Principles in Pilon Fracture Management
Revisiting Rüedi and Allgöwer Concepts

Christian Bastias, MD[a,b,]*, Leonardo Lagos, MD[a,b]

KEYWORDS

• Pilon fracture • Tibial plafond • Distal tibia columns • Rüedi and allgöwer

KEY POINTS

• The concepts of Rüedi and Allgöwer are still valid, but with modifications concerning a better understanding of the anatomy and mechanics of this fracture.
• Fibular fixation is not always the first stage, depending on the pattern and complexity of the fracture.
• In the presence of severe intra-articular comminution, the quality of joint reduction can be sacrificed to prioritize stability and alignment.
• Bone grafting is reserved for cases of substantial metaphyseal bone loss, and in general, in a delayed stage.
• Not only does the medial column have to be stabilized, but all damaged pilars in the pilon fracture.

INTRODUCTION

Fractures of the distal tibia with joint involvement are infrequent, less than 1% of fractures of the lower limb, but one of the most challenging injuries in their treatment to be able to achieve good results.[1] Initially called "tibial pilon" by Destot in 1911, it was Bonin who coined the term "tibial plafond" in 1950, as a way of describing the alteration of the ankle ceiling.[2]

The described injury mechanism presents 2 significant variants. One torsional of relatively low energy, associated with falls in sports activities, and another of high energy in which the talus impacts axially on the distal tibia producing fractures with comminution at different levels, usually associated with falls from a height and automobile accidents.[2] The fracture pattern is determined by the position of the foot, and therefore the talus at the time of injury.

[a] Foot and Ankle Unit, Hospital Mutual de Seguridad, Avenida Alameda 4848, Estación Central, 9160000 Santiago de Chile; [b] Foot and Ankle Unit, Clínica Santa María, Santiago de Chile
* Corresponding author.
E-mail address: cibastias@gmail.com

Foot Ankle Clin N Am 25 (2020) 505–521
https://doi.org/10.1016/j.fcl.2020.08.004
1083-7515/20/© 2020 Elsevier Inc. All rights reserved.

CLASSIFICATION

Various classifications have described over the years. Lauge Hansen described them as a pronation–dorsiflexion fracture with a 4-stage progression. Rüedi and Allgöwer, in their 1969 publication, described 3 groups based on joint and metaphyseal comminution and displacement.[3]

Müller, in 1987 described the most widely used classification to date, adopted by the AO, which is associated with a prognostic factor. It is divided into 3 groups: group A extra-articular, group B partial articular, and group C total articular. Each one is divided consecutively into subgroups, through which the prognosis worsens and the complexity of the fracture increases.

All these classifications suffer from the problem of being based on radiographic images, which does not allow us to have a real idea of the fracture pattern. In this regard, in 2017, Leonetti presented a new computed tomography (CT) scan-based classification, with 4 main groups and respective subgroups.[4] The classification is based on the number of fragments displaced in the different sections of the CT scan, ranging from type 1 (not displaced) to type 4 (with ≥ 4 fragments and high comminution). It is a classification that has prognostic value, is reproducible, and better guides the surgical treatment.

TREATMENT CONCEPTS
Staged Treatment

Tibial pilon fractures, particularly high-energy ones, involve bone and significant soft tissue damage. Given the high rate of soft tissue complications associated with immediate open reduction and internal fixation (ORIF), it is since the 1990s, and particularly after Sirkin's work in 1999, treatment considers 2 stages: an initial external fixation for fracture alignment and stabilization and a second delayed stage, once the soft tissue is in good condition, for reduction and osteosynthesis of the fracture.[5]

Although staggered management is most widely used currently, there are some cases where there is no soft tissue compromise and immediate resolution of the fracture is feasible, even within the first 72 hours, without increasing the risk of complications.[6,7]

Rüedi and Allgöwer

At the time of skeletal stabilization, the good results described by Rüedi and Allgöwer in their publications in 1969 and 1973[3,8] give rise to the treatments that remain in use today. They are sequential principles regarding fracture fixation, the objectives of which are to achieve anatomic reduction and stable osteosynthesis. They are:

1. Recovery of the fibular length.
2. Reconstruction of the articular surface.
3. Bone graft to the metaphyseal region.
4. Stabilization of the tibial fracture with a medial plate.

Anatomic Concepts: Columns and Articular Fragments

The concepts defined by Rüedi and Allgöwer, although current, were stated based on studies carried out with radiographs, but after the advent of CT scans in recent decades, we have better understood the morphology and patterns of fractures, which has given rise to anatomic concepts that better guide treatment. In his 2013 study, which is based on CT images of C3 AO tibial pilon fractures, Cole describes a constant fracture pattern at the articular level (>90% of cases); we found 3 main fragments:

medial, anterolateral, and posterolateral, with a base Y shape at the level of the fibular notch. In turn, the areas of greatest comminution are usually central, coinciding with the central point of the talus, and anterolateral.[9] (**Fig. 1**).

Concerning the columns or pilars, it refers to an anatomic continuum between the articular or epiphyseal fragments, with their respective metaphyseal and diaphyseal zones. Assal and coworkers,[10] in 2015, describes 3 columns, exclusively tibial: medial, lateral, and posterior.

More recent works already consider 4 columns, when adding the distal fibula as one more column, which provides reduction and stability[11] (**Fig. 2**). These 4 columns are:

- Lateral column: distal fibula
- Posterior column: posterior part of the articular fragment and one-third of the distal portion of the posterior tibia
- Anterior column: anterior part of the articular fragment and distal one-third of the anterior tibia
- Medial column: one-third of the medial portion of the articular fragment and distal tibia.

The importance of these anatomic concepts is that recognizing the articular areas and columns of most considerable comminution allows us to plan more accurately where we should use our implants to stabilize the fracture. In the same way, we can plan the approaches we require for surgery.

We analyze the Rüedi and Allgöwer principles, one by one, to assess their current validity and whether they have been modified.

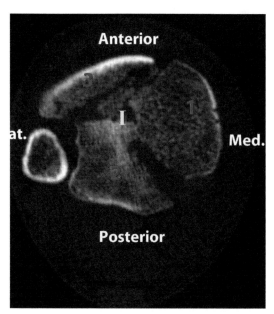

Fig. 1. Articular fragments in a pilon fracture. Note the (1) medial, (2) posterolateral, and (3) anterolateral fragments of the pilon fracture. Anterolateral comminution is observed. (*From* Cole P, Merle R, Bhandari M, Zlowodski M. The pilon map: fracture lines and comminution zones in OTA/AO Type 43C3 pilon fractures. J Orthop Trauma. 2013; 27: 152 – 156; with permission.)

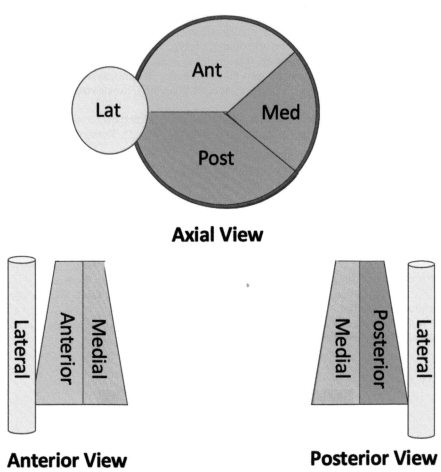

Fig. 2. The 4 columns of the tibial pilon. (*From* Chen H, Cui X, Ma B, Rui Y, Li H. Staged procedure protocol based on the four-column concept in the treatment of AO/OTA type 43-C3.3 pilon fractures. J Int Med Res. 2019; 47: 2045-2055; with permission.)

RECOVERY OF THE FIBULAR LENGTH

Fibula fracture occurs in 90% of tibial pilon fractures,[12] and many authors agree that fibular fixation is crucial in this type of fracture.

- It gives stability to the lateral column, which would avoid valgus displacement and reduces angular displacement.[13]
- It helps us to reduce the tibia concerning length, alignment, and translation. The syndesmotic ligaments insertions help to reduce the anterolateral and posterolateral tibial articular fragments.[14]
- It helps us with stability and syndesmosis reduction if it is injured.[15,16]

Sommer and associates,[17] in their prospective work, showed a relationship between correct fibular reduction and good functional results.

Despite what previously established, recently Kurylo and colleagues[18] did not find differences between tibial pilon fractures with or without fibular fixation with respect to the final alignment achieved; they argue that fibular fixation may not be necessary, especially in fractures in that anatomic reduction of the fibula is not achieved and therefore does not help us to reduce the tibia. Some studies also show that fibular fixation can be associated with nonunion, higher withdrawal of osteosynthesis, and an increased incidence of superficial infection.[19,20] Despite what these latter authors have expressed, most of the studies support the need for fibular fixation in fractures of the tibial pilon.

We can perform fibular fixation in 2 moments:

- Emergency in conjunction with external fixation as part of staged management, and
- Along with the definitive osteosynthesis of the fracture.

The emergency fibular fixation, in conjunction with the external fixator, corresponds with the initial phase of treatment in stages,[14] where the objective of fibular fixation is to give adequate stability to the lateral column. In contrast, medial stability is given by the fixator. Several studies support emergency fibular fixation owing to the benefits already discussed and because it would help to decrease operating time in definitive surgery.

In contrast, and taking into account what is the real clinical context every day, we have to consider that the emergency management of this type of fracture is often carried out by a general orthopedist, who will not perform the definitive treatment. In this scenario, many times there are various factors not considered, such as approaches and types of implants to be used later. In this way, emergency fibular fixation can result in a procedure that hinders the definitive management of the fracture.

What Problems Can We Have with Emergency Fibular Fixation?

- Malreduction in complex or comminuted fractures, resulting in recurvatum, shortening, and rotation of the fibula, which influence the tibial reduction when we are going to perform definitive management. Borrelli and Catalano,[21] in their study, showed that even leaving a long fibula can cause a varus deformity of the tibia and overload of the lateral plafond region (**Fig. 3**).
- It affects us in the planning of the approaches, because in some cases for the type of fracture we require an anterolateral approach that we can no longer

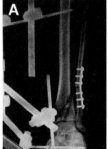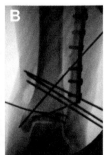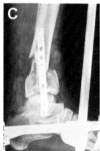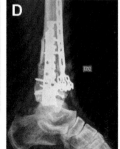

Fig. 3. Example of 2 patients who underwent emergency fixation of the fibula. One case resulting in valgus (*A, B*) and the other in recurvatum (*C, D*). Both stabilizations were revised at the time of definitive surgery. *From* Chen H, Cui X, Ma B, et al. Staged procedure protocol based on the four-column concept in the treatment of AO/OTA type 43-C3.3pilon fractures. J Int Med Res. 2019; 47(5):2045-2055; with permission.

perform if it has a direct lateral approach, because of the high risk of soft tissue complications.

- In cases of great tibial comminution, fixing the fibula and maintaining its length would not allow us to perform a certain degree of shortening to achieve contact of the tibial metaphyseal region.

Currently, we suggest not performing emergency fibular fixation, but to place a delta external fixation system to achieve stability, length, and proper alignment, to allow soft tissue healing and allow time for adequate planning.

When facing the final fixation of the fracture, we suggest starting with the fibula when we know that we can achieve anatomic reduction (simple fractures or low comminution) and stable fixation, which facilitates the reduction of the tibial fragments (**Fig. 4**). However, in some instances, when the fibular fracture is very comminuted and we cannot achieve an anatomic reduction for length and rotation, or it prevents us from reducing the tibia adequately, we suggest starting with the tibial reduction (**Fig. 5**).

Regarding the OTS, we suggest a third-tube plate with simple fractures, but in cases of comminution, a more rigid plate, such as reconstruction or locked. Be careful to attach the plate well in the area where the lateral cortex of the fibula presents a torsion because otherwise, we leave an inadequate reduction in the rotational plane. We recommend the use of an endomedullary fixation (percutaneous technique) in case of severe soft tissue damage in the approach area or cases of patients with significant comorbidity. In the presence of simple transverse fractures, a Steinman may be sufficient, but if the fracture has a complex pattern, we recommend new endomedular devices, like fibular nails.

We believe that this first principle of Rüedi and Allgöwer is fundamental to achieve in most cases, but it is not always the first. It should not be performed as an emergency

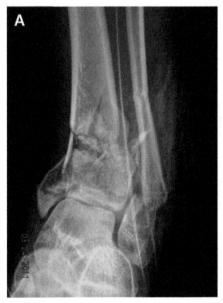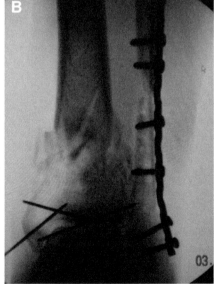

Fig. 4. (*A*) Tibial plafond fracture with great tibial and segmental fibular comminution. (*B*) We achieved an anatomic fixation, and this helps us a lot with tibial reduction.

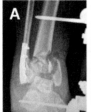
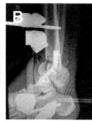
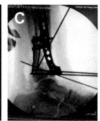
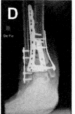
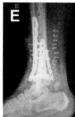

Fig. 5. (*A, B*) 41-year-old female patient with a comminuted tibia fracture and a previously operated ankle fracture. With the refracture of the fibula, we did not have a good reference point to achieve anatomic reduction; it had consolidated in recurvatum. (*C*) We preferred to start with the tibia reducing a large posterior fragment. (*D, E*) After that, we fixed the rest of the tibia, and finally, the fibula.

as part of the first stage of treatment. In definitive surgery, you need a plate that provides adequate stability, especially in cases of comminution.

RECONSTRUCTION OF THE ARTICULAR SURFACE

Although we can obtain an optimal result in this type of fracture for joint reduction and alignment, and also without infections or soft tissue problems, the results are not always as expected. In high-energy fractures, there is irreversible damage to the articular cartilage and the structures that surround and give stability to the ankle.[22] Murray and colleagues[23] demonstrated the death of chondrocytes in joint fractures with a high impact, and this death of the chondrocyte increases as more energy is involved in the fracture.[24] It is known that in addition to the initial injury, severe joint injuries leave damage to the extracellular matrix and chondrocyte metabolism, which triggers a cascade of events that leads to joint degeneration.[25]

Although we know that we have these factors against us, we must never forget our objectives to achieve in surgery, adequate stability, correct alignment of the axes, and anatomic articular reduction.

One of the most critical objectives emphasized in joint fractures is the anatomic reduction of the joint surface; several authors have reinforced this finding.[3,26–28] Rüedi evaluated fracture types, surgical modalities, and quality of reduction, and only found significance in the last one concerning good functional scores. De Las Heras Romero and associates[29] showed that joint reduction was the only factor that could be modified by the surgeon. Williams and colleagues[30] related joint reduction and injury severity with signs of radiologic osteoarthritis, but not directly with functional results. Recently, Sommer and associates,[17] in a multicenter and prospective study, showed a relationship between fibular length and functional results but did not find a relationship between the reduction of the articular surface and good functional results.

The reduction of the articular surface must always be one of our main objectives in this type of fracture, although we know that it is not the only one. Still, it must be taken with good clinical judgment in cases of high-energy trauma with significant soft tissue involvement. Trying to achieve an anatomic reduction sometimes means making large incisions, excessive periosteal stripping, placing large implants, and a longer operative time, which increases the possibilities of complications and poor functional results. Therefore, in these cases, the joint reduction must be sacrificed to avoid complications, but in pursuit of the objective of stability and correct alignment of the fracture.

Regarding the reduction of the articular surface, we suggest:

- In fractures where we have the possibility of reduction, we commence with a sizable metaphyseal fragment (column or pillar), generally posterior or medial, and fix it with Kirschner wires in a temporary form or plate. Then we proceed to reduce the articular surface taking the already reduced column as a reference.
- In the case of fractures with great metaphyseal comminution, where we have no reference to reduce any pillar or column, we must reduce the articular surface first. Then, we reduce this large articular block to the tibial metaphysis and diaphysis with anatomic plates, worrying about leaving a correct alignment (**Fig. 6**).
- In cases where we have an extensive soft tissue injury, and the ORIF is not an option, we suggest performing a percutaneous reduction of the joint with compression screws and arthroscopic assistance when we have large articular fragments. Then external fixation or percutaneous plate is used to stabilize the rest of the pillars. We know in these cases that we are sacrificing joint reduction for a greater good (**Fig. 7**).

Analyzing this second principle, we believe that the best possible reduction should be obtained, but not at the expense of soft tissue damage or devascularization of the bone fragments. We know that leaving a perfect reduction improves, but does not ensure, a good functional result. In complex fractures, many of them sometimes with nonreconstructible joints, achieving adequate stability and alignment, which allows consolidation while avoiding complications, becomes more critical than anatomic reduction.

BONE GRAFT SUPPLY AT THE METAPHYSEAL REGION

Metaphyseal involvement can be our great headache in these fractures. Depending on the energy involved in the trauma, we can find simple fractures, the comminution of 1 or 2 metaphyseal pillars, comminution of all the pillars, or even segmental loss.

It is known that the posterior pillar is the one that generally does not present comminution. It is followed by the medial and, finally, the anterolateral pillar. This is due to the resistance of the cortices in this anatomic area and influenced by the mechanism of

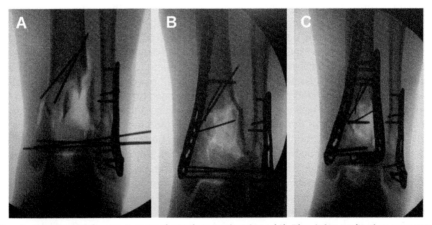

Fig. 6. Fracture with great metaphyseal comminution. (*A*) The joint reduction was performed first. (*B, C*) Then this articular block was united to the diaphysis using an anatomic medial and anterolateral plate.

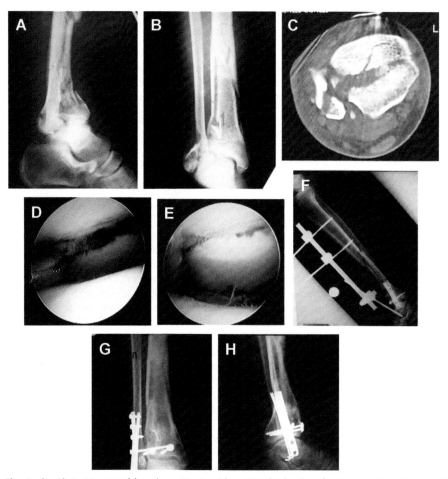

Fig. 7. (*A–C*) A 45-year-old male patient with a C3 tibial pilon fracture, with diaphyseal extension and soft tissue involvement. (*D, E*) The joint reduction performed with arthroscopic assistance. (*F*) The rest of the fracture stabilized with an external fixator for 3 months. (*G, H*) Consolidation and excellent results achieved.

trauma (the position of the foot, and therefore the talus at the moment of impact on the tibial plafond, determines which pillar is the most compromised).[9–11]

Metaphyseal comminution alone is a big problem, but it can be even worse for the following reasons:

- In severe compromise of all the pillars, anatomic references are difficult to identify. In this case reduction must start with joint reduction and then metaphyseal alignment, avoiding shortening, ante or recurvatum and misalignments in varus–valgus. It must be stabilized with an anatomic locking medial plate.
- In the case of open fractures, the wound is generally transverse medially and is directly related to the comminution zone, so it adds a considerable risk of infection, nonunion and makes the option of a stable synthesis in the area impossible for at least the first weeks, or until coverage is achieved with a flap in cases it is required.

- A lack of bone stock (comminution) and compromise of local coverage (soft tissue injury) makes this area at risk of nonunion, which can lead to OTS failure and varus misalignment.[5]

Multiple studies share Ruedi's principle of providing bone graft to fill the metaphyseal bone defect. Still, based on this discussion, we believe that this is not always the case and should be evaluated on a case-by-case basis, as we explain.

- When we are faced with comminution of a metaphyseal column, we generally do not place a bone graft, we only fill it with the same fracture fragments and achieve good stability with locking plates.
- In case of having 2 or more columns compromised, with minor soft tissue damage that allows ORIF, we suggest providing bone grafting. We usually use cancellous bone graft taken from the ipsilateral proximal tibia or an allograft with osteoinductive and osteoconductive properties. There are no studies that validate that the use of one or the other is better.
- Another scenario is the presence of a sizable metaphyseal defect with significant soft tissue involvement. In these cases, an open approach will increase the risk of infection and complications, so we prefer NOT to perform ORIF. It is better to operate with external fixation and minimal or percutaneous OTS to the joint, and also consider percutaneous medial plate to the tibia. We defer the supply of bone graft for a few weeks until soft tissue is in good condition, and we do it through a small anterior incision.
- Finally, we have the case of an open fracture, generally medial, with great comminution or loss of bone stock. Our planning is surgical debridement plus external fixation, and we fill the defect with bone cement with antibiotics. It helps us to provide stability and decrease the risk of infection. We wait for soft tissue improvement until definitive fixation with whatever technique is considered for the case. At around 6 weeks, we performed cement removal and bone graft delivery, using the Masquelet technique.[31] We have also performed this technique in patients susceptible to ORIF, but with a significant metaphyseal segmental defect, here we believe that the contribution of cement helps us to stabilize and creates a better biological environment for the integration of the graft in the future and with a lower risk of infection (**Fig. 8**).

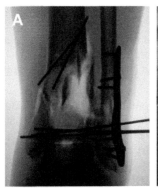
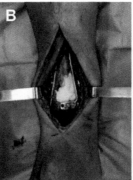
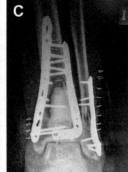

Fig. 8. (*A*) Fracture with significant metaphyseal defect. (*B, C*) At the time of the definitive synthesis, it is filled with bone cement, which between 4 and 8 weeks later, will be removed for bone graft, following the Masquelet technique.

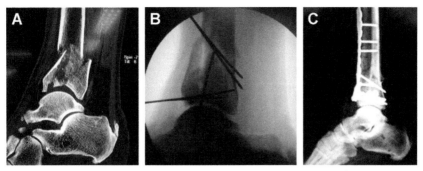

Fig. 9. (*A, B*) Reduction of the posterior column via an anterior approach, and temporary fixation with Kirschner wires. (*C*) Then screw fixation through the anterior plate.

Acute shortening of the metaphyseal segment and subsequent reconstruction by distraction osteogenesis or vascularized graft is also an option.

This third principle is the one we perform least at the time of definitive surgery. Not all cases require bone grafting. In the case of a large metaphyseal comminution, the best option would be fixation with a percutaneous technique and deferring the contribution of grafting, if necessary.

STABILIZATION OF THE TIBIAL FRACTURE WITH A MEDIAL PLATE

Proper planning is essential for tibial pilon fracture treatment and thus deciding what type of approach and synthesis we carry out, taking into account the type of fracture and the state of soft tissue. To achieve a good understanding of the fracture, we

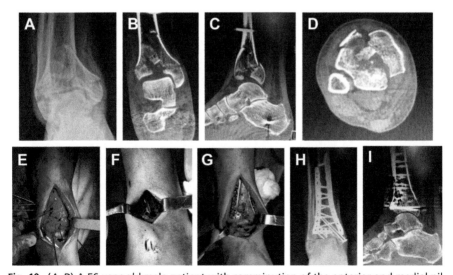

Fig. 10. (*A–D*) A 56-year-old male patient with comminution of the anterior and medial pillars. The posterior column presents a large fragment. (*E, G*) Double plate fixation performed by the anterior approach. (*F*) Small posteromedial approach to achieve the reduction of the posterior fragment and percutaneous placement of the medial plate. (*H, I*) Satisfactory reduction was achieved.

believe that it is vitally important to evaluate the compromised column or columns, at the articular and metaphyseal level, and the failure in tension or compression presented by these pillars, as explained by Assal and associates.[10]

Along with this, we must know the implants currently available, which have evolved considerably. We have specific anatomic plates with angular stability for the medial, anterolateral and posterior pillars. They facilitate the fixation of fragments and provide adequate stability for them.

In their study, Penny and colleagues[32] showed that the placement of an anterolateral plate alone does not achieve a good fixation of the medial fragment, and a medial alone does not achieve a good fixation of the anterolateral fragment, which is why it suggests the placement of 2 plates to achieving stable fixation of the typical articular fragments of the tibial pilon, the same reinforced by the study by Aneja and colleagues.[33]

Oken and associate[34] in 43 C1 fractures showed no difference in stability given by medial and anterolateral plate in isolation. The same had shown in the study carried out by Yenna and cowrkers[35] in plastic bones. Ketz and Sanders,[36] in their study, showed the usefulness of fixation of the posterior pillar and fibula by a posterolateral approach in a first stage, and then the anterior reconstruction with a plate to achieve an anatomic reduction of the articular surface. Haller and colleagues,[37] in their study, showed a higher risk of nonunion by not stabilizing the medial column.

We suggest the analysis of the degree of comminution of each column, both metaphyseal and articular, to decide the most appropriate synthesis:

- If we have anterior column comminution (articular and metaphyseal fragments), we suggest a locked anterolateral plate. If this fragment is large and without comminution only a third plate of tube and screws is needed.

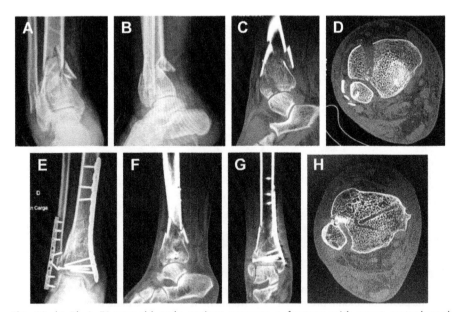

Fig. 11. (A–D) A 51-year-old male patient presents a fracture with great metaphyseal comminution of all the pillars and a simple articular fracture. (E–H) Percutaneous synthesis performed with a medial plate and screws to the joint.

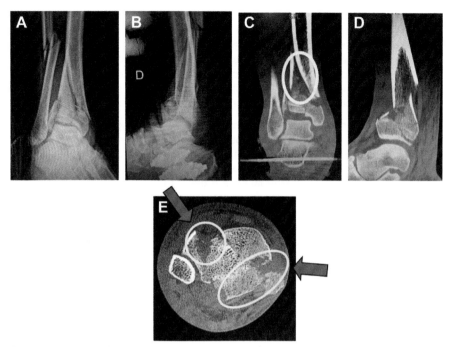

Fig. 12. A 50-year-old patient with a pilon fracture after fall from a height. External fixation in the acute setting. Definitive fixation planning as follows. (*A–E*) Fracture with comminution of the anterior and posterior pillars. The medial pillar presents a large fragment of the tibial malleolus. The *circles* show the "key" areas that we should see directly to achieve anatomic reduction. The *arrows* show the approaches chosen for this case (anterolateral and modified posteromedial approach).

- Regarding the medial pillar, we believe that it always requires plate stabilization. If it is comminuted, we suggest a medial locked plate, which can be with a minimally invasive or open technique, depending on the case. If it is a large fragment, we can use a less rigid plate such as a one-third tubular or reconstruction.
- In the case of the posterior column, which is generally a sizable noncomminuted fragment, we always try to perform an indirect reduction of this by an anterior

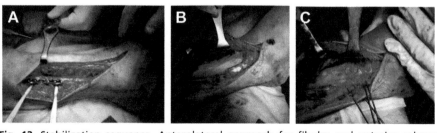

Fig. 13. Stabilization sequence. Anterolateral approach for fibular and anterior column reduction and fixation. (*A*) Fibular fixation. (*B*) Metaphyseal reduction and screw fixation of the anterolateral column. (*C*) Anterolateral joint reduction and Kirschner wires temporary fixation.

approach. We maintain it with Kirschner wires, we reduce the rest of the surface and fix it through the anterior plate (**Fig. 9**). We believe that deperiostizing the posterior and anterior region of the tibia is not a good idea owing to the tremendous vascular damage that we can cause and the risk of nonunion.[38] We reserve the posterior plate, which we place by a posteromedial approach, for very selected cases, when it is impossible for us to achieve a good reduction owing to the most commonly used standard approaches.

If we analyze the compromised columns together, we can suggest that in fractures where there is a compromise of all the metaphyseal and articular columns, the use of 2 or even 3 plates becomes essential to achieve adequate stability and thus avoid future nonunion and malunion. The pillars that we usually fix directly with plates are medial and anterolateral; we only directly fix (with a plate) the posterior column when it is not comminuted, but we cannot reduce and fix it indirectly (**Fig. 10**). When all the articular and metaphyseal columns have comminution, we suggest the use of external fixation. In cases of fracture with metaphyseal comminution but simple and large joint fragments, we could consider a medial plate (open or percutaneous) + OTS with screws or small plates at the joint (**Fig. 11**).

About this fourth principle expounded by Rüedi and Allgöwer, the fixation of the medial column, in our opinion, is fundamental and should be carried out always. The possibility of future nonunion and varus failure is quite high, and it increases if there is comminution. Still, indeed we must currently add to this principle the stable fixation of the other committed columns as the case may be.

Finally, with this case, we want to illustrate the concepts that guide our choice for the surgical approaches, concerning the areas of most significant bone conflict of our fracture ("key zones"). These areas require anatomic reduction and stable fixation (**Figs. 12–14**).

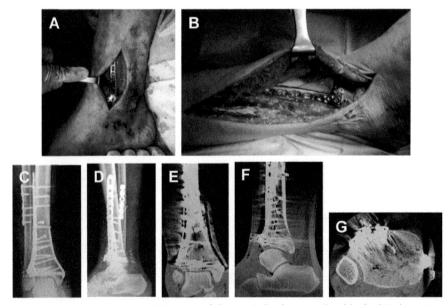

Fig. 14. (*A*) Reduction and stabilization of the medial column with a blocked T-plate, via a modified posteromedial approach. (*B*) Final fixation of the anterior pillar with a locking anterolateral plate. (*C–G*) Good postoperative result.

SUMMARY

The tibial pilon fracture is a very complex fracture that require us to maximize our criteria and experience. Staged management is perhaps the gold standard of treatment of these lesions, although some authors have published excellent results with immediate ORIF.[6,7]

At the time of determining definitive management of the fracture, the principles of Rüedi and Allgöwer are still valid, but they have undergone modifications. The reconstitution of the fibular length is not always the first step to perform. The reconstruction of the articular surface is not the most essential factor to achieve excellent results. Many times, the articular prognosis is already sealed, therefore avoiding further soft tissue injury, achieving adequate stability and alignment becomes the most important. Bone graft filling is only required in selected cases, and finally, the stabilization of the medial column is still essential, but it must be associated with the stabilization of at least one other column in complex pilons.

CLINICS CARE POINTS

- Always plan your surgery based on a CT study; it allows an adequate understanding of the fracture that is, not feasible only with a radiograph.
- Fibular fixation is not recommended at the time of external fixation as a part of the first stage of step management. If so, it should then be performed by the same surgeon who will perform the final fixation as part of well-designed planning.
- At the time of ORIF, start fixation by the fibula only if you are sure to regain length, alignment, and rotation. In cases of much fibular comminution, it is sometimes better to start from the tibia.
- Always try to achieve an anatomic joint reduction (it is an element that improves functional prognosis) unless soft tissue damage or comminution does not allow this to be possible.
- The use of bone grafting is not always necessary, particularly with the development of percutaneous techniques that offer better soft tissue care.
- Not only must the medial column of the fracture be stabilized, but all that is compromised, particularly in the presence of metaphyseal comminution must be stabilized.

DISCLOSURE

C. Bastias: Speaker. Johnson & Johnson, Depuy Synthes. L. Lagos: Nothing to disclose.

REFERENCES

1. Barei D, Nork S. Fractures of the tibial plafond. Foot Ankle Clin N Am 2008;13: 571–91.
2. Chen D, Li B, Aubeeluck A, et al. Open reduction and internal fixation of posterior pilon fractures with buttress plate. Acta Orthop Bras 2014;22:48–53.
3. Rüedi TP, Allgöwer. Fractures of the lower end of the tibia into the ankle joint. Injury 1969;1:92–9.
4. Leonetti D, Tigani D. Pilon fractures: a new classification system based on CT scan. Injury 2017;48:2311–7.
5. Sirkin M, Sanders R, DiPasquale T, et al. A staged protocol for soft tissue management in the treatment of complex pilon fractures. J Orthop Trauma 1999;13: 78–84.

6. White T, Kennedy S, Cooke C, et al. Primary internal fixation of AO type C pilon fractures is safe. Orthopaedic Trauma Association Proceedings. Phoenix, October 5 - 7, 2006.

7. Guy P, White T, Cooke C, et al. The results of early primary open reduction and internal fixation for treatment of AO C-type tibial pilon fractures: a cohort study. J Orthop Trauma 2010;24:757–63.

8. Rüedi TP, Allgöwer M. Fractures of the lower end of the tibia into the ankle joint: result 9 years after open reduction and internal fixation. Injury 1973;5:130–4.

9. Cole P, Merle R, Bhandari M, et al. The pilon map: fracture lines and comminution zones in OTA/AO Type 43C3 pilon fractures. J Orthop Trauma 2013;27:152–6.

10. Assal M, Ray A, Stern R. Strategies and surgical approaches in open reduction internal fixation of pilon fractures. J Orthop Trauma 2015;29:69–79.

11. Chen H, Cui X, Ma B, et al. Staged procedure protocol based on the four-column concept in the treatment of AO/OTA type 43-C3.3 pilon fractures. J Int Med Res 2019;47:2045–55.

12. Barei DP, Nork SE, Bellabarba C, et al. Is the absence of an ipsilateral fibular fracture predictive of increased radiographic tibial pilon fracture severity? J Orthop Trauma 2006;20:6–10.

13. Kumar A, Charlebois SJ, Cain EL, et al. Crates JM "Effect of fibular plate fixation on rotational stability of simulated distal tibial fractures treated with intramedullary nailing". J Bone Joint Surg Am 2003;85:604–8.

14. Helfet DL, Koval K, Pappas J, et al. Intraarticular "pilon" fracture of the tibia. Clin Orthop Relat Res 1994;298:221–8.

15. Torino D, Mehta S. Fibular fixation in distal tibia fractures: reduction aid or nonunion generator? J Orthop Trauma 2016;30(Suppl 4):S22–5.

16. Haller JM, Githens M, Rothberg D, et al. Syndesmosis and syndesmotic equivalent injuries in tibial plafond fractures. J Orthop Trauma 2019;33(Number 3):e74–8.

17. Sommer C, Nork SE, Graves M, et al. Quality of fracture reduction assessed by radiological parameters and its influence on functional results in patients with pilon fractures—a prospective multicentre study. Injury 2017;48:2853–63.

18. Kurylo JC, Datta N, Iskander KN, et al. Does the fibula need to be fixed in complex pilon fractures? J Orthop Trauma 2015;29:424–7.

19. Williams TM, Marsh JL, Nepola JV, et al. External fixation of tibial plafond fractures: is routine plating of the fibula necessary? J Orthop Trauma 1998;12:16–20.

20. Avilucea FR1, Triantafillou K, Whiting PS, et al. Suprapatellar intramedullary nail technique lowers rate of malalignment of distal tibia fractures. J Orthop Trauma 2016;30:557–60.

21. Borrelli J Jr, Catalano L. Open reduction and internal fixation of pilon fractures [current controversies in orthopaedic trauma]. J Orthop Trauma 1999;13:573–82.

22. McKinley TO, Rudert MJ, Koos DC, et al. Incongruity versus instability in the etiology of posttraumatic arthritis. Clin Orthop Relat Res 2004;423:44–51.

23. Murray MM, Zurakowski D, Vrahas MS. The death of articular chondrocytes after intra-articular fracture in humans. J Trauma 2004;56:128–31.

24. Jeffrey JE, Gregory DW, Aspden RM. Matrix damage and chondrocyte viability following a single impact load on articular cartilage. Arch Biochem Biophys 1995;10:87–96.

25. Milentijevic D, Rubell F, Liew AS, et al. An in vivo rabbit model for cartilage trauma: a preliminary study of the influence of impact stress magnitude on chondrocyte death and matrix damage. J Orthop Trauma 2005;19:466—73.

26. Ovadia DN, Beals RK. Fractures of the tibial plafond. J Bone Joint Surg Am 1986; 68:543–51.
27. Korkmaz A, Ciftdemir M, Özcan M, et al. The analysis of the variables, affecting outcome in surgically treated tibia pilon fractured patients. Injury 2013;44: 1270–4.
28. Babis GC, Vayanos ED, Papaioannou N, et al. Results of surgical treatment of tibial plafond fractures. Clin Orthop Relat Res 1997;341:99–105.
29. De-las-Heras-Romero J, Lledo-Alvarez A, Lizaur-Utrilla A. Quality of life and prognostic factors after intra-articular tibial pilon fracture. Injury 2017;48:1258–63.
30. Williams TM1, Nepola JV, DeCoster TA, et al. Factors affecting outcome in tibial plafond fractures. Clin Orthop Relat Res 2004;423:93–8.
31. Masquelet A, Kanakaris NK, Obert L, et al. Bone repair using the Masquelet technique. J Bone Joint Surg Am 2019;101:1024–36.
32. Penny P1, Swords M, Heisler J, Cien A. Ability of modern distal tibia plates to stabilize comminuted pilon fracture fragments: is dual plate fixation necessary? Injury 2016;47:1761–9.
33. Aneja A, Luo TD, Liu B, et al. Anterolateral distal tibia locking plate osteosynthesis and their ability to capture OTAC3 pilon fragments. Injury 2018;49:409–13.
34. Oken OF, Yildirim AO, Asilturk M. Finite element analysis of the stability of AO/OTA 43-C1 type distal tibial fractures treated with distal tibia medial anatomic plate versus anterolateral anatomic plate. Acta Orthop Traumatol Turc 2017;51:404–8.
35. Yenna ZC1, Bhadra AK, Ojike NI, et al. Anterolateral and medial locking plate stiffness in distal tibial fracture model. Foot Ankle Int 2011;32:630–7.
36. Ketz J, Sanders R. Staged posterior tibial plating for the treatment of Orthopaedic Trauma Association 43C2 and 43C3 tibial pilon fractures. J Orthop Trauma 2012; 26:341–7.
37. Haller J, Githens M, Rothberg D, et al. Risk factors for tibial plafond nonunion: medial column fixation may reduce nonunion rates. J Orthop Trauma 2019;33: 443–9.
38. Chan DS, Balthrop PM, White B, et al. Does a staged posterior approach have a negative effect on OTA- 43C fracture outcomes? J Orthop Trauma 2016; 31:90–4.

High-Energy Pilon Fractures: Role of External Fixation in Acute and Definitive Treatment. What are the Indications and Technique for Primary Ankle Arthrodesis?

Michael P. Swords, DO[a],*, Brian Weatherford, MD[b,c,d]

KEYWORDS

- Pilon fracture • Plafond • External fixation • Arthrodesis • Ankle

KEY POINTS

- Most of the tibial pilon fractures benefit from a staged protocol with initial external fixation and delayed internal fixation with direct reduction of the articular surface.
- Reduction techniques performed to achieve restoration of mechanical axis during application of external fixation are a key component to successful pilon fracture management.
- The use of an external fixator, with or without limited internal fixation, can be useful in patients with significant soft tissue compromise.
- Primary arthrodesis can be considered in patients with nonreconstructable articular injuries, delayed presentation, significant medical comorbidities, or peripheral neuropathy.

INTRODUCTION

The management of tibial pilon fractures remains a significant challenge for orthopedic surgeons. Historically these injuries have been associated with significant complications including high rates of infection and wound compromise.[1,2] Advances in the understanding of soft tissue management with the use of temporary bridging external fixators have significantly decreased the rate of soft tissue complication.[3,4] Staged treatment with a spanning external fixator followed by delayed definitive reconstruction has become the standard for these injuries. High-energy fractures of the distal

[a] Michigan Orthopedic Center, 2815 South Pennsylvania Avenue, suite 204, Lansing MI 48901, USA; [b] Orthopaedic Trauma, Reconstructive Foot and Ankle Surgery; [c] Illinois Bone and Joint Institute, 2401 Ravine Way, Glenview, IL 60025, USA; [d] University of Chicago Pritzker School of Medicine, Chicago, IL, USA
* Corresponding author.
E-mail address: foot.trauma@gmail.com

Foot Ankle Clin N Am 25 (2020) 523–536
https://doi.org/10.1016/j.fcl.2020.08.005
1083-7515/20/© 2020 Elsevier Inc. All rights reserved.

tibia still routinely result in long-term pain and dysfunction despite appropriate treatment.[5,6]

The use of techniques including definitive external fixation or primary arthrodesis is typically reserved for patients with significant soft tissue compromise, unreconstructable injuries, or severe underlying comorbidities. In these select patients, these alternative techniques are required to restore a functional limb, while minimizing the risk of further complications.

ACUTE EXTERNAL FIXATION AS PART OF STAGED MANAGEMENT

In patients presenting with a tibial pilon fracture, a thoughtfully applied external fixator is an essential component of initial management. The decision-making is straight forward. All significant injuries resulting in loss of limb or articular alignment will benefit from timely application of external fixation to restore limb alignment. Very rarely does the external fixator need to be applied rapidly in a "damage control" scenario. The use of an external fixator with tibial pilon fractures should be considered the first stage of a 2-stage reconstruction of the limb. A well thought out and applied external fixator will reestablish essential length, alignment, and rotation, greatly aiding the staged reconstruction of the articular injury when the soft tissues allow. Ideally, frame application should be done by surgeons who will ultimately treat the injury. If not possible, they should at a minimum be familiar with the fixation philosophy of the individual/institution that will provide definitive care. The fibula should be left alone if the surgeon will not be ultimately managing the overall care of the injury. If the first stage is done poorly, it makes it significantly more challenging to execute the second stage. Barei and colleagues[7] found that 40 of 42 patients with provisional external fixation of a pilon fracture transferred to a tertiary referral trauma center required revision before definitive treatment, most commonly secondary to tibial malreduction. Several key components should be considered when applying a spanning external fixator for a tibial pilon fracture:

- Restoration of adequate length is essential. The relationship of the lateral process of the talus to the distal fibula can be a guide to appropriate restoration of length.
- The talus must be centered under the tibial shaft on all views. If the talus is not under the tibia, the limb is malaligned and the construct should be revised.
- Pin placement should be clear of any planned surgical incisions. Draw out planned incisions and anticipate plate locations before placing the external fixator.
- The construct must be stable enough to maintain alignment during the anticipated soft tissue recovery. Consider secondary pin placement in the foot to aid with stability.
- Pins should be placed carefully and in the correct plane to aid in reduction with the frame.
  - Tibia pins perpendicular to the long axis of the tibia
  - Calcaneus pins parallel to the top of the talar dome and perpendicular to the long axis of the foot
  - Cuneiform pin perpendicular to the long axis of the foot

Delta Frame

The most commonly used method of ankle spanning external fixation for pilon fractures is a "delta frame" construct typically composed of anterior tibial half pins connected to a centrally threaded transcalcaneal pin. Historically fixation of the fibula was advocated at the time of initial external fixation application. Appropriate reduction

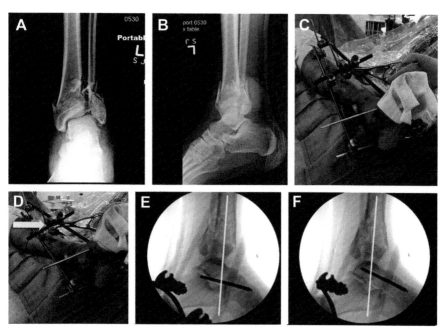

Fig. 1. Anteroposterior (AP) (*A*) and lateral radiographs of a high-energy tibial pilon fracture with compressive failure of the lateral tibia and fibula. (*B*) Clinical photo demonstrating placement of a fixed clamp and lamina spreader before correction of sagittal deformity. (*C*) Clinical photo demonstrating utilization of a fixed clamp and lamina spreader to correct sagittal alignment. Note increased space of lamina spreader corresponding with posterior translation of the tibia. (*D*) Lateral fluoroscopic image of the previous patient demonstrating posterior translation of the distal segment with apex anterior deformity. The yellow line highlights the posterior translation of the talus relative to the mid-axis of the tibia. (*E*) Lateral fluoroscopic image demonstrating improved sagittal alignment using a second tibial pin with lamina spreader to correct tibial alignment. The yellow line now bisects the talar dome, indicating appropriate alignment (*F*).

of the fibula can assist with stability, indirect reduction of the limb, and maintenance of reduction. Fixation of the fibula at the time of initial external fixation or even definitive treatment is controversial.[8] Malreduction of the fibula or a poorly placed incision can significantly hinder the definitive treatment of the tibial fracture. The authors recommend against fixation of the fibula if the surgeon performing external fixation will not be performing the definitive treatment. The incision for fixation of the fibula must be considered as part of the global treatment plan of the injury and if not correctly placed, may compromise the overall fixation strategy. In addition, malreduction may require revision at the time of definitive treatment, increasing the complexity of the reconstruction and the risk of complications.

Several adjuncts can be useful to assist with maintenance of stability and alignment during placement of ankle spanning external fixation. When using a delta frame construct, reduction of the tibia in the sagittal plane can be challenging. In most of the pilon fracture patterns there is compressive failure of the anterior plafond with anterior instability or extrusion of the talus. Therefore, the anterior to posterior vector from the anterior tibial half pins to the posterior transcalcaneal pin assists with reduction. However, in patterns with posterior instability this vector can accentuate the deformity. This deformity can be corrected using a standardized sequence of reduction (**Fig. 1**).[9]

Reduction sequence for delta frame external fixation

1. Coronal plane alignment is established first between the proximal tibial pin and calcaneal pin.
2. The sagittal plane can then be reduced by placing a lamina spreader between the distal tibia half pin and a fixed point (a clamp or T-handled chuck) to dial in the sagittal plane reduction.

Medial Frame

An alternative frame construct is a medial-based frame. This frame is in line with the long axis of the tibia shaft and is at times preferable in fractures with more extensive posterior comminution or shaft extension. A 5-mm half pin is placed well proximal to the anticipated plate needed for definitive fixation. A second 5-mm pin is placed in the calcaneus, parallel to the superior surface of the talar dome. Distraction between these 2 pins allows for restoration of overall alignment. Frame stability is improved by adding an additional pin through a clamp between the first 2 pins inserted. This pin can be used to aid in reduction of the shaft and correction of varus or valgus malalignment. In cases with an open medial wound, the pin is used to push the tibia away from the compromised soft tissues before locking the clamp to aiding in soft tissue recovery. The foot is then held in a neutral position by placing a 4-mm cuneiform pin. The pin is predrilled in the proximal (to avoid penetration into the second tarsometatarsal joint) and upper half of the cuneiform (to avoid placing the pin under the middle cuneiform) from medial to lateral. Incorporating the midfoot into the fixation construct will increase stability of the frame construct as well as prevent ankle equinus. Several commercially available external fixation systems have distraction instruments included in the set. These devices can be used to increase the amount of distraction across the ankle joint.

Reduction Tips with Acute External Fixation

1. Always place tibia pins perpendicular to the long axis of the tibia.
2. The calcaneal pin should be placed parallel to the talar dome and perpendicular to the long axis of the foot.
3. Distraction device may be used to gain additional distraction.
4. The foot position under the tibia can be adjusted using a T-handle chuck and a mallet to translate the foot medial or lateral relative to the tibia (**Fig. 2**).
5. A Schanz pin may be placed into the tibia through a clamp and then using a T-handle chuck the pin can be "pushed" or "pulled" and then locked to the frame to correct varus or valgus alignment or to relieve tension on compromised soft tissues or open wounds (**Fig. 3**).

EXTERNAL FIXATION FOR DEFINITIVE TREATMENT

Numerous series have evaluated the definitive use of external fixation for definitive management of pilon injuries. Most of these studies are comparative, with limitations in design, including small sample size, retrospective nature, and selection of treatment method in a nonrandomized fashion.

External fixation may be used as a definitive treatment in conjunction with limited internal fixation and joint reduction or by external fixation alone, usually as circular small wire fixation.

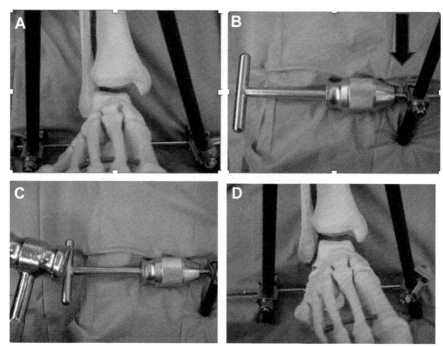

Fig. 2. Malalignment of the talus under the tibia in the coronal plane is present with the center of the talus 5 mm lateral relative to the mechanical axis of the tibia (*A*). A T-handle chuck is placed equidistance (5 mm) from the clamp on the opposite side of the frame (*B*). The clamp is unlocked from the calcaneal pin, and a mallet is used to gently correct the translational deformity (*C*). The clamp is tightened after correct alignment of the talus under the tibia is achieved (*D*).

EXTERNAL FIXATION WITH LIMITED INTERNAL FIXATION FOR DEFINITIVE TREATMENT

Select fractures may be treated successfully with a combination of external fixation with limited internal fixation, and this may be done in low fractures with minimal to no metadiaphyseal extension or comminution and in partial articular fractures. The goals of initial external fixation are the same. The talus should be centered under the tibia on both anteroposterior and lateral views and the tibia mechanical axis, length, and rotation restored. Computed tomography scanning allows for detailed planning of the articular reduction, which may be performed with a series of percutaneous placed reduction clamps and followed by screw insertion (**Fig. 4** right injury).[10,11] In addition, mini fragment fixation may be used to add additional stability to the fracture fixation construct. The general articular injury in AO/Orthopedic Trauma Association (OTA) 43C pilon fractures has been well described.[12] Successful treatment of this fracture pattern typically requires 2 plates to sufficiently maintain reduction over time.[13] The external fixator may also be used to stage plate fixation (see **Fig. 4** left injury). If there is severe soft tissue injury medially, the articular surface may be approached and reduced using an anterolateral approach and plate. The medial fracture segment can be stabilized with screws and the external fixator

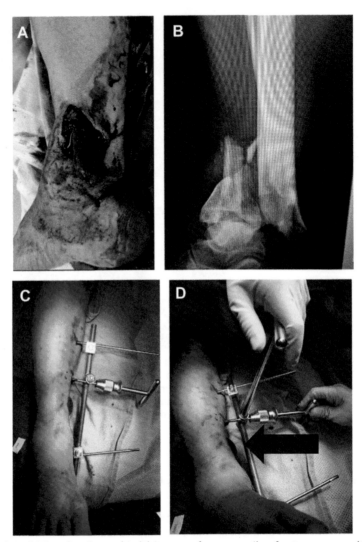

Fig. 3. Clinical (*A*) and radiographic (*B*) images of an open pilon fracture as a result of a fall from a ladder. A medial external fixator is used to obtain alignment and stabilize the injury. (*C*) A pin is placed through a clamp and inserted into the tibia. After insertion into the tibia an axial load is placed on the pin "pushing" the tibia away from the traumatized soft tissues before the clamp is tightened to the frame construct (*D*).

maintained after reduction. The patient can be returned to the operating room for medial plate placement and external fixation removal after the medial soft tissues have recovered. Bone grafting may be performed at the same time if necessary. Use of an ankle spanning external fixator used with limited fixation for the articular surface is associated with ankle stiffness, loss of reduction, malunion, and inferior outcomes when compared with standard open techniques.[11,14] Despite these risks, this treatment method is an option for select fractures that are not amenable to standard open reduction and internal fixation (ORIF).

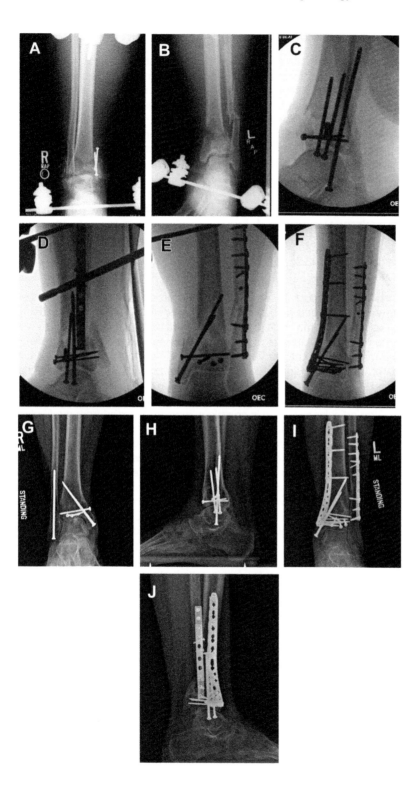

CIRCULAR EXTERNAL FIXATION FOR DEFINITIVE TREATMENT OF PILON FRACTURES

Circular external fixation of a pilon fracture is a technically demanding surgical procedure. Pilon fractures are among the most difficult traumatic injuries to manage surgically. Familiarity with circular external fixation techniques is a prerequisite for attempting management of high-energy pilon fractures with this method of fixation. Circular constructs allow for management of the injury with less disruption to the soft tissue envelope. In addition, frame constructs are rigid enough to allow early weight bearing. With the possibility of gradual correction over time with computer-assisted correction, frames also allow for fine tuning fracture alignment beyond what is achieved during the surgical event.

FRAME ESSENTIALS FOR PRIMARY MANAGEMENT OF PILON FRACTURES WITH CIRCULAR EXTERNAL FIXATION

1. Proximal ring block above the fracture with rings perpendicular to the tibia
2. Periarticular ring with small wires to control the articular injury at the ankle level
3. Foot ring

The proximal ring block is assembled to the leg above the level of the fracture. Smooth wires are placed distally to control the articular surface. Knowledge of the capsular reflections of the ankle joint are important, as intraarticularly placed wires increase the risk of development of joint infection. The posterior capsular reflection is roughly 2 mm with the anterior capsular reflection extending as high as 12.2 mm.[15] The mean capsular extension is a distance of 3.8 mm proximal to the dome of the tibial plafond.[16] The articular fracture components may be manipulated percutaneously for reduction or reduced by small incision techniques and provisionally held with standard K wires. After articular reduction is complete, a wire is inserted from the fibula to the anteromedial portion of the distal tibia. A smooth wire is then advanced from the posterior portion of the medial distal tibia just anterior to the posterior tibial tendon and advanced out the anterolateral aspect of the tibia. Transverse wires may be added to increase frame stability to the articular block as needed. In fractures with minimal metadiaphyseal comminution or extension, the periarticular ring can be connected to the proximal ring block with threaded bolts. More complicated fracture patterns may require telescopic struts that allow for gradual correction or fine tuning of fracture alignment over time. In addition, angular shortening and deformity may be used to allow closure of traumatic wounds or bone deficits then corrected gradually over time (**Fig. 5**).[17–19]

A foot ring is incorporated in the frame, which allows immobilization of the ankle decreasing pin complications at the distal tibia ring caused by soft tissue movement

◀————————————————————————————

Fig. 4. AP image of the right (*A*) and left (*B*) demonstrated severe low pilon injuries from a fall from fourth floor of a parking garage. Note the old medial malleolar screws. Operative views of the right (*C*) and left (*D*) ankle demonstrating congruent articular reductions. The patient was treated with percutaneous reduction and limited fixation for the articular injuries combined with external fixation due to severity of soft tissue injury and poor general medical condition. Medial metadiaphyseal bone loss and ankle varus due to lack of buttress are visible on the intraoperative image of the left ankle (*E*). A medial plate for buttress and bone grafting was performed on the left injury at 8 weeks when both frames were removed (*F*). Mortise (*G*) and lateral (*H*) views of the right and mortise (*I*) and lateral radiographs (*J*) of the left ankle 7 years postinjury.

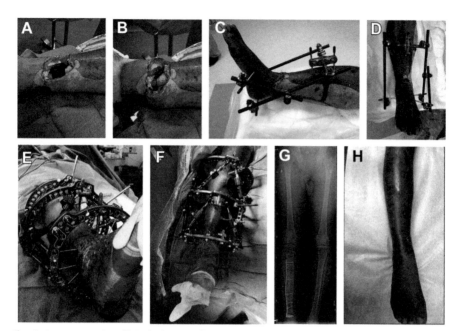

Fig. 5. Intraoperative clinical photos of a patient with a high-energy open pilon fracture. The patient had a significant bone defect with soft tissue loss. (*A*) Intentional shortening of the limb was performed to minimize the soft tissue defect. (*B*), (*C*), and (*D*) are clinical photos following aggressive debridement and closure of the traumatic wound with initial standard delta frame external fixator. (*E*) and (*F*) are clinical photos following conversion to circular external fixator with proximal corticotomy and gradual distraction osteogenesis to restore limb length. Note the density of thin wire fixation to stabilize the short distal segment. Standing alignment radiograph demonstrating restoration of limb length with healing of distal tibia and proximal tibia regenerate. (*G*) Patient was converted to internal fixation to shorten time in external fixator. Clinical photo demonstrating well-healed soft tissue envelope following removal of external fixation. (*H*).

associated with ankle dorsiflexion and plantarflexion. A foot ring also allows a walker ring to be added for weight bearing. The foot portion of the frame can be left on for the entirety of the treatment course or removed part way through treatment to allow for ankle range of motion. More complex fractures with additional metadiaphyseal or shaft components may require additional rings to allow for more accurate management and control of additional fracture segments.

Richards reported a series of 60 patients treated either with definitive external fixation or with delayed ORIF.[20] The groups did not differ in smoking status, OTA fracture classification, age, or number of open fractures. No difference in quality of articular reduction or deep infection was noted. Nonunion and delayed union were seen more frequently in the external fixation group. The ORIF group was noted to have improved Iowa Ankle Scores and SF-36 scores at both 6 and 12 months postinjury. Bacon, in a retrospective analysis, found no statistically significant difference in complication rates, deep infection, time to union, malunion, and delayed union in fractures treated either with open plating or with Ilizarov techniques.[21] Watson and colleagues[22] developed a treatment protocol based on severity of soft tissue injury. Eighty-one percent of patients in the external fixation group and 75% in the open plating group had good or excellent results. C-type fractures had poorer results regardless of treatment. Plate fixation was associated with higher rates of nonunion, malunion, and severe wound complications as compared with patients treated with external fixation.

THE AUTHORS' INDICATIONS FOR CONSIDERATION OF SMALL WIRE FIXATION AS DEFINITIVE TREATMENT

1. Severe soft tissue compromise
2. Infection
3. Bone loss
4. Inability to comply with non–weight-bearing requirements

PRIMARY ARTHRODESIS FOR ACUTE PILON FRACTURES

Primary arthrodesis for pilon fracture is reserved for select situations. Patients with high-energy injuries that are deemed nonreconstructable due to extreme comminution or loss of articular surface from open injury may be managed with primary arthrodesis. Additional patients to consider primary arthrodesis include neuropathic patients and patients with multiple medical comorbidities. Ankle arthrodesis increases the risk of arthritis to the adjacent joints in the hindfoot and midfoot.[23] Ankle arthrodesis also leads to decrease in gait velocity, cadence, and stride length when compared with age-matched controls.[24] Treatment options for primary arthrodesis for severe pilon injuries include plates and screws, Hindfoot nailing, and external fixation. Zelle and colleagues[25] reported on 17 patients with nonreconstructable pilon injuries treated with primary arthrodesis with a posterior blade plate. Union was achieved at an average of 132 days. One patient required revision of a nonunion with a circular frame. At an average of 7.2 years of follow-up all patients were walking without assist devices. There were no deep infections. Similarly, Bozic treated a series of 14 patients with nonreconstructable pilon injuries with posterior blade plate and iliac crest graft. All patients went on to union.[26] There was one deep infection. The investigators have reported good outcomes with hindfoot arthrodesis nails for treatment of pilon injuries with arthrodesis.[27–29] Hindfoot arthrodesis nails alter the subtalar joint, resulting in loss of function of the hindfoot, as inversion and eversion are necessary for improved function. In addition, hindfoot arthrodesis nails do not have the flexibility to modify the fixation to the individual fracture pattern due to the limited proximal and distal locking options with essentially no fragment-specific fixation at the joint level. Because of these shortcomings, arthrodesis with a hindfoot nail is recommended only in low- demand patients and those with fractures with minimal shaft extension.

CIRCULAR EXTERNAL FIXATION FOR PRIMARY ARTHRODESIS FOR ACUTE PILON FRACTURES

The concepts for frame construction previously described for circular external fixation for definitive treatment of pilon injuries are the starting point for extending the use of frames to include primary arthrodesis of the ankle for more severe injuries. Arthrodesis is recommended in cases where comminution is severe or articular bone loss is present (**Fig. 6**). The articular cartilage is carefully removed after relative articular reduction is achieved. If the fracture is closed and without contamination, bone grafting may be done acutely. In cases of open fractures consideration should be made to delay bone grafting 6 to 8 weeks to ensure no infection develops. The main difference between the frame for primary care for treatment of a pilon fracture and the frame

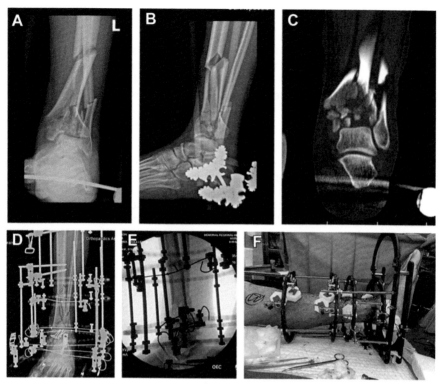

Fig. 6. Mortise (*A*) lateral radiographs (*B*) and CT (*C*) demonstrating a severely comminuted high-energy pilon fracture with associated tibial shaft fracture. Mortise (*D*), lateral (*E*), and clinical images (*F*) demonstrating small wire frame construct used to definitively treat all components of the fracture and perform a primary arthrodesis of the ankle. (*Courtesy of S. Steinlauf, MD, Hollywood, FL.*)

used to achieve ankle arthrodesis is the addition of compression between the articular block and the foot ring. This is most commonly achieved using threaded bolts with compression added acutely at the time of surgery once the frame is assembled on the limb in the operating room.

FRAME ESSENTIALS FOR PRIMARY MANAGEMENT OF PILON FRACTURES WITH PRIMARY ARTHRODESIS

1. Proximal ring block above the fracture
2. Periarticular ring with small wires to control the articular injury at the ankle level
3. Foot ring to control the foot and use to compress across the ankle to achieve arthrodesis

Beaman and Gellman reported on a series of 63 pilon fractures, 12 of which were treated with primary arthrodesis.[30] Two patients were treated with ring fixation only, whereas the remaining 10 patients were treated with anterior arthrodesis plating in conjunction with ring fixation to address shaft extension or to provide additional stability. Average time to union was 4.4 months, and 88% of patients achieved an excellent or good result.

SUMMARY

Utilization of external fixation is both indicated and necessary in the management of high-energy tibial pilon injuries. The wide variability of soft tissue and osseus injury requires treatment to be catered to the individual case. Temporizing external fixation, external fixation with limited articular fixation, small wire fixation for definitive management, and arthrodesis techniques with external fixation all play a role in the management of these difficult injuries.

CLINICS CARE POINTS

- Staged treatment with ankle spanning external fixation has dramatically reduced the rate of soft tissue complications with tibial pilon fractures.
- Definitive external fixation with limited internal fixation has inferior outcomes compared with open reduction; however, it can be used in select circumstances.
- Small wire circular external fixators are useful to manage pilon fractures with significant soft tissue compromise or metadiaphyseal bone loss and demonstrate similar outcomes compared with open techniques.
- Primary arthrodesis of tibial pilon fractures is indicated only in patients with unreconstructable articular injuries, neuropathic fractures, or patients who require early weight bearing due to inability to follow precautions or underlying medical conditions.

DISCLOSURE

The authors have nothing to disclose.

REFERENCES

1. Kellam JF, Waddell JP. Fractures of the distal tibial metaphysis with intra-articular extension–the distal tibial explosion fracture. J Trauma 1979;19(8):593–601.
2. Teeny SM, Wiss DA. Open reduction and internal fixation of tibial plafond fractures. Variables contributing to poor results and complications. Clin Orthop Relat Res 1993;(292):108–17.
3. Patterson MJ, Cole JD. Two-staged delayed open reduction and internal fixation of severe pilon fractures. J Orthop Trauma 1999;13(2):85–91.
4. Sirkin M, Sanders R, DiPasquale T, et al. A staged protocol for soft tissue management in the treatment of complex pilon fractures. J Orthop Trauma 1999; 13(2):78–84.
5. Pollak AN, McCarthy ML, Bess RS, et al. Outcomes after treatment of high-energy tibial plafond fractures. J Bone Joint Surg Am 2003;85(10):1893–900.
6. Marsh JL, Weigel DP, Dirschl DA. Tibial plafond fractures. How do these ankles function over time? J Bone Joint Surg Am 2003;85(2):287–95.
7. Barei DP, Gardner MJ, Nork SE, et al. Revision of provisional stabilization in pilon fractures referred from outside institutions. Orthopaedic Proceedings 2011;93-B: 264–5.
8. Kurylo JC, Datta N, Iskander KN, et al. Does the fibula need to be fixed in complex pilon fractures? J Orthop Trauma 2015;29(9):424–7.
9. Liskutin T, Bernstein M, Summers H, et al. Surgical technique: achieving anatomic alignment with temporizing, ankle-spanning external fixation. J Orthop Trauma 2018;32(Suppl 1):S38–9.

10. Blauth M, Bastian L, Krettek C, et al. Surgical options for the treatment of severe tibial pilon fractures: a study of three techniques. J Orthop Trauma 2001;15(3): 153–60.
11. Dickson KF, Montgomery S, Field J. High energy plafond fractures treated by a spanning external fixator initially and followed by a second stage open reduction internal fixation of the articular surface: a preliminary report. Injury 2001;32(Suppl 4):SD92–8.
12. Cole PA, Mehrle RK, Bhandari M, et al. The pilon map: fracture lines and comminution zones in OTA/AO 43C pilon fractures. J Orthop Trauma 2013;27(7):e152–6.
13. Penny P, Swords MP, Heisler J, et al. Ability of modern distal tibia plates to stabilize comminuted pilon fracture fragments: is dual plate fixation necessary? Injury 2016;47(8):1761–9.
14. Pugh KJ, Wolinsky PR, McAndrew MP, et al. Tibial pilon fractures: a comparison of treatment methods. J Trauma 1999;47(5):937–41.
15. Vora AM, Haddad SL, Kadakia A, et al. Extracapsular placement of distal tibia transfixation wires. J Bone Joint Surg Am 2004;86(5):988–93.
16. Lee PT, Clarke MT, Bearcraft PW, et al. The proximal extent of the ankle capsule and safety for the insertion of percutaneous fine wires. J Bone Joint Surg Br 2005; 87(5):668–71.
17. Gulsen M, Ozkan C. Angular shortening and delayed gradual distraction for the treatment of asymmetrical bone and soft tissue defects of tibia: a case series. J Trauma 2009;66(5):E61–6.
18. Lahoti O, Findlay I, Shetty S, et al. Intentional deformation and closure of a soft tissue defect in open tibial fractures with a taylor spatial frame- asimple technique. J Orthop Trauma 2013;27(8):451–6.
19. Nho SJ, Helfet DL, Rozbruch SR. Temporary intentional leg shortening and deformation to facilitate wound closure using the Ilizarov/Taylor spatial frame. J Orthop Trauma 2006;20(6):419–24.
20. Richards JE, Magill M, Tressler MA, et al. External fixation versus. ORIF for distal intra-articular tibia fractures. Orthopedics 2012;35(6):e862–7.
21. Bacon S, Smith WR, Morgan SJ, et al. A retrospective analysis of comminuted intra-articular fractures of the tibial plafond. Open reduction and internal fixation versus external Ilizarov fixation. Injury 2008;39(2):196–202.
22. Watson JT, Moed BR, Karges DE, et al. Pilon fractures. Treatment protocol based on severity of soft tissue injury. Clin Orthop Relat Res 2000;375:78–90.
23. Coester LM, Saltzman CL, Leupold J, et al. Long-term results following ankle arthrodesis for post-traumatic arthritis. J Bone Joint Surg Am 2001;83-A(2): 219–28.
24. Thomas R, Daniels TR, Parker K. Gait analysis and functional outcomes following ankle arthrodesis for isolated ankle arthritis. J Bone Joint Surg Am 2006;88(3): 526–35.
25. Zelle BA, Gruen GS, McMillen RL, et al. Primary arthrodesis of the tibiotalar joint in severely comminuted high-energy pilon fractures. J Bone Joint Surg Am 2014; 96(11):e91.
26. Bozic V, Thordarson DB, Hertz J. Ankle fusion for definitive management of non-reconstructable pilon fractures. Foot Ankle Int 2008;29(9):914–8.
27. Al-Ashhab ME. Primary ankle arthrodesis for severely comminuted tibial pilon fractures. Orthopedics 2017;40(2):e378–81.
28. Hsu AR, Szatkowski JP. Early tibiotalocalcaneal arthrodesis with intramedullary nail for treatment of a complex pilon fracture (AO/OTA 43C). Foot Ankle Spec 2015;8(3):220–5.

29. Nikura T, Miwa M, Sakai Y, et al. Ankle arthrodesis using antegrade intramedullary nail for salvage of nonreconstructable tibial pilon fractures. Orthopedics 2009; 32(8). https://doi.org/10.3928/01477447-20090624-26.
30. Beaman DN, Gellman R. Fracture reduction and primary ankle arthrodesis: a reliable approach for severely comminuted tibial pilon fracture. Clin Orthop Relat Res 2014;472(12):3832–4.

Induced Membrane Technique (Masquelet) for Bone Defects in the Distal Tibia, Foot, and Ankle: Systematic Review, Case Presentations, Tips, and Techniques

Paul Andrzejowski, BMBS, MRCS[a], Alain Masquelet, MD[b], Peter V. Giannoudis, MD, FRCS[a],*

KEYWORDS

- Induced membrane • Masquelet • Reconstruction • Defect • Foot • Ankle • Tibia
- Hindfoot

KEY POINTS

- Preparation is the key. By ensuring a thorough work-up of the patient and targeted therapy using the diamond concept, this approach increases the chances of success.
- Respect for soft tissues is paramount. Unless soft tissues are respected throughout the procedure, the chances of success are significantly diminished.
- Thorough and repeated debridement is essential. Where inadequate initial and subsequent debridement is not aggressively performed, persisting devitalized tissue creates high risk of infection: any procedure is doomed to failure.
- Success when a full approach is followed. Where all of the principles of the diamond concept are followed, and principles of Masquelet included in management, this article shows that outcomes are very favorable.
- Further work is needed. Numbers of focused studies for the Masquelet procedure in foot and ankle and outcomes are small: large-scale studies are needed to fully assess this.

Conflict of interest: No benefits in any form have been received or will be received from a commercial party related directly or indirectly to the subject of this article.
[a] Academic Department of Trauma & Orthopaedics, School of Medicine, University of Leeds, Leeds General Infirmary, Clarendon Wing, Floor D, Great George Street, Leeds LS1 3EX, UK;
[b] Department of Orthopaedic Surgery, Avicenne Hospital AP–HP, 123, route de Stalingrad, Bobiny 93009, France
* Corresponding author.
E-mail address: pgiannoudi@aol.com

Foot Ankle Clin N Am 25 (2020) 537–586
https://doi.org/10.1016/j.fcl.2020.08.013

foot.theclinics.com

APPROACH

- There may be cases where the approach is made challenging, such as fragile tissue or extensive scarring over the anterior or medial aspect of the tibia. In these cases, clinicians can undertake an extended bypass intertibiofibular graft to bridge the tibial defect.[1]

DEBRIDEMENT

- The importance of debridement, in the second stage as well as the first, was emphasized in a recent review of complications following the Masquelet procedure. Poor results are likely to follow if this advice is ignored.[2]
- Multiple samples must be sent at both stages, to fully assess infective load.
- Ensure that antibiotic prophylaxis is withheld until samples are taken.

CEMENT APPLICATION

- In order for the antibiotic in the cement to be effective, measures must be taken to maximize its porosity so that it can leach out into the surrounding area. To achieve this, make sure that it is added last to the mixture, and avoid suction/vacuum mixing of cement.
- The cement must overlap the edges of the defect by at least 1 cm, to ensure that the membrane is produced away from the defect itself, which significantly improves outcomes.
- When using external fixation in the first stage, which is less rigid, the authors recommend using the molding method to place the cement around a 2-mm Kirschner wire, which is inserted through the defect and into the medullary canals of the 2 opposing bone ends in order to prevent displacement.
- Polymethylmethacrylate (PMMA) cement sets with a powerful exothermic reaction, which is harmful to living cells nearby. To avoid cell lysis from thermal necrosis, the authors recommend separating this area from the other tissues using a surgical glove, and constantly irrigating the area with saline, while the cement sets. Furthermore, any antibiotic chosen must be heat stable.

SECOND-STAGE FIXATION

- In order for a fracture or bone defect to heal by the second stage, the mechanical environment must be considered equally alongside the biological environment, with the ultimate osteosynthesis chosen providing adequate stability to facilitate osseous growth and integration with the graft (**Fig. 1**).[1,3]

RESPECT FOR SOFT TISSUES

- A rich vascular network is essential for osseous healing, allowing abundant nutrients, growth factors, and cells to transform the defect area into new bone. The surrounding soft tissues, periosteum, and endothelial structures, which have been shown to have their own intrinsic regenerative capacity, must be protected and respected throughout, as must the induced membrane, which shares similar properties. Otherwise, the chance of success diminishes (see **Fig. 1**).[1,3,4]

CONTAINMENT

- Unless clinicians ensure that the potent osteogenic recipe that has been achieved through the Masquelet technique is kept together in 1 place, or

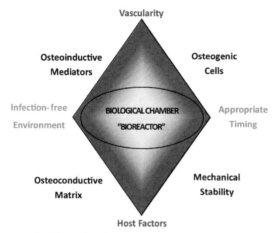

Fig. 1. Diamond concept of bone healing.

contained, then success is likely to be limited. It has been shown, especially for defects larger than 5 cm, that there is a high rate of graft resorption, nullifying clinicians' extensive efforts to repair them. Therefore, it is crucial that the membrane is used to keep everything together in a biological chamber, or bioreactor (see **Fig. 1**).[1,3,4]

POSTOPERATIVE REGIME

- Ensure that all patients receive suitable thromboprophylaxis, such as low-molecular-weight heparin (LMWH), for at least 6 weeks.
- For tibial injuries, mobilize touch-toe weight bearing only and, for defects of the foot and ankle, avoid weight bearing altogether at this stage. Provide a frame or crutches.
- Wound inspection at 2 weeks, then radiograph follow-up at 6 weeks.
- Further follow-up until radiological signs of union and pain-free mobilization (**Figs. 2**I, J and **3**H).

JUSTIFICATION

There have not been any systematic reviews that focus on the Masquelet technique being used specifically distal tibia, foot, and ankle, despite this being an area of interest for surgeons managing large bone defects there. Our objectives were to perform a comprehensive appraisal of all the original literature available on the subject, which specifically focused on the distal third tibia, foot, and ankle. We wanted to explore the whole area where the induced membrane technique was used, from background patient characteristics to the specific technique, final surgical outcomes, and union/consolidation. Preferred Reporting Items for Systematic Reviews and Meta-Analyses (PRISMA) guidelines were consulted throughout.[5,6]

INTRODUCTION

Bone defects involving the distal one-third of the tibia, ankle, and foot usually present following trauma, debridement secondary to infection, nonunion, and tumor excision.[1] Their management can be challenging and long lasting. Different techniques have been described in the literature for their management, including distraction

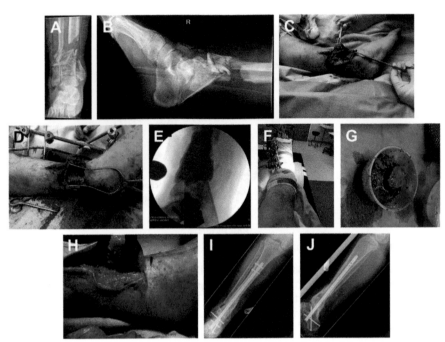

Fig. 2. (*A*) Admission ankle anteroposterior (AP) radiograph in a 40-year-old man who sustained an open distal tibial intraarticular fracture in a motorbike accident. (*B*) Admission ankle lateral radiograph. (*C*) Intraoperative (first stage) image showing extent of soft tissue damage before debridement. (*D*) Intraoperative (first stage) image following external fixator and cement application. (*E*) Intraoperative lateral radiograph (first stage) following cement spacer. (*F*) Postoperative appearance (first stage) with external fixator in situ, and bandages around leg. (*G*) Second stage: reamer-irrigator-aspirator (RIA) autograft harvested, ready for implantation. (*H*) Implanted augmented RIA autograft (with bone marrow aspirate concentrate, bone morphogenetic protein -2, demineralized bone matrix) in cavity formed by induced membrane (IM) nail, following further debridement. (*I*) Fifteen months postoperative AP radiograph showing osseous healing of the defect area. (*J*) Fifteen months postoperative lateral radiograph showing bone union.

osteogenesis, free fibula vascularized graft, titanium cages, intramedullary lengthening devices, and the Masquelet or induced membrane (IM) technique.[1]

Since its inception in 1986, the IM technique has become a well-established method for restoring areas of critical bone loss. It has shown excellent results where a strict treatment regime is followed, providing a positive solution to difficult problems.[1] It is based on a 2-stage principle. The first stage allows eradication of any infective organisms and formation of an osteoinductive membrane around a cement spacer, which involves debridement, temporary or permanent bridging or in-line fixation, and cement spacer packing, plus any required soft tissue reconstruction. Following a period of 6 to 8 weeks, the second stage can take place, consisting of removal of the cement spacer and insertion of bone graft in the defect area.[1]

The IM technique can be used in all areas of the body, including the foot, ankle, and tibia, which is the focus of this article, providing an overview of the basic science, practical technique, evidence of its success through a detailed literature review, and direction for future research.

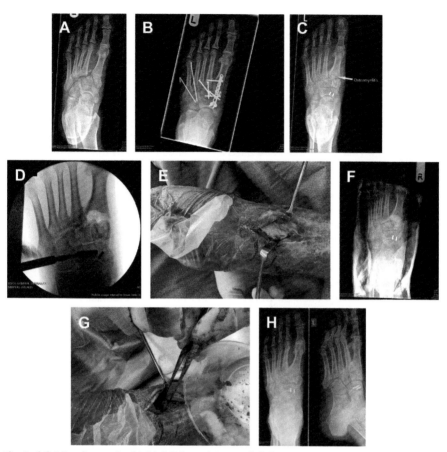

Fig. 3. (*A*) AP radiograph of initial Lisfranc injury to left foot in male patient 35 years old. (*B*) AP radiograph following initial repair of injury. (*C*) AP radiograph showing osteomyelitis to left midfoot, before Masquelet. (*D*) Intraoperative AP radiograph. Debridement of region, first-stage Masquelet procedure. (*E*) Intraoperative image of cement insertion into defect following debridement. (*F*) Postoperative AP radiograph, with cement spacer in situ. (*G*) Intraoperative image of second-stage composite grafting, into cavity formed by IM, following further debridement. (*H*) Twenty-one months following bone graft (second stage); AP (*left*)/oblique (*right*) radiographs.

INDICATIONS FOR THE INDUCED MEMBRANE TECHNIQUE

The IM technique can be considered in the treatment of bone defects in the foot and ankle greater than 2 cm, and more than 3 cm for the distal tibia.[1,3,7,8] In the foot specifically, it has been used following trauma, nonunion (aseptic or septic), osteomyelitis in Charcot foot, tuberculosis (TB) infection, and for management of defect left after erosive gouty tophus.[7,9–11] Interestingly, the IM technique has been used successfully in defects of long bones up to 25 cm.[1]

PRINCIPLES

In order to optimize the chances of healing, clinicians must address all of the factors in a systematic fashion, through meticulous planning before surgery.[1,12] An infected environment must be converted to an aseptic one in order to promote a successful healing response. Clinicians must adhere strictly to the principles of the diamond concept, which describes the elements required for optimal revascularization and osseous healing of the affected environment (see **Fig. 1**).[3,4] The Non-Union Scoring System could also be considered when assessing what to focus on.[13,14]

INITIAL ASSESSMENT

The surgeon should take a meticulous history of the presenting complaint, in particular ascertaining the energy of the insult, extent of any open fracture, and associated soft tissue defects. This stage should be used as a chance to review management so far, assess whether all appropriate guidelines have been followed, and optimize care where needed. A thorough clinical examination is important; in the acute context, assess the extent of soft tissue injury, presence of fracture blisters, and likely need/method for repair; all open fractures should be discussed preoperatively with the plastic surgery team where possible.[15] In the more chronic context, infection must always be assumed in the case of nonunion until proved otherwise.[16,17] In all cases, clinicians must assess for any obvious rotational deformity, limb/extremity shape or length discrepancy, peripheral neurovascular status (which must include assessment of sensation and power), and peripheral pulses, as well as the skin condition. Extended bedside investigations such as Doppler testing and ankle-brachial pressure index assessment must be considered where appropriate in cases of vasculopathy or neuropathy.

A detailed past medical, drug, and social history should be obtained, in order to allow optimization of the patient (host) to reduce global risk factors for nonunion, with particular attention paid to management of systemic disease such as infection, diabetes, vasculopathy, osteoporosis, nephropathy, and all chronic inflammatory diseases alongside smoking cessation and nutritional supplementation (calcium and vitamin D), as well as review of any medication that may inhibit osteogenesis.[4] It also helps with organizing rehabilitation following surgery to enable optimal outcome, which should always be the aim. Early discussion with other medical specialties, and coordination of a holistic approach, is an essential tenet of care.

Biochemical (C-reactive protein, erythrocyte sedimentation rate, vitamin D, thyroid function, bone chemistry, and so forth) and radiological investigations (plain radiographs, computed tomography [CT] scan, MRI, PET scan, and so forth) should be part of the initial assessment, providing essential information to dictate the appropriate surgical plan on a personalized basis.

TECHNIQUE

The technique consists of 2 stages. This article presents 2 cases, along with final long-term radiographs. Patient A presented with a Gustillo grade IIIB distal pilon fracture following a fall from height, which had united by 4 months (see **Fig. 2A–J**). Patient B presented following a septic nonunion of a Lisfranc injury repair (**Fig. 3A–C**), which had united by 3 months (**Fig. 3D–H**).

FIRST STAGE
Step 1: Debridement

The whole of the defect area must be thoroughly inspected and aggressively debrided. Any foreign material, devitalized bone, or tumor must be removed. Bone ends must be taken back to healthy-looking, bright, bleeding tissue. Utmost care should be taken to respect the soft tissue envelope throughout this process, and not to damage essential neurovascular structures (see **Figs.** 2C and 3D).

It is important at this stage to take multiple samples of fluid and tissue to send for microscopy, culture, and sensitivities plus or minus histology as indicated. Before this point, it is best practice to avoid intravenous antibiotic prophylaxis, especially if this is the first time samples are being taken, so as not to obscure the results. Results of these tests must be used to guide antimicrobial therapy. Intraoperative image-intensifier radiograph guidance must be used here too, to make sure that sufficient material has been debrided and all obvious foreign bodies have been removed.

Pearls and pitfalls are discussed later.

Step 2: Fixation

For stage 1, the method of fixation applied depends on the nature of the injury/defect, both of the bone and soft tissues; whether there is overt evidence of infection; and whether this is a revision procedure and a method of osteosynthesis has already been used. In this case, the suitability of this implant needs to be evaluated, and possibly revised. Internal or external methods of fixation are suitable, as long as the construction is stable enough to allow minimal disturbance to the cement spacer and induce formation of the membrane, without introducing risk of infection (see **Fig.** 2D–F).

Pearls and pitfalls are discussed later.

Step 3: Cement Spacer

Most exponents of the technique use PMMA bone cement loaded with antibiotics. In our unit, we include 2 g of vancomycin per cement sachet (see **Figs.** 2D and 3E–F).

Pearls and pitfalls are discussed later.

Step 4: Soft Tissue Coverage

This is an essential step, and, for all cases, a discussion must take place with plastic surgery colleagues in the planning phase of the procedure. If any form of flap or tissue transfer is required, it must be done at this stage. This step is crucial to encourage optimal membrane vitality.

Pearls and pitfalls are discussed later.

Step 5: Closure

A tension-free closure around the area must now be performed, in layers, while ensuring a good seal. Close attention needs to be paid to the soft tissue envelope and neurovascular structures throughout.

Step 6: Interim Plus or Minus Return to Start

This step can be considered an extension of the first stage. Patients must be pre-scribed appropriate systemic antibiotics if there is any suspicion of infection, and these must be guided by the culture results from intraoperative tissue samples. Usu-ally this is for a minimum period of 6 weeks; however, this depends on advice from microbiology colleagues. Further imaging or investigation is also required if there is new evidence of local recurrence of infection, which may also precipitate return to the beginning of the process: this requires repeat debridement and removal of the IM. Repeated debridement and antibiotic therapy must continue until subsequent tis-sue samples and inflammatory markers indicate resolution of infection.

SECOND STAGE: AT 6 TO 8 WEEKS
Step 1: Incision and Inspection

- Using the previous scar, incise longitudinally. Incise the membrane in the same direction, taking care not to tear beyond this or cause damage to a soft tissue flap that may have been used, ensuring to keep away from the vascular pedicle anastomosis.
- Look closely for any sign of persisting infection, and, if present, redebride (including IM), send tissue samples, and return to stage 1.

Step 2: Removal of Cement

The cement must be removed. Even if the area appears clean, it is advisable to send some sterile samples to confirm eradication of infection.

Step 3: Bone Edge Debridement

Bone should then be redebrided back to bleeding bone surfaces, and any bone that does not look fully vital following this must be removed or else risk harboring infection.
    The same should be done for medullary canal, to encourage endosteal communication to the graft. Tissue samples must be sent to microbiology.

Step 4: Autologous Bone Graft Harvest

- Iliac crest bone graft is considered the gold standard. Approximately up to 26 cm^2 can be obtained from the anterior iliac crest, and up to 33 cm^2 from the posterior iliac crest.[18]
- The reamer-irrigator-aspirator device can be used to obtain up to 80 cm^2 of cancellous autograft, and is useful for larger defects[19] (see **Fig. 2**G).

Step 5: Assess/Revise Fixation

In cases where a temporary external fixator has been used in the first stage, this now has to be revised to definitive fixation, which could include an internal plate or intramedullary nail, or converted to a more permanent circular frame externally.

Step 6: Bone Graft Expanders

In cases where the volume of the autologous graft harvested is not adequate, graft expanders can be used to increase the graft volume.

- The autologous bone graft can be expanded by using, xenograft, allograft, or calcium triphosphate. Ensure that at least 60% to 70% of this is autograft.
- Osteoinductivity is enhanced by adding bone morphogenetic protein (BMP)-2, or demineralized bone matrix (DBM), or platelet-rich plasma, which is obtained via a peripheral blood sample and centrifuged.
- Bone marrow aspirate concentrate (BMAC) can also be added, which can be obtained through aspiration of the iliac crest of 60 mL, and centrifugation, providing a powerful osteogenic potential through a concentrated source of multipotent stem cells (MSCs).

Step 7: Graft Implantation

- The bone graft can now be implanted carefully into the defect cavity, within the IM and between the edges of fresh bleeding bone. Apply just enough to fill the defect, but do not overpack the area, otherwise closure of the membrane will be difficult, impairing both containment and revascularization (see **Figs. 2**H and **3**G).

Step 8: Closure

- The membrane must be closed over the packed area, using a tension-free technique, but in such a way as to contain everything inside well.
- The surrounding area should be closed in layers, to form a tight seal around the defect to reinforce the containment of graft material within the IM, to maximize the regenerative potential.

Pearls and pitfalls are discussed later.

Systematic Review Methods

The authors performed a systematic literature review, paying close attention to PRISMA guidelines.[5] All original studies were considered. Review articles were excluded but kept for reference. All studies that specified either in the title/abstract/full article outcomes for the distal tibia, foot, or ankle where the IM Masquelet technique had been used were included. OVID Medline (PubMed) and Embase classic and Embase databases were interrogated. All articles published or nonindexed/in print and Web e-publication ahead of print, daily, and daily versions from 1946 to 13 March 2020 were considered. The following search was run through both Embase and Medline databases: "foot or ankle or distal tibia or hindfoot or midfoot or forefoot or metatarsal or calcaneum or talus AND [Masquelet OR Induced Membrane]." The search yielded 144 articles; when deduplicated, this was 82. A further 17 articles were selected for review from the bibliographies of 2 recent review articles (Mi and colleagues,[2] Masquelet and colleagues[1]).

All titles and abstracts were screened from this. If there was no reference to the distal tibia/foot/ankle within the title/abstract, the full article was downloaded and thoroughly checked for any specific results. Only original research/results were considered. Review articles or editorials were kept for reference purposes only. All articles were read and selected by the primary author (P.A.), and verified by the senior author (P.V.G.). Following this process, 21 articles met inclusion criteria. A table was created using Microsoft Excel to ensure systematic collection of all relevant data, which was completed by P.A. and verified by P.V.G. (**Fig. 4**).

RESULTS: SYSTEMATIC REVIEW

Overall, our systematic review included 103 defects, comprising the following anatomic sites: distal tibia, 62; ankle only, 2; hindfoot, 1; midfoot, 17; forefoot, 16; foot/ankle nonspecified area, 5. The studies were all case reports and retrospective cohorts, of level IV and V evidence respectively (**Table 1**, Appendix 1–3).

DISCUSSION

A recent review of 677 cases found that, overall, the technique has mainly been used in the tibia (59.12%) and femur (22.65%), with use in the foot including the metatarsal (1.03%), calcaneus (0.88), and talus (0.15%).[2] Our review uncovered various ways the IM technique has been used in the foot and ankle, some of which have not previously been included in large reviews because small case series are often excluded. However, we think it is important to consider these because multiple large series have yet to be published.

Liu and colleagues[11] used the technique successfully in 11 patients with defects secondary to erosive gouty tophus, ranging from 3 to 6 cm in length. Uric acid levels were optimized preoperatively, the area debrided in a similar fashion to that described herein, and Kirschner wires used instead of an external fixator during the first stage.

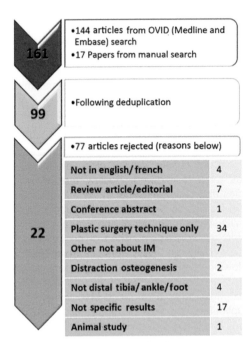

Fig. 4. Systemic review search/selection strategy.

Complete fusion was seen in all cases at 2.3 to 3.6 months (mean, 3 months) after surgery, with average Maryland scores increasing from 27.8 to 74.1. Significant improvement was seen in all but 1 patient, who developed transfer metatarsalgia. The investigators noted the utility of the technique, especially in cases where amputation would otherwise have been considered.[11]

Mak and colleagues[10] were successfully able to reconstruct almost the whole midfoot (lateral, second/third cuneiforms, all cuboids) in a diabetic patient with Charcot foot with osteomyelitis and associated massive ulcer to the plantar aspect of his foot. The IM technique was used successfully in combination with medial and lateral column reconstruction to achieve a plantigrade with a 3-level percutaneous tenotomy of the Achilles tendon to correct the ankle equinus deformity and reduce mechanical stresses on the midfoot. The investigators emphasized the importance of making multiple perforations in the surrounding metatarsals, navicular, and calcaneus to induce bleeding. By 25 months after surgery, the graft had assumed a normal cortical appearance.[10]

Qu and colleagues[30] successfully treated 4 patients who had stage IV foot and ankle TB with sinus tracts, using a delayed first-stage technique, which they termed a 3-stage process. Patients were left for 7 days with a vacuum dressing in situ after the initial debridement before insertion of cement, in order to assess inflammatory markers and culture results for more focused antibiotic-loaded cement. The investigators cautioned that, in many cases, a mixed bacterial picture is present, which further complicates treatment. Good results were obtained, with average union seen at 3.7 months, and American Orthopaedic Foot and Ankle Society (AOFAS) score increasing from 51.8 ± 15 to 81.8 ± 6.3.[30] Zou and colleagues[34] used the technique for 14 patients with midfoot TB (8 with stage IV TB, 6 with stage III). All patients achieved successful union, at an average time of 3.8 months, with Short-form 36

Table 1
Summarized results from systematic review

Author, Year	n	Age (y)	Body Region	DM?	Indication	Defect Size (Mean)	First-stage Fixation	Time Between Stages (wk)	Second-stage Fixation	Bone Graft Composition	% Union	Time to Union/ Consolidation (mo)	Cx
Abdulazim et al,[20] 2019	1	45	Talus	No	Trauma: Gustillo IIIC	5 cm	ExFix	6	IMN fusion	RIA	100	9	None
Demirri et al,[21] 2018	1	33	Distal one-third tibia	No	Trauma: Gustillo IIIB	6 cm	IMN	12	Exchange IMN	RIA	100	13	Delayed second stage as malaligned
Giannoudis et al,[3] 2016	3	30 (19–53)	MT	NP	2: trauma 1: TMTJ septic NU	2: 2 cm 1: 5 cm	Plates/ cement only	6–8	Plate left in situ	ICBG/RIA ± BMP/ BMAC/ orthos	100	3.6 (2–6)	None
Huffman et al,[9] 2012	1	26	First MT, first c'form, navicular	No	Trauma: gunshot	NP	Cement only	Several months	Proximal humeral plate	RIA	100	12	None
Largey et al,[7] 2009	1	24	90% c'form first MT, ATFL/CFL	No	Trauma: Gustillo IIB	9 × 5 cm	ExFix, K-wires	8	Screws, K-wires	ICBG	100	19	None
Liu et al,[11] 2018	11	33 (23–43)	First MT	NP	Erosive gouty tophus	3–6 cm (4.6 cm)	K-wires	6	Waveform locking plate	ICBG ± bone allograft	100	3 (2.3–5.6)	One foot infected, healed following VAC therapy. Transfer metatarsalgia in 1 patient
Luo et al,[22] 2017	19	31 ± 11	Distal one-third tibia	NP	OM	6.35 cm ± 6.35 cm	Locking plate	8	IMN	ICBG	100	5.9 ± 2.02	IC morbidity (2), further debridement (3), ankle dysfunction (8), delayed stress # (1)
Ma et al,[23] 2017	13	53 (35–72)	Distal one-third tibia	NP	Recalcitrant NU	NP	External locking plate	6–8	Plate left in situ	ICBG	100	6.5 (5–12)	Pin tract infection in 3, broken screw in 1, angular deformity in 2 patients of 7–10°
Mak et al,[10] 2015	1	50	Lateral cuboid, 1–3 c'forms	Yes	OM (WG3), midfoot (BG1)	3 × 6 cm	Frame, screws	6	Screws	ICBG	100	25	Delay until final stage because of infection

(continued on next page)

Table 1
(continued)

Author, Year	n	Age (y)	Body Region	DM?	Indication	Defect Size (Mean)	First-stage Fixation	Time Between Stages (wk)	Second-stage Fixation	Bone Graft Composition	% Union	Time to Union/Consolidation (mo)	Cx
Makridis et al,[24] 2014	1	53	First MT defect, 2-3 MT#	No	Trauma: Gustillo IIIB	5 cm	ExFix, K-wires	6	2 locking plates	RIA, orthos, BMP-7, BMAC	100	5	First MTPJ and TMTJ fusion of MTPJ at 10 m, better after 4 m
Mathieu et al,[25] 2019	3	35 (27–55)	Distal tibia	NP	Trauma: crash Gustillo IIIB	5 cm (4–6 cm)	ExFix, 2; plate, 1	6	ExFix, 2; plate, 1	ICBG ± RIA ± allograft	100	10.3 (9–12)	1 patient required repeat debridement and ITFG after stage 2 but went onto union
McCammon et al,[26] 2016	1	58	Ankle #	Yes	Septic NU	5.5 cm	Circular frame	7	Circular frame	ICBG + DBM + allograft + PRP	100	17	1 pin site infection, recovered with no issues
Morris et al,[27] 2017	3	47 (16–48)	Distal one-third tibia	NP	Open #	4.3 cm (3–7 cm)	NP	35–89	IMN/plate/TSF	RIA ± BMP-7 (unclear)	66	NP	2 out of 3 ongoing infection. 1 required BKA. Cx as poor first debridement
Oh et al,[28] 2019	1	32	Ankle pilon and osteochondral fragment	No	Trauma: Gustillo IIIB	~5 cm	ExFix	4	IMN	ICBG and TCP, also cortical graft	100	12	Long time taken until final stage because of ongoing infection
Pelissier et al,[29] 2002	1	71	Foot dorsum and 1–2 MT	Yes	Trauma: gunshot	10 × 12 cm	ExFix	8	ExFix/POP	ICBG and HA	100	9	Oozing leg eczema postoperatively at 8 wk in WB cast: switched to WB with sticks
Qu et al,[30] 2019	5	57 (33–81)	Foot and ankle	NP	TB OM	NP	ExFix, K-wires	12–36	Plates, screws	ICBG ± homolateral fibula graft	80	NP	Distal tibia # (1): refused progression to final stage, but TB had been eliminated
Ronga et al,[31] 2019	3	31 (27–53)	Distal one-third tibia	No	Trauma: 3B open #	6–7 cm	ExFix	12	Plate/frame (1), IMN (2)	RIA + BMP ± allograft/xenograft	100	4, 6, 23	Infected nonunion (1): graft debrided; converted to circular frame. Ankle pain: required fusion (1)
Siboni et al,[32] 2018	14	51 (24–88)	Distal tibia	Yes (3)	Septic NU	6.1 cm (1–18 cm)	ExFix/POP	7.9	Plate, 7; POP 4; ExFix, 3	ICBG ± allograft	93	14 (4–32)	Ongoing sepsis (3). Amputation (1). Further revision for union (8). Cx as inadequate initial wound care

Study													
Sivakumar et al,[33] 2016	1	15	Distal one-third tibia	No	Septic NU, Gustillo IIIB	7 cm	LRS	6	LRS	ICBG	100	12	None
Zoller et al,[8] 2017	5	35 (22–53)	Distal one-third tibia	NP	Open #. 2: trauma, 1 aseptic NU, 2 septic NU	6 cm (3–10 cm)	ExFix	10 (4–19.7), o/l at 33w	IMN/plate	RIA ± allograft	100	5.55 (1.8–9.1), o/l at 26.6	1 infection that resolved, 1 infection following initial union that resulted in amputation
Zou et al,[34] 2016	14	59 (50–70)	Midfoot	NP	TB OM	NP	K-wires, ExFix to lateral side	24	Locking plates	ICBG ± allogenic bone graft	100	3.8 (3–6)	None

Abbreviations: AB, antibiotic; ATFL, anterior tibiofibular ligament; BG1, Charcot Brodsky grade 1; BMAC, Bone Marrow Aspiration Cytology; BMP, Bone Morphogenic Protein; CFL, calcaneofibular ligaments; c'form, cuneiform; CW, contaminated wound; Cx, complications; DBM, Demineralised bone matrix; DM, n with diabetes mellitus; ExFix, external fixator; HA, hydroxyapatite; IC, iliac crest; ICBG, Iliac Crest Bone Grafting; ITFG, Inter TibioFibular Graft; IMN, intramedullary nail; K-wire, Kirschner wire; LRS, Ilizarov limb reconstruction system monorail; MT, Metatarsal; MTPJ, Metatarso-Phalangeal Joint NA, not applicable; NP, not provided; NU, nonunion; o/l, outlier; OM, osteomyelitis; orthos, scaffold material (Orthobiologics, UK); PRP, Platelet Rich Plasma; RIA, reamer-irrigator-aspirator; TCP, tricalcium phosphate; TMTJ, tarsometatarsal joint; TSF, Taylor spatial frame; WB, weight bearing; WG3, Wagner grade 3 ulcer; #, Fracture.

Data from Refs.[3,7–11,20–34]

(SF-36) scores increasing from 46.1 ± 6.1 to 83.1 ± 5.4. Both studies used a combination of vancomycin and streptomycin in the cement. Neither describe augmenting the graft with MSCs or BMP. They describe a slightly different method to that recommended in this article, leaving it 3 months and 6 months, respectively, to start the final stage, which, given the nature of the long treatment time for the granulomatous mycobacterium TB, is understandable.[30,34]

The procedure has also been used for reconstruction following massive foot trauma. Makridis and colleagues[107] reported on a patient with severe polytrauma following a motorcycle accident, for a grade 3b open fracture to his left first-third metatarsals. He required a radial forearm flap, K-wiring of second and third metatarsals, with Masquelet procedure to repair the 5-cm bone defect to his first metatarsal. BMP-7 and BMAC were used to augment the graft in the second stage. He underwent subsequent arthrodesis of his tibiotalar and first metatarsophalangeal (MTP) joint with screws and hindfoot nailing 10 months later. At 14-month follow-up, there was good healing and integration of the defect.[107] Giannoudis and colleagues[3] were able to successfully repair 3 metatarsal defects from 2 to 5 cm using a standard 2-stage approach, and augmenting the graft with BMP and BMAC, with union seen between 2 and 6 weeks. Huffman and colleagues[9] describe a patient with multiple gunshot wounds, with comminuted fractures to the first metatarsal, medial cuneiform, and navicular. A radial forearm flap was used to cover the defect, with a proximal humeral locking plate applied for internal fixation (to avoid risk of pin tract infection), and the second stage performed several months later. Good healing was achieved and the patient had returned to normal function 1 year later.[9] Pelissier and colleagues[29] achieved successful regeneration of second and third metatarsal loss in a diabetic patient following a 10 × 12-cm contaminated gunshot wound to the dorsum of his foot, using a bi-Masquelet procedure, supramalleolar island flap to cover the soft tissue defect, as well as the IM technique. Despite not following the procedure rigorously (ie, they did not overlap the cement to bony ends, and used hydroxyapatite instead of allograft) union was achieved by 9 months.[29] Largey and colleagues[7] were able to reconstruct a massive traumatic compound defect of the medioplantar foot with 90% cuneiform loss through use of a saphenous cross-leg flap and 2-stage Masquelet procedure with grafting and internal fixation at 2 months. After a period of 2 months' immobilization, CT scan confirmed good integration with bone. The patient returned to normal professional and sporting activities by 24 months.[7] Oh and colleagues[28] used the technique successfully in a difficult case of distal tibiofibular open 3B pilon fracture, and used a modified technique, choosing not to entirely enclose the membrane for the second stage but use the cortical area of Iliac Crest Bone Graft for the anterior aspect of the defect. Union was seen at 12 months.[28] Abdulazim and colleagues[20] were able to reconstruct a talus following a Gustillo IIIB injury with vascular stripping of the posterior tibial artery, which required a primary talectomy.

The technique has also been used in cases of traumatic infected nonunion. McCammon and colleagues[26] managed an infected nonunion of an open right trimalleolar ankle fracture sustained in open water, with a 5.5-cm area of bone loss, in a diabetic patient. They required several procedures until the final spacer could be inserted because of lingering infection. The graft was augmented with stem cell DBM and PRP, and the fragile overlying fascia reinforced with a 2.5 × 2.5-cm amniotic tissue graft layer. A circular frame was used for fixation. Complete consolidation was confirmed at 17 months, and the patient had returned to normal activity.

When considering the distal tibia, studies that specifically referred to this area used the IM technique to treat acute trauma, nonunion (both aseptic and infective), and osteomyelitis. Because most of the studies that reported their results using the IM procedure did not provide outcomes for the distal tibia specifically, these had to be excluded from the review. It is therefore likely that there is an overrepresentation of good results in the review undertaken, because it is known that the distal third of the tibia has the worst blood supply of any long bone, and has previously been reported as showing worse outcomes with a higher risk of nonunion.[4,108,109] A recent review found overall union in the tibia was 55.1%, with persisting deep infection seen in 50.91% of cases.[2] In our review, there was an overall excellent rate of union/consolidation of distal tibia defects. However, 2 studies showed lower rates of union in this region. Siboni and colleagues[32] reported a union rate of 93% when treating septic nonunion, with 8 out of 14 patients requiring further procedures after the second stage before union, and 1 ultimately requiring amputation. Morris and colleagues[27] reported union in 2 out of 3 distal tibia defects, with the overall rate of union being 5 out of 12, including patients in the wider study, and 1 noncompliant patient requiring an amputation. Siboni and colleagues[32] also noted that patients who were immobilized with plaster of Paris for their second-stage operations took longer to achieve union. Both investigators attribute most of the issues to inadequate debridement throughout the process, especially at the first stage. Mathieu and colleagues[25] reported outcomes in a military population, where the standard technique is to perform serial debridement during the first stage, and slower overall progress, with union taking up to 12 months in an otherwise fit and healthy population. These cases emphasize the importance of debridement, which should be a priority in both the primary and secondary stages in order to remove avascular, devitalized bone that may harbor pathogenic bacteria, and also encourage adequate revascularization and therefore host integration of the bone graft implant.[1,2,27]

Timing of the second stage of the procedure is important. Studies suggest that the peak vascular and osteoinductive period of the membrane is at 4 weeks; Aho and colleagues[112] further showed that a 40% reduction in growth factors was seen by 2 months, and vascularization had decreased by 60% at 3 months.[110–112] However, several studies show good results can be achieved even in cases where the second stage is performed outside of the recommended 6-week to 8-week time frame: in such cases, the authors recommend augmentation of the graft in every case, to optimize the bioactivity and chance of healing.

When choosing between sources of bone graft, the gold standard is considered to be morcelized pelvic autograft, taken either from the anterior or posterior iliac crest, which is also rich in MSCs. The reamer-irrigator-aspirator (RIA) can also be used for this purpose, especially for larger defects because up to 80 cm^3 of cancellous bone can be obtained; however, in our experience, most of the intrinsic MSCs are washed away through this process. Graft expanders such as bovine xenograft or tricalcium phosphate are also a viable option to include for large defects as volume expanders. DBM can also be used, and has the advantage of retaining some intrinsic osteoinductive BMPs.[1,3,4] Through investigation, the authors have previously found that, in patients more than 55 years of age, the iliac crest pelvic bone marrow has a significantly lower concentration of MSCs, which are less potent.[113] It is even more important in cases of elderly patients or when using RIA to augment the graft with BMAC/BMP, while being mindful of the respective contraindications.[114–116]

Most investigators choose to include antibiotics in the cement; however, the original technique described did not require this, and achieved good results without it. Some investigators argue that it potentially selects out resistant organisms, which can cause further issues. When managing infective cases in particular, it is a sensible course of action and can achieve local minimum bacterial inhibitory concentration of 3 to 10 times, to help manage infection.[1] Interestingly, the antibiotics in cement have been shown to have an independently beneficial effect on bone healing by upregulating osteoprotegerin , which counteracts receptor activator of nuclear factor kappa-B ligand (RANK), an osteoclast inducer.[117]

SUMMARY

This article explains how to optimize the Masquelet procedure for the distal tibia, foot, and ankle. The available evidence shows that, for the foot and ankle, the technique can be very successful in the right patients and performed in the correct way, with close attention to debridement and respect for soft tissues and bearing in mind the principles of the diamond concept throughout. Further work is needed to investigate specific outcomes for the proximal/medial/distal thirds of the tibia where the technique is used, in order to obtain a clearer overall view of success in these regions.

CLINICS CARE POINTS

Approach
- There may be cases where the approach is made challenging, such as fragile tissue or extensive scarring over the anterior or medial aspect of the tibia. In these cases, clinicians can undertake an extended bypass intertibiofibular graft to bridge the tibial defect.[1]

Debridement
- The importance of debridement, in the second stage as well as the first, was emphasized in a recent review of complications following the Masquelet procedure. Poor results are likely to follow if this advice is ignored.[2]
- Multiple samples must be sent at both stages, to fully assess infective load.
- Ensure that antibiotic prophylaxis is withheld until samples are taken.

Cement application
- In order for the antibiotic in the cement to be effective, measures must be taken to maximize its porosity so that it can leach out into the surrounding area. To achieve this, make sure that it is added last to the mixture, and avoid suction/vacuum mixing of cement.
- The cement must overlap the edges of the defect by at least 1 cm, to ensure that the membrane is produced away from the defect itself, which significantly improves outcomes.
- When using external fixation in the first stage, which is less rigid, the authors recommend using the molding method to place the cement around a 2-mm Kirschner wire that is inserted through the defect and into the medullary canals of the 2 opposing bone ends in order to prevent displacement.
- PMMA cement sets with a powerful exothermic reaction, which is harmful to living cells nearby. To avoid cell lysis from thermal necrosis, the authors recommend separating this area from the other tissues using a surgical glove, and constantly irrigating the area with saline, while the cement sets. Furthermore, any antibiotic chosen must be heat stable.

Second-stage fixation
- In order for a fracture or bone defect to heal by the second stage, the mechanical environment must be considered equally alongside the biological environment, with the ultimate osteosynthesis chosen providing adequate stability to facilitate osseous growth and integration with the graft (see **Fig. 1**).[1,3]

Respect for soft tissues
- A rich vascular network is essential for osseous healing, allowing abundant nutrients, growth factors, and cells to transform the defect area into new bone. The

surrounding soft tissues, periosteum, and endothelial structures, which have been shown to have their own intrinsic regenerative capacity, must be protected and respected throughout, as must the IM, which shares similar properties. Otherwise, the chance of success diminishes (see **Fig. 1**).[1,3,4]

Containment

- Unless clinicians ensure that the potent osteogenic recipe that has been achieved through the Masquelet technique is kept together in 1 place, or contained, then success is likely to be limited. It has been shown, especially for defects larger than 5 cm, that there is a high rate of graft resorption, nullifying clinicians' extensive efforts to repair them. Therefore, it is crucial that the membrane is used to keep everything together in a biological chamber, or bioreactor (see **Fig. 1**).[1,3,4]

Postoperative regime

- Ensure that all patients receive suitable thromboprophylaxis, such as LMWH for at least 6 weeks.
- For tibial injuries, mobilize touch-toe weight bearing only and, for defects of the foot and ankle, avoid weight bearing altogether at this stage. Provide a frame or crutches.
- Wound inspection at 2 weeks, then radiograph follow-up at 6 weeks.
- Further follow-up until radiological signs of union and pain-free mobilization (see **Figs. 2**I–J and **3**H).

REFERENCES

1. Masquelet A, Kanakaris NK, Obert L, et al. Bone Repair Using the Masquelet Technique. J Bone Joint Surg Am 2019;101(11):1024–36.

2. Mi M, Papakostidis C, Wu X, et al. Mixed results with the Masquelet technique: A fact or a myth? Injury 2020;51(2):132–5.

3. Giannoudis PV, Harwood PJ, Tosounidis T, et al. Restoration of long bone defects treated with the induced membrane technique: protocol and outcomes. Injury 2016;47(Suppl 6):S53–61.

4. Andrzejowski P, Giannoudis PV. The 'diamond concept' for long bone non-union management. J Orthop Traumatol 2019;20(1):21.

5. Moher D, Liberati A, Tetzlaff J, et al. Reprint–preferred reporting items for systematic reviews and meta-analyses: the PRISMA statement. Phys Ther 2009; 89(9, 873):e1000097.

6. Tricco AC, Lillie E, Zarin W, et al. PRISMA extension for scoping reviews (PRISMA-ScR): checklist and explanation. Ann Intern Med 2018;169(7):467.

7. Largey A, Faline A, Hebrard W, et al. Management of massive traumatic compound defects of the foot. Orthop Traumatol Surg Res 2009;95(4):301–4.

8. Zoller SD, Cao LA, Smith RA, et al. Staged reconstruction of diaphyseal fractures with segmental defects: Surgical and patient-reported outcomes. Injury 2017;48(10):2248–52.

9. Huffman LK, Harris JG, Suk M. Using the bi-masquelet technique and reamer-irrigator-aspirator for post-traumatic foot reconstruction. Foot Ankle Int 2009; 30(9):895–9.

10. Mak MF, Stern R, Assal M. Masquelet technique for midfoot reconstruction following osteomyelitis in charcot diabetic neuropathy: a case report. JBJS Case Connect 2015;5(2):e281–5.

11. Liu F, Huang R-k, Xie M, et al. Use of Masquelet's technique for treating the first metatarsophalangeal joint in cases of gout combined with a massive bone defect. Foot Ankle Surg 2018;24(2):159–63.

12. Giannoudis PV, Faour O, Goff T, et al. Masquelet technique for the treatment of bone defects: tips-tricks and future directions. Injury 2011;42(6):591–8.

13. Calori GM, Phillips M, Jeetle S, et al. Classification of non-union: Need for a new scoring system? Injury 2008;39(SUPPL.2):S59–63.

14. Calori GM, Colombo M, Mazza EL, et al. Validation of the Non-Union Scoring System in 300 long bone non-unions. Injury 2014;45(Suppl 6):S93–7.

15. Elniel AR, Giannoudis PV. Open fractures of the lower extremity: Current management and clinical outcomes. EFORT Open Rev 2018;3(5):316–25.

16. Ciaccia L. Fundamentals of surgery. 1. Inflammation. Nurs Times 2011;62(43):1421–65.

17. Ulug M, Ayaz C, Celen MK, et al. Are sinus-track cultures reliable for identifying the causative agent in chronic osteomyelitis? Arch Orthop Trauma Surg 2009;129(11):1565–70.

18. Burk T, Del Valle J, Finn RA, et al. Maximum quantity of bone available for harvest from the anterior iliac crest, posterior iliac crest, and proximal tibia using a standardized surgical approach: a cadaveric study. J Oral Maxillofac Surg 2016;74(12):2532–48.

19. Zalavras CG, Sirkin M. Treatment of long bone intramedullary infection using the RIA for removal of infected tissue: Indications, method and clinical results. Injury 2010;41(SUPPL. 2):S43–7.

20. Abdulazim AN, Reitmaier M, Eckardt H, et al. The Masquelet technique in traumatic loss of the talus after open lateral subtalar dislocation-A case report. Int J Surg Case Rep 2019;65:4–9.

21. Demitri S, Vicenti G, Carrozzo M, et al. The Masquelet technique in the treatment of a non-infected open complex fracture of the distal tibia with severe bone and soft tissue loss: A case report. Injury 2018;49(Suppl 4):S58–62.

22. Luo F, Wang X, Wang S, et al. Induced membrane technique combined with two-stage internal fixation for the treatment of tibial osteomyelitis defects. Injury 2017;48(7):1623–7.

23. Ma C-H, Chiu YC, Tsai KL, et al. Masquelet technique with external locking plate for recalcitrant distal tibial nonunion. Injury 2017;48(12):2847–52.

24. Makridis KG, Theocharakis S, Fragkakis EM, et al. Reconstruction of an extensive soft tissue and bone defect of the first metatarsal with the use of Masquelet technique: A case report. Foot Ankle Surg 2014;20(2):e19–22.

25. Mathieu L, Bilichtin E, Durand M, et al. Masquelet technique for open tibia fractures in a military setting. Eur J Trauma Emerg Surg 2019. https://doi.org/10.1007/s00068-019-01217-y.

26. McCammon M, Pinney S, McGlamry M. Masquelet technique for reconstruction of the ankle following a traumatic infected nonunion: a case presentation. Decatur (GA): The Podiatry Institute; 2016.

27. Morris R, Hossain M, Evans A, et al. Induced membrane technique for treating tibial defects gives mixed results. Bone Joint J 2017;99-B(5):680–5.

28. Oh Y, Yoshii T, Okawa A. Ankle arthrodesis using a modified Masquelet induced membrane technique for open ankle fracture with a substantial osteochondral defect: A case report of novel surgical technique. Injury 2019;50(11):2128–35.

29. Pelissier P, Bollecker V, Martin D, et al. [Foot reconstruction with the "bi-Masquelet" procedure]. Ann Chir Plast Esthet 2002;47(4):304–7.

30. Qu W, Wei C, Yu L, et al. Three-stage masquelet technique and one-stage reconstruction to treat foot and ankle tuberculosis. Foot Ankle Int 2020;41(3): 331–41.

31. Ronga M, Cherubino M, Corona K, et al. Induced membrane technique for the treatment of severe acute tibial bone loss: preliminary experience at medium-term follow-up. Int Orthop 2019;43(1):209–15.

32. Siboni R, Joseph E, Blasco L, et al. Management of septic non-union of the tibia by the induced membrane technique. What factors could improve results? Orthop Traumatol Surg Res 2018;104(6):911–5.

33. Sivakumar R, Mohideen MG, Chidambaram M, et al. Management of large bone defects in diaphyseal fractures by induced membrane formation by masquelet's technique. J Orthop Case Rep 2016;6(3):59–62.

34. Zou J, Shi Z, Mei G, et al. Two-stage operation to treat destructive midfoot tuberculosis: 14 cases experience. Orthop Traumatol Surg Res 2016;102(8):1075–80.

35. Ballmer FT, Hertel R, Noetzli HP, et al. The medial malleolar network: a constant vascular base of the distally based saphenous neurocutaneous island flap. Surg Radiol Anat 1999;21(5):297–303.

36. Beck M, Touzard R, Masquelet AC. Metatarso-cuboid impingement following malunion of a Jones fracture: Case report and review of the literature. Foot Ankle Surg 1997;3(3):143–6.

37. Begue T, Masquelet AC, Nordin JY. Anatomical basis of the anterolateral thigh flap. Surg Radiol Anat 1990;12(4):311–3.

38. Belfkira F, Forli A, Pradel P, et al. [Distally based sural neurocutaneous flap: clinical experience and technical adaptations. Report of 60 cases]. Experience clinique et adaptations techniques du lambeau neurocutane sural a pedicule distal. Ann Chir Plast Esthet 2006;51(3):199–206.

39. Bernstein M, Fragomen A, Rozbruch SR. Tibial bone transport over an intramedullary nail using cable and pulleys. JBJS Essent Surg Tech 2018;8(1):e9.

40. Beveridge J, Masquelet AC, Romana MC, et al. Anatomic basis of a fasciocutaneous flap supplied by the perforating branch of the peroneal artery. Surg Radiol Anat 1988;10(3):195–9.

41. Blondel B, Launay F, Jacopin S, et al. Limb lengthening using ankle joint distraction (arthrodiastasis) followed by arthrodesis. Experience with one case. Orthop Traumatol Surg Res 2011;97(4):438–42.

42. Caglioni C, Manca G. Distal-based sural flaps treatment of 17 lesions of the distal third of the lower extremity. Riv Ital Chir Plast 1998;30(4):275–81.

43. Charrois O, Bégué T, Muller GP, et al. [Plantar dislocation of the tarso-metatarsal articulation (Lisfranc articulation). Apropos of a case]. Rev Chir Orthop Reparatrice Appar Mot 1998;84(2):197–201.

44. Cho AB, Pohl PH, Ruggiero GM, et al. The proximally designed sural flap based on the accompanying artery of the lesser saphenous vein. J Reconstr Microsurg 2010;26(8):501–8.

45. Azi ML, Teixeira AAA, Cotias RB, et al. Induced-membrane technique in the management of posttraumatic bone defects. JBJS Essent Surg Tech 2019; 9(2):e22.

46. Costa MLR, Azevedo L, Zenha H, et al. The posterior arm flap-our department's experience. Eur J Plast Surg 2011;34(2):119–24.

47. Costa-Ferreira A, Reis J, Pinho C, et al. The distally based island superficial sural artery flap: clinical experience with 36 flaps. Ann Plast Surg 2001;46(3): 308–13.

48. Dumont CE, Masquelet AC. A reverse triangular soleus flap based on small distal communicating arterial branches. Ann Plast Surg 1998;41(4):440–3.

49. Durand S, Sita-Alb L, Ang S, et al. The flexor digitorum longus muscle flap for the reconstruction of soft-tissue defects in the distal third of the leg: anatomic considerations and clinical applications. Ann Plast Surg 2013;71(5):595–9.

50. El-Alfy B, Abulsaad M, Abdelnaby WL. The use of free nonvascularized fibular graft in the induced membrane technique to manage post-traumatic bone defects. Eur J Orthop Surg Traumatol 2018;28(6):1191–7.

51. Fitoussi F, Bajer B, Bégué T, et al. [The medial saphenous hetero (cross leg) flap in coverage of soft tissue defects of the leg and foot]. Rev Chir Orthop Reparatrice Appar Mot 2002;88(7):663–8.

52. Jonard B, Dean E. Posttraumatic reconstruction of the foot and ankle in the face of active infection. Orthop Clin North Am 2017;48(2):249–58.

53. Karger C, Kishi T, Schneider L, et al. Treatment of posttraumatic bone defects by the induced membrane technique. Orthop Traumatol Surg Res 2012;98(1):97–102.

54. Klaue K, Hansen ST, Masquelet AC. Clinical, quantitative assessment of first tarsometatarsal mobility in the sagittal plane and its relation to hallux valgus deformity. Foot Ankle Int 1994;15(1):9–13.

55. Le Nen D, Beal D, Person H, et al. Anatomical basis of a fascio-cutaneous pedicle flap based on the infero-lateral collateral artery of the leg. Surg Radiol Anat 1994;16(1):3–9.

56. Levante S, Masquelet AC, Nordin JY. [Coverage of chronic osteomyelitis of the ankle and the foot using a soleus muscle island flap, vascularized with retrograde flow on the posterior tibial artery. A seven cases report]. Ann Chir Plast Esthet 2009;54(6):523–7.

57. Li Z, Tang S, Wang J, et al. Masquelet technique combined with tissue flap grafting for treatment of bone defect and soft tissue defect. Zhongguo Xiu Fu Chong Jian Wai Ke Za Zhi 2016;30(8):966–70.

58. Louisia S, Masquelet AC. The medial and inferior calcaneal nerves: an anatomic study. Surg Radiol Anat 1999;21(3):169–73.

59. Madison RD, Nowotarski PJ. The reamer-irrigator-aspirator in nonunion surgery. Orthop Clin North Am 2019;50(3):297–304.

60. Mainard D, Wépierre G, Cronier B, et al. [Double use of sural fascio-cutaneous flap with distal pedicle to cover loss of substance of ankle or heel]. Rev Chir Orthop Reparatrice Appar Mot 1995;80(1):73–7.

61. Masquelet AC, Penteado CV, Romana MC, et al. The distal anastomoses of the medial plantar artery: Surgical aspects (2.10.1987). Surg Radiol Anat 1988;10(3):247–9.

62. Masquelet AC. [Repair of the soft tissues and the skin covering: recovery]. Soins Chir 1992;(138–139):20–8.

63. Masquelet AC. [Surgical reconstruction of post-traumatic tissue loss of the weight-bearing sole of the foot]. Ther Umsch 1991;48(12):842–8.

64. Masquelet AC, Beveridge J, Romana C, et al. The lateral supramalleolar flap. Plast Reconstr Surg 1988;81(1):74–81.

65. Masquelet AC, Gilbert A, Restrepo J. [The plantar flap in reconstructive surgery of the foot]. Presse Med 1984;13(15):935–6.

66. Masquelet AC, Kishi T, Benko PE. Very long-term results of post-traumatic bone defect reconstruction by the induced membrane technique. Orthop Traumatol Surg Res 2019;105(1):159–66.

67. Masquelet AC, Nordin JY, Guinot A. Vascularized transfer of the adductor magnus tendon and its osseous insertion: a preliminary report. J Reconstr Microsurg 1985;1(3):169–76.
68. Masquelet AC, Rinaldi S, Mouchet A, et al. The posterior arm free flap. Plast Reconstr Surg 1985;76(6):908–13.
69. Masquelet AC, Romana MC. The medialis pedis flap: a new fasciocutaneous flap. Plast Reconstr Surg 1990;85(5):765–72.
70. Masquelet AC, Romana MC. [External supramalleolar flap in the reconstructive surgery of the foot]. J Chir (Paris) 1988;125(5):367–72.
71. Massin P, Romana C, Masquelet AC. Anatomic basis of a pedicled extensor digitorum brevis muscle flap. Surg Radiol Anat 1988;10(4):267–72.
72. Motamed S, Yavari M, Mofrad HR, et al. Distally based sural artery flap without sural nerve. Acta Med Iran 2010;48(2):127–9.
73. Muller GP, Masquelet AC. [Chronic compartment syndrome of the foot. A case report]. Rev Chir Orthop Reparatrice Appar Mot 1995;81(6):549–52.
74. Namiki Y, Torii S, Hayashi Y, et al. Experiences with reverse-flow lateral supramalleolar flaps. JPN J PLAST RECONSTR SURG 1989;32(8):787–93.
75. Navissano M, Malan F, Raiteri E, et al. The reconstruction of the lower third of the leg by lateral supramalleolar flap. [in Italian] RIV ITAL CHIR PLAST 1996;28(3):341–4.
76. Neumayer F, Djembi YR, Gerin A, et al. Closed rupture of the tibialis anterior tendon: a report of 2 cases. J Foot Ankle Surg 2009;48(4):457–61.
77. Oberlin C, Azoulay B, Bhatia A. The posterolateral malleolar flap of the ankle: a distally based sural neurocutaneous flap–report of 14 cases. Plast Reconstr Surg 1995;96(2):400–7.
78. Ogun TC, Arazi M, Kutlu A. An easy and versatile method of coverage for distal tibial soft tissue defects. J Trauma 2001;50(1):53–9.
79. Pannier S. Congenital pseudarthrosis of the tibia. Orthop Traumatol Surg Res 2011;97(7):750–61.
80. Qiu X, Chen Y, Qi X, et al. [Effectiveness analysis of induced membrane technique in the treatment of infectious bone defect]. Zhongguo Xiu Fu Chong Jian Wai Ke Za Zhi 2017;31(9):1064–8.
81. Rincon-Cardozo DF, Camacho-Casas JA, Reyes-Nunez VA. [Dislocation and necrosis of the first, second and third wedges. Management with the Masquelet technique. A case report]. Acta Ortop Mex 2013;27(1):55–9.
82. Romana MC, Masquelet AC, Klaue K. [Soft tissue preservation and reconstruction in non-supporting foot parts]. Ther Umsch 1991;48(12):836–41.
83. Saxer F, Eckardt H. [Reconstruction of osseous defects using the Masquelet technique]. Orthopade 2017;46(8):665–72.
84. Scholz AO, Gehrmann S, Glombitza M, et al. Reconstruction of septic diaphyseal bone defects with the induced membrane technique. Injury 2015;46(Suppl 4):S121–4.
85. Tremp M, Largo RD, Borens O, et al. Bone propeller flap: a staged procedure. J Foot Ankle Surg 2014;53(2):226–31.
86. Valenti P, Masquelet AC, Romana C, et al. Technical refinement of the lateral supramalleolar flap. Br J Plast Surg 1991;44(6):459–62.
87. Vesely R, Procházka V, Kocis J, et al. [Reconstruction of soft tissue defects of lower leg, ankle and foot using sural flap]. Rozhl Chir 2007;86(3):134–8.
88. Viateau V, Guillemin G, Calando Y, et al. Induction of a barrier membrane to facilitate reconstruction of massive segmental diaphyseal bone defects: an ovine model. Vet Surg 2006;35(5):445–52.

89. Voche P, Stussi JD, Merle M. [The supramalleolar flap. Our experience in 35 cases]. Le lambeau supramalleolaire lateral. Ann Chir Plast Esthet 2001;46(2): 112–24.

90. Wang X, Luo F, Huang K, et al. Induced membrane technique for the treatment of bone defects due to post-traumatic osteomyelitis. Bone Joint Res 2016;5(3): 101–5.

91. Assal M, Stern R. The masquelet procedure gone awry. Orthopedics 2014; 37(11):e1045–8.

92. Apard T, Bigorre N, Cronier P, et al. Two-stage reconstruction of post-traumatic segmental tibia bone loss with nailing. Orthop Traumatol Surg Res 2010;96(5): 549–53.

93. Cambon-Binder A, Revol M, Hannouche D. Salvage of an osteocutaneous thermonecrosis secondary to tibial reaming by the induced membrane procedure. Clin Case Rep 2017;5(9):1471–6.

94. Cho JW, Kim J, Cho WT, et al. Circumferential bone grafting around an absorbable gelatin sponge core reduced the amount of grafted bone in the induced membrane technique for critical-size defects of long bones. Injury 2017; 48(10):2292–305.

95. Kombate NK, Walla A, Ayouba G, et al. Reconstruction of traumatic bone loss using the induced membrane technique: preliminary results about 11 cases. J Orthop 2017;14(4):489–94.

96. Olesen UK, Eckardt H, Bosemark P, et al. The Masquelet technique of induced membrane for healing of bone defects. A review of 8 cases. Injury 2015; 46(Suppl 8):S44–7.

97. Masquelet AC, Fitoussi F, Begue T, et al. [Reconstruction of the long bones by the induced membrane and spongy autograft]. Ann Chir Plast Esthet 2000; 45(3):346–53.

98. Masquelet AC. Muscle reconstruction in reconstructive surgery: soft tissue repair and long bone reconstruction. Langenbecks Arch Surg 2003;388(5): 344–6.

99. Stafford PR, Norris BL. Reamer-irrigator-aspirator bone graft and bi Masquelet technique for segmental bone defect nonunions: a review of 25 cases. Injury 2010;41(Suppl 2):S72–7.

100. Tetsworth K, Isaacs J, Glatt V. Patient specific 3D printed titanium truss strut implants combined with the masquelet technique: a novel strategy to reconstruct massive segmental bone loss. J Orthop Res 2017;35(Supple 1).

101. Gupta G, Ahmad S, Mohd Zahid fnm, et al. Management of traumatic tibial diaphyseal bone defect by "induced-membrane technique. Indian J Orthop 2016;50(3):290–6.

102. Liu C, You JX, Chen YX, et al. Effect of induced membrane formation followed by polymethylmethacrylate implantation on diabetic foot ulcer healing when revascularization is not feasible. J Diabetes Res 2019;2019:2429136.

103. Muhlhausser J, Winkler J, Babst R, et al. Infected tibia defect fractures treated with the Masquelet technique. Medicine (Baltimore) 2017;96(20):e6948.

104. Taylor BC, Hancock J, Zitzke R, et al. Treatment of bone loss with the induced membrane technique: techniques and outcomes. J Orthop Trauma 2015; 29(12):554–7.

105. Wong TM, Wing Lau T, Li X, et al. Masquelet technique for treatment of posttraumatic bone defects. ScientificWorldJournal 2014;2014:710302.

106. Zhang C, Zhu C, Yu G, et al. Management of infected bone defects of the lower extremities by three-stage induced membrane technique. Med Sci Monit 2020; 26:e919925.

107. Makridis KG, Ahmad MA, Kanakaris NK, et al. Reconstruction of iliac crest with bovine cancellous allograft after bone graft harvest for symphysis pubis arthrodesis. Int Orthop 2012;36(8):1701–7.

108. Santolini E, West R, Giannoudis PV. Risk factors for long bone fracture non-union: a stratification approach based on the level of the existing scientific evidence. Injury 2015;46(Suppl 8):S8–19.

109. Santolini E, Goumenos SD, Giannoudi M, et al. Femoral and tibial blood supply: A trigger for non-union? Injury 2014;45(11):1665–73.

110. Wang X, Wei F, Luo F, et al. Induction of granulation tissue for the secretion of growth factors and the promotion of bone defect repair. J Orthop Surg Res 2015;10:147.

111. Jin F, Xie Y, Wang N, et al. Poor osteoinductive potential of subcutaneous bone cement-induced membranes for tissue engineered bone. Connect Tissue Res 2013;54(4–5):283–9.

112. Aho OM, Lehenkari P, Ristiniemi J, et al. The mechanism of action of induced membranes in bone repair. J Bone Joint Surg Am 2013;95(7):597–604.

113. Ganguly P, El-Jawhari JJ, Giannoudis PV, et al. Age-related changes in bone marrow mesenchymal stromal cells: a potential impact on osteoporosis and osteoarthritis development. Cell Transplant 2017;26(9):1520–9.

114. Devine JG, Dettori JR, France JC, et al. The use of rhBMP in spine surgery: is there a cancer risk? Evid Based Spine Care J 2012;3(2):35–41.

115. Beachler DC, Yanik EL, Martin BI, et al. Bone morphogenetic protein use and cancer risk among patients undergoing lumbar arthrodesis. J Bone Joint Surg Am 2016;98(13):1064–72.

116. James AW, LaChaud G, Shen J, et al. A review of the clinical side effects of bone morphogenetic protein-2. Tissue Eng Part B Rev 2016;22(4):284–97.

117. Shah SR, Smith BT, Tatara AM, et al. Effects of local antibiotic delivery from porous space maintainers on infection clearance and induction of an osteogenic membrane in an infected bone defect. Tissue Eng 2017;23(3–4):91–100.

118. Mi M, Papakostidis C, Wu X, et al. Mixed results with the Masquelet technique: A fact or a myth? Injury 2020;51(2):132–5.

119. Masquelet A, Kanakaris NK, Obert L, et al. Bone Repair Using the Masquelet Technique. J Bone Joint Surg Am 2019;101(11):1024–36.

Appendix 1
Full systematic review

Author, Year	Study Type, EL	Study Size (n)	Age (y)	Men	Body Region	DM?	Indication
Abdulazim et al,[20] 2019	CR, 5	1	45	1	Talus	No	Trauma: Gustillo IIIC
Demitri et al,[21] 2018	CR, 5	1	33	0	Distal one-third tibia	No	Trauma: 3B open #
Giannoudis et al,[3] 2016	RCH, 4	3	2, 19; 1, 53	3	MT	NP	2, trauma; 1, infection (previous Lisfranc ORIF)
Huffman et al,[9] 2012	CR, 5	1	26	1	First MT, first cuneiform, navicular	No	Trauma: gunshot wound, foot, medial aspect
Largey et al,[7] 2009	CR, 5	1	24	1	Cuneiform, first MT	No	Trauma: motorcycle accident. Gustillo IIB. Polytrauma
Liu et al,[11] 2018	RCH, 4	11	33.1 (23–43)	7	First MT	NP	Erosive gouty tophus
Luo et al,[22] 2017	RCH, 4	19	31.96 ± 11.45	Whole study: 58 out of 67	Distal one-third tibia	NP	Osteomyelitis: traumatic, 19; hematogenous, 3
Ma et al,[23] 2017	RCH, 4	13	53.5 (35–72)	12	Distal one-third tibia	1 of 17	Recalcitrant nonunion
Mak et al,[10] 2015	CR, 5	1	50	1	Lateral cuboid, 1–3 cuneiforms	Yes	Ulcerative osteomyelitis (WG3) in Charcot midfoot (BG1)
Makridis et al,[24] 2014	CR, 5	1	53	1	First MT defect, 2–3 MT#	No	Trauma: motorcycle accident. Soft tissue and bone loss. Gustillo IIIB. Polytrauma
Mathieu et al,[25] 2019	RCH, 4	3	35 (27–55)	NP	Distal tibia	NP	Trauma: crash. 3× IIIB open #
McCammonet al,[26] 2016	CR, 5	1	58	1	Ankle	Yes	Infected nonunion of trimalleolar ankle #
Morris et al,[27] 2017	RCH	3	47 (16–48)	2	Distal one-third tibia	NP	Open #
Oh et al,[28] 2019	CR, 5	1	32	1	Ankle pilon	No	Trauma: fall. Gustillo IIIB open #. Large osteochondral fragment from distal tibia/fibula lost (extruded)
Pelissier et al,[29] 2002	CR, 5	1	71	1	Foot	Yes	Trauma: gunshot wound foot dorsum
Qu et al,[30] 2019	RCH, 4	5	56.7 (33–81)	6	Foot and ankle	NP	TB osteomyelitis

Author, Year	Infection Present at Start? (N)	Defect Size (Mean) (cm)	First-Stage Fixation	Time Between Stages 1 and 2 (wk)	Second-Stage Fixation	Graft	Delayed First Stage?	Flap/Skin Graft	Notes on Technique/Study	PROMs: Before/After (Change)
Ronga et al,[31] 2019	RCH	3	31 (27-53)	3		Distal one-third tibia		No		Trauma: 3B open #	
Siboni et al,[32] 2018	RCH, 4	14	51 (24-88)	11		Distal tibia				3 of 14 Septic nonunion	
Sivakumar et al,[33] 2016	CR, 5	1	15	1		Distal one-third tibia		No		Infected area at site of malunited Gustillo IIIB fracture that had been managed with a triangular frame ExFix	
Zoller et al,[8] 2017	RCH, 4	5	35 (22-53)	5		Distal one-third tibia		NP		Open fractures. 2, trauma; 1 aseptic nonunion, 2 septic nonunion	
Zou et al,[34] 2016	RCH, 4	14	58.9 (50-70)	9		Midfoot		NP		TB osteomyelitis	
Abdulazim et al,[20] 2019	No, but CW	5	ExFix	6	IMN fusion	RIA	No	Free gracilis	Posterior tibial artery stripped. After initial debridement and spacer, VAC put in situ, then flap 7 d later	NP
Demitri et al,[21] 2018	No, but CW	6	IMN	12	Exchange IMN	RIA	Yes	No	NB. Delayed first stage (16 d) after VAC/Debridement	AOFAS ADL score 92% at end

(continued on next page)

Appendix 1
(continued)

Author, Year	Infection Present at Start? (N)	Defect Size (Mean) (cm)	First-Stage Fixation	Time Between Stages 1 and 2 (wk)	Second-Stage Fixation	Graft	Delayed First Stage?	Flap/Skin Graft	Notes on Technique/Study	PROMs: Before/After (Change)
Giannoudis et al,[3] 2016	Yes (1)	2, 2 cm; 1, 5 cm	Plates, trauma; cement only, infection	6–8	Plates in trauma cases	ICBG/RIA, ±BMP/BMAC/orthos	No	No	For patient with larger defect, graft fully augmented. Patient with infection, BMAC added. third patient: no augmentation	NP
Huffman et al,[9] 2012	No, but CW	NP	Cement only	Several months	Proximal humeral locking plate	RIA	Yes	Radial forearm	Delayed first stage: 2 wk of internal stabilization with humeral locking plate following initial debridement before first stage of Masquelet, when this was removed. At second stage: mid/hindfoot arthrodesis	NP

Largey et al,[7] 2009	No, but CW	9 × 5cm	ExFix, K-wires	8	Screws, K-wires	ICBG	No	Yes	Cuneiform 90% loss. Comminuted # first MT. ATFL/CFL torn. Saphenous cross-leg fasciocutaneous flap with proximal pedicle: delayed for 5 d by using VAC therapy to confirm no superinfection. Midfoot arthrodesis at second stage	NP
Liu et al,[11] 2018	None	3–6 (4.6)	K-wires	6	Waveform locking plate	ICBG ± bone allograft	No	No	—	Maryland Foot Score: 27.8 out of 74.1 (46.3)
Luo et al,[22] 2017	Yes (19)	6.35 ± 6.35	Locking plate	8	IMN	ICBG	No	No	First stage: locking plate (internal ExFix), also covered in AB cement. At second stage internal ExFix removed and replaced. NB: plates covered with AB cement	NP

(continued on next page)

Appendix 1 (*continued*)

Author, Year	Infection Present at Start? (N)	Defect Size (Mean) (cm)	First-Stage Fixation	Time Between Stages 1 and 2 (wk)	Second-Stage Fixation	Graft	Delayed First Stage?	Flap/Skin Graft	Notes on Technique/Study	PROMs: Before/After (Change)
Ma et al,[23] 2017	None	NP	External locking plate as fixator	6–8	Plate left in situ	ICBG	No	No	NB use of locking plate ExFix left for long time. Unclear how removed	Iowa: 83 (68–91)
Mak et al,[10] 2015	Yes (1)	3 × 6 cm	Partial ring fixator, medial column screw	6	Screws	ICBG	Yes	No	Initial debridement and ring fixator, 2 wk VAC therapy, further debridement, and AB cement. Fixator and cement removed. Repeat microbiological testing confirmed the area was sterile (no microorganisms), a medial column reconstruction and antibiotic cement was then inserted. 6 wk later: grafting and definitive fixation,	NP

Study										
Makridis et al,[24] 2014	No, but CW	5 cm	ExFix, K-wires	6	2 locking plates	RIA, orthos, BMP-7, BMAC	No	Yes: radial forearm flap at first stage	lateral column and hindfoot stabilization/ arthrodesis, percutaneous 3 l evel tenotomy of Achilles tendon, good plantigrade, ulcer-free result	ExFix to first MT, K-wires to 2–3 MT. K-wire within cement	NP
Mathieu et al,[25] 2019	No, but CW	5 (4–6)	ExFix, 2; Plate, 1	6	ExFix, 2; plate, 1	ICBG ± RIA ± allograft	Yes	Yes: free ALT	Military injuries. Stage 1 delayed 7– 48 d, depending on devitalized/ infection load l ocally. VAC therapy used during interim. ALT flaps used in preference where possible	NP

(continued on next page)

Appendix 1
(continued)

Author, Year	Infection Present at Start? (N)	Defect Size (Mean) (cm)	First-Stage Fixation	Time Between Stages 1 and 2 (wk)	Second-Stage Fixation	Graft	Delayed First Stage?	Flap/Skin Graft	Notes on Technique/Study	PROMs: Before/After (Change)
McCammon et al,[26] 2016	Yes: open ulcer	5.5 cm	Circular frame	7	Circular frame	ICBG + DBM + allograft + PRP	Yes	No	Delayed first stage: initial debridement and VAC. Cement placed at a later date. Unclear when. Amniotic tissue graft used at final stage to reinforce extensor retinaculum. After this, frame compressed for a further 6 mo	NP
Morris et al,[27] 2017	No, but CW	4.3 (3–7)	NP	35–89	IMN/plate/TSF	RIA ± BMP-7 (unclear which were augmented)	Yes	Yes, but unclear what for each patient	Delay to first stage (4–31d). Quality of debridement at peripheral district general hospitals of variable quality, investigators speculate as source of ongoing infection in some cases	NP

Study									
Oh et al,[28] 2019	No, but CW	~5	ExFix	4	IMN	ICBG and TCP, also cortical graft	Yes	FTSG	Delayed first stage of 2 wk after debridement. Ongoing infection at 6 mo. Cement removed, radical debridement, and new cement. Second stage done 4 mo after this. Membrane not fully closed to anterior aspect: wide layer of cortical bone graft kept at this point	NP
Pelissier et al,[29] 2002	No, but CW	10 × 12	ExFix	8	ExFix	ICBG and HA	No	Yes: lateral supramalleolar 8 × 10 cm	ExFix left in situ because of infection risk and not to injure flap	NP
Qu et al,[30] 2019	Yes: TB stage IV	NP	ExFix, K-wires	12–36	Locking plates, screws, hindfoot arthrodeses	ICBG ± homolateral fibula graft	Yes	No	Method described as 3 stage by investigators. In reality = delayed first stage. Initially, debridement and VAC therapy, repeat if biochemical markers worsening,	AOFAS: 51.8/81.8 (30) VAS: 5.4/1.0 (5.3)

(continued on next page)

Appendix 1
(continued)

Author, Year	Infection Present at Start? (N)	Defect Size (Mean) (cm)	First-Stage Fixation	Time Between Stages 1 and 2 (wk)	Second-Stage Fixation	Graft	Delayed First Stage?	Flap/Skin Graft	Notes on Technique/Study	PROMs: Before/After (Change)
									ExFix, then AB cement (streptomycin/vancomycin cement) and K-wires. Second (third) stage: grafting, f ixation, and arthrodesis. NB: often mixed bacterial infection	
Ronga et al,[31] 2019	No, but CW	6-7 cm	ExFix	12	1 patient, plate later replaced with circular frame, 2 patients: IMN	RIA + BMP ± allograft/ xenograft	No	Yes: 2 latissimus dorsi free flap, 1 gracilis free flap	—	NP
Siboni et al,[32] 2018	Yes: all	6.1 (1–18)	ExFix/POP	7.9	Locking plate, 7; plaster	ICBG ± allograft	No	No	Patients put in POP after stage 2 did less well: not stable enough, and unable	Mean WOAC after

			cast, 4; ExFix, 3						union: 23 ± 22
Sivakumar et al,[33] 2016	Yes	7	LRS fixator	6	LRS) fixator	ICBG	No	No	LRS kept for 2 mo, then replaced by POP for a further month	NP	to WB. Smokers had a negative trend associated with healing. Union: without further procedure, 10.8 (4–32), Those requiring further procedures: 19 (10–27)
Zoller et al,[8] 2017	Yes: in 2 cases	6 (3–10)	ExFix	10 (4–19.7), o/l at 33w	IMN/plate	RIA ± allograft	No	No	In aseptic nonunion case (6 cm defect), both IMN and plate used	LEFS: 53.1 after fixation
Zou et al,[34] 2016	Yes: TB (8 stage IV, 6 stage III)	NP	K-wires, ExFix to lateral side	24	Locking plates	ICBG ± allogenic bone graft	No	No	Standard procedure. streptomycin/ vancomycin cement	SF-36: 46.1 out of 83.1;; AOFAS 51.7 out of 82.9; VAS, 6.1 out of 1.4

Author, Year	% Union	Time to Union/ Consolidation (mo)	NWB Period	PWB Period	Rehabilitation Complete (Mean, mo)	Complications
Abdulazim et al,[20] 2019	100	9	TTWB 6 mo	3 mo	12	None
Demitri et al,[21] 2018	100	13	NP	NP	13	At initial attempt at second stage: exchange nailing and improved reduction required because of malalignment. Another 3 mo left before final second stage
Giannoudis et al,[3] 2016	100	3.6 (2–6)	6–8 wk	NP	12	None
Huffman et al,[9] 2012	100	12	NP	NP	12	None
Largey et al,[7] 2009	100	19	2	10	24	None
Liu et al,[11] 2018	100	3 (2.3–5.6)	—	—	NP	One foot infected, healed following VAC therapy. Transfer metatarsalgia in 1 patient

Luo et al,[22] 2017	100	5.9 ± 2.02	4	From 4 wk	NP	Iliac crest donor morbidity in 2, 3 required further debridement, 8 had ankle joint dysfunction, 1 had delayed stress #
Ma et al,[23] 2017	100	6.5 (5–12)	None	5–12 mo	NP	Pin tract infection in 3, broken screw in 1, angular deformity in 2 patients of 7–10°
Mak et al,[10] 2015	100	25	12	12	25	Delay until final stage because of infection
Makridis et al,[24] 2014	100	5	NP	NP	18	Instability of first MTPJ: residual pain. At 10 mo, fusion of MTPJ and tibiotalar joint performed. Painless by 4 mo afterward
Mathieu et al,[25] 2019	100	10.3 (9–12)	NP	NP	NP	1 patient required repeat debridement and ITFG after stage 2 but went on to union
McCammon et al,[26] 2016	100	17	24	None	24	1 pin site infection, recovered with no issues
Morris et al,[27] 2017	66	NP	NP	NP	NP	2 of 3 patients had infection that delayed progress. 1 of these was lost to initial follow-up and represented with severe infection: ultimately required BKA. Overall series had high rate of infection, which investigators attribute to poor quality of initial debridement

(continued on next page)

Appendix 1
(continued)

Author, Year	% Union	Time to Union/ Consolidation (mo)	NWB Period	PWB Period	Rehabilitation Complete (Mean, mo)	Complications
Oh et al,[28] 2019	100	12	2	5	36	Long time taken until final stage because of ongoing infection
Pelissier et al,[29] 2002	100	9	0	8	9	Oozing leg eczema postoperatively at 8 wk in WB cast: switched to WB with sticks
Qu et al,[30] 2019	80	NP, but follow-up ranged 6–57 mo	Until partial union	At partial union	NP	1 patient sustained a fracture of distal tibia, and refused progression to third stage, but TB had been eliminated
Ronga et al,[31] 2019	100	4, 6, 23	NP	5	Up to 23	1 patient had an infected nonunion, and compound graft debrided: converted to Ilizarov circular frame (23 mo union). Another required ankle fusion because of pain
Siboni et al,[32] 2018	93	14 (4–32)	8	NP	NP	2
Sivakumar et al,[33] 2016	100	12	16	NP	12	None

| Zoller et al,[8] 2017 | 100 | Defects: 3–6 cm, 4.4 mo (1.8–9.1 mo); 10 cm, 26.6 mo | Protected until radiographic signs of union: mean, 4.5 mo | — | 18 | 1 infection that resolved, 1 infection following initial union that resulted in amputation |
| Zou et al,[34] 2016 | 100 | 3.8 (3–6) | 4 | At 4 wk, NP how long for | NP | None |

Data from Refs.[3,7–11,20–34]

Appendix 2
Methodology (parts A and B)

Topic[5,6]	Description
Eligibility criteria	All original studies were considered. Review articles excluded but kept for reference. All studies that specified either in the title/abstract/full article outcomes for the distal tibia, foot, or ankle where the IM Masquelet technique had been used
Information sources	OVID Medline (PubMed) and Embase classic and Embase databases. All articles published or nonindexed/in print and Web e-publication ahead of print, daily and daily versions from 1946 to 13 March 2020 were considered
Search	The following search was run through both Embase and Medline databases: "Foot or ankle or distal tibia or hindfoot or midfoot or forefoot or metatarsal or calcaneum or talus AND [Masquelet OR Induced Membrane]"
Study selection	The search yielded 144 articles; when deduplicated this was 82. A further 17 articles were selected for review from the bibliographies of 2 recent review articles (Mi[118] et al, Masquelet[119] et al) All titles and abstracts were screened from this. If there was no reference to the distal tibia/foot/ankle within the title/abstract, the full article was downloaded and thoroughly checked for any specific results Only original research/results were considered. Review articles or editorials were kept for reference purposes only All articles were read and selected by the primary author (P.A.), and verified by the senior author (P.V.G.) Following this process, 21 articles met inclusion criteria
Data collection process	A table was created using Microsoft Excel to ensure systematic collection of all relevant data, which was completed by P.A. and verified by P.V.G.

Data Items Sought for Systematic Review[5,6]	Description
Author, year	Primary author of the publication and year
Study type, evidence level	Evidence levels: case report, level 5; retrospective study, level 4
Study size (n)	Number of relevant defects included
Age	Average age of participants

(continued on next page)

Appendix 2 (continued)	
Data Items Sought for Systematic Review[5,6]	**Description**
Men/Women	Gender demographics
Body region	Distal third tibia/ankle/foot: unless the outcomes for each specific area were clear in the article, it was excluded
Presence of diabetes	Significant in foot and ankle for disorder in general, and also affects rate and success of osseous healing
Indication for Masquelet	Divided into acute trauma, septic and aseptic nonunion
Infection present at start? (n)	To make it clear, and, for some open fractures, to state that infection may not have been present, but that the wound was contaminated
Defect size, mean (cm)	Either the longitudinal size of the defect or the area of the defect
First-stage fixation method	The method of fixation used (temporary or permanent) in the first stage
Time (weeks) between stages 1 and 2	No assumptions were made here. As per the text in the article
Second stage fixation method	Definitive fixation method used at the second stage
Bone graft composition	Where this is from, and whether it has been augmented (and with what)
Delayed first stage?	This is common, and we wanted to quantify its use
Flap/skin graft required (and what type)?	What extra soft tissue cover was required?
Notes on technique/study	To make notes on interesting ways the investigators dealt with problems, or did things in a unique way
PROMs: before/after surgery	PROMs to benchmark different studies alongside each other
% Union or consolidation of patients in study	The relative amounts of defects that went on to complete union/consolidation
Time to union/consolidation: (mo)	How long it took for union on average to occur: as stated by investigators
Non–weight-bearing period	How long it is stated that patients were asked not to weight bear
Partially weight-bearing period	How long it is stated that patients were asked to partially weight bear
Mean rehabilitation period complete at what time period? (mo)	If stated, how long patients took to make a full recovery
Cx in study	Cx as per stated in the article
Risk of bias in individual studies	Risk of bias was assessed on a study-by-study basis, and we include reference to this in the text

(continued on next page)

Appendix 2 *(continued)*	
Data Items Sought for Systematic Review[5,6]	**Description**
Summary measures	Total number of defects included and within each category by location and outcomes
Synthesis of results	The overall outcomes are combined as investigated for each body area

Data from Moher, D., et al., Preferred Reporting Items for Systematic Reviews and Meta-Analyses: The PRISMA Statement. PLoS Medicine, 2009. 6(7): p. e1000097 and Tricco, A.C., et al., PRISMA Extension for Scoping Reviews (PRISMA-ScR): Checklist and Explanation. Annals of Internal Medicine, 2018. 169(7): p. 467.

Appendix 3
Complete list of rejected articles and summarized rationale

Not in English/French	Review Article/Editorial	Conference Abstract	Plastic Surgery Technique Only (Not IM)	Other Not About IM	Distraction Osteogenesis	Not Lower Tibia/Ankle/Foot	Not Specific Enough in Results	Animal Study	Total
4	7	1	34	7	2	4	17	1	77

Article Title	First Author	Reference	Reason Article Rejected
Induced-membrane technique in the management of posttraumatic bone defects	Azi ML[45]	JBJS Essential Surgical Techniques. 9(2):e22, 2019 Jun 26	RV: NA
The medial malleolar network: a constant vascular base of the distally based saphenous neurocutaneous island flap	Ballmer FT[35]	Surgical & Radiologic Anatomy. 21(5):297–303, 1999	Plastics flap
Metatarso-cuboid impingement following malunion of a Jones fracture: Case report and review of the literature	Beck M[36]	Foot and Ankle Surgery. 3 (3) (pp 143–146), 1997. Date of publication: 1997	No IM technique described
Anatomical basis of the anterolateral thigh flap	Begue T[37]	Surgical & Radiologic Anatomy. 12(4):311–313, 1990	Plastics flap
Distally based sural neurocutaneous flap: clinical experience and technical adaptations. Report of 60 cases [French]	Belfkira F[38]	Annales de Chirurgie Plastique et Esthetique. 51(3):199–206, 2006 Jun	Plastics flap
Subspecialty procedures: Tibial bone transport over an intramedullary nail using cable and pulleys	Bernstein M[39]	JBJS Essential Surgical Techniques. 8 (1) (no pagination), 2018. Article Number: e9. Date of publication: 2018	Distraction osteogenesis

(continued on next page)

Appendix 3
(continued)

Article Title	First Author	Reference	Reason Article Rejected
Anatomic basis of a fascio-cutaneous flap supplied by the perforating branch of the peroneal artery	Beveridge J[40]	Surgical & Radiologic Anatomy. 10(3):195–199, 1988	Plastics flap
Limb lengthening using ankle joint distraction (arthrodiastasis) followed by arthrodesis. Experience with one case	Blondel B[41]	Orthopaedics and Traumatology: Surgery and Research. 97 (4) (pp 438–442), 2011. Date of publication: June 2011	Distraction osteogenesis
Distal-based sural flaps treatment of 17 lesions of the distal third of the lower extremity [Italian]	Caglioni C[42]	Rivista Italiana di Chirurgia Plastica. 30 (4) (pp 275–281), 1998. Date of publication: 1998	Plastics flap
Plantar dislocation of the tarso-metatarsal articulation (Lisfranc articulation). Apropos of a case [French]	Charrois O[43]	Revue de Chirurgie Orthopedique et Reparatrice de l Appareil Moteur. 84(2):197–201, 1998 Apr	No IM technique described
The proximally designed sural flap based on the accompanying artery of the lesser saphenous vein	Cho AB[44]	Journal of Reconstructive Microsurgery. 26(8):501–8, 2010 Oct	Plastics flap
The posterior arm flap: Our department's experience	Costa MLR[46]	European Journal of Plastic Surgery. 34 (2) (pp 119–124), 2011. Date of publication: April 2011	Forearm
The distally based island superficial sural artery flap: clinical experience with 36 flaps	Costa-Ferreira A[47]	Annals of Plastic Surgery. 46(3):308–13, 2001 Mar.	Plastics flap
A reverse triangular soleus flap based on small distal communicating arterial branches	Dumont CE[48]	Annals of Plastic Surgery. 41(4):440–443, 1998 Oct	Plastics flap
The flexor digitorum longus muscle flap for the reconstruction of soft-tissue	Durand S[49]	Annals of Plastic Surgery. 71(5):595–599, 2013 Nov	Plastics flap

	Description	Citation	Notes
	defects in the distal third of the leg: anatomic considerations and clinical applications		
El-Alfy B[50]	The use of free nonvascularized fibular graft in the induced membrane technique to manage posttraumatic bone defects	European Journal of Orthopaedic Surgery & Traumatology. 28(6):1191-1197, 2018 Aug	Middle tibia and proximal to this only
Fitoussi F[51]	The medial saphenous hetero (cross leg) flap in coverage of soft tissue defects of the leg and foot [French]	Revue de Chirurgie Orthopedique et Reparatrice de l Appareil Moteur. 88(7):663–668, 2002 Nov	Plastics flap
Fitoussi F	The cross-leg flap in soft tissue defects of the leg and foot [French]	Revue de Chirurgie Orthopedique et Reparatrice de l'Appareil Moteur. 88 (7) (pp 663–668), 2002. Date of publication: November 2002	Plastics flap
Giannoudis PV[12]	Masquelet technique for the treatment of bone defects: Tips-tricks and future directions	Injury. 42 (6) (pp 591–598), 2011. Date of publication: June 2011	NA: review
Jonard B[52]	Posttraumatic reconstruction of the foot and ankle in the face of active infection	Orthopedic Clinics of North America. 48 (2) (pp 249–258), 2017. Date of publication: 01 Apr 2017	Review article
Karger C[53]	Treatment of posttraumatic bone defects by the induced membrane technique	Orthopaedics & Traumatology, Surgery & Research. 98(1):97–102, 2012 Feb	Did not specify distal tibia in article. No foot or ankle specific #
Klaue K[54]	Clinical, quantitative assessment of first tarsometatarsal mobility in the sagittal plane and its relation to hallux valgus deformity	Foot & Ankle International. 15(1):9–13, 1994 Jan	No IM technique described
Le Nen D[55]	Anatomical basis of a fascio-cutaneous pedicle flap based on the infero-lateral collateral artery of the leg	Surgical & Radiologic Anatomy. 16(1):3–8; discussion 9, 1994	Plastics flap

(continued on next page)

Appendix 3 (*continued*)

Article Title	First Author	Reference	Reason Article Rejected
Coverage of chronic osteomyelitis of the ankle and the foot using a soleus muscle island flap, vascularized with retrograde flow on the posterior tibial artery. A seven cases report [French]	Levante S[56]	Annales de Chirurgie Plastique et Esthetique. 54(6):523–527, 2009 Dec	Plastics flap
Masquelet Technique Combined with Tissue Flap Grafting for Treatment of Bone Defect and Soft Tissue Defect [Chinese]	Li Z[57]	Chung-Kuo Hsiu Fu Chung Chien Wai Ko Tsa Chih/Chinese Journal of Reparative & Reconstructive Surgery. 30(8):966–970, 2016 Aug 08	Chinese
The medial and inferior calcaneal nerves: an anatomic study	Louisia S[58]	Surgical & Radiologic Anatomy. 21(3):169–173, 1999	Anatomic study
The reamer-irrigator-aspirator in nonunion surgery	Madison RD[59]	Orthopedic Clinics of North America. 50 (3) (pp 297–304), 2019. Date of publication: July 2019	NA: RV
Double use of sural fascio-cutaneous flap with distal pedicle to cover loss of substance of ankle or heel [French]	Mainard D[60]	Revue de Chirurgie Orthopedique et Reparatrice de l Appareil Moteur. 80(1):73–77, 1995	Plastics flap
The distal anastomoses of the medial plantar artery: Surgical aspects (2.10.1987)	Masquelet AC[61]	Surgical and Radiologic Anatomy. 10 (3) (pp 247-249), 1988. Date of publication: 1988	Plastics flap
Repair of the soft tissues and the skin covering: recovery [French]	Masquelet AC[62]	Soins - Chirurgie. (138-139):20-8, 1992 Aug-Sep	Plastics flap
Surgical reconstruction of post-traumatic tissue loss of the weight-bearing sole of the foot [German]	Masquelet AC[63]	Therapeutische Umschau. 48(12):842–848, 1991 Dec	Plastics flap
The lateral supramalleolar flap	Masquelet AC[64]	Plastic & Reconstructive Surgery. 81(1):74–81, 1988 Jan	Plastics flap

The plantar flap in reconstructive surgery of the foot [French]	Masquelet AC[65]	Presse Medicale. 13(15):935–936, 1984 Apr 07	Plastics flap
Very long-term results of post-traumatic bone defect reconstruction by the induced membrane technique	Masquelet AC[66]	Orthopaedics & Traumatology, Surgery & Research. 105(1):159–166, 2019 02	Article does not give distal tibia results. All results are joined together in groups. No individual data provided
Vascularized transfer of the adductor magnus tendon and its osseous insertion: a preliminary report	Masquelet AC[67]	Journal of Reconstructive Microsurgery. 1(3):169–176, 1985 Jan	Plastics flap
The posterior arm free flap	Masquelet AC[68]	Plastic & Reconstructive Surgery. 76(6):908–913, 1985 Dec	Plastics flap
The medialis pedis flap: a new fasciocutaneous flap	Masquelet AC[69]	Plastic & Reconstructive Surgery. 85(5):765–772, 1990 May	Plastics flap
External supramalleolar flap in the reconstructive surgery of the foot [French]	Masquelet AC[70]	Journal de Chirurgie. 125(5):367–372, 1988 May	Plastics flap
Anatomic basis of a pedicled extensor digitorum brevis muscle flap	Massin P[71]	Surgical & Radiologic Anatomy. 10(4):267–272, 1988	Plastics flap
Distally based sural artery flap without sural nerve	Motamed S[72]	Acta Medica Iranica. 48(2):127–129, 2010 Mar–Apr	Plastics flap
Chronic compartment syndrome of the foot. A case report [French]	Muller GP[73]	Revue de Chirurgie Orthopedique et Reparatrice de l Appareil Moteur. 81(6):549–5-52, 1995	No IM technique described
Experiences with reverse-flow lateral supramalleolar flaps [Japanese]	Namiki Y[74]	Japanese Journal of Plastic and Reconstructive Surgery. 32 (8) (pp 787–793), 1989. Date of publication: 1989	Plastics flap
The reconstruction of the lower third of the leg by lateral supramalleolar flap [Italian]	Navissano M[75]	Rivista Italiana di Chirurgia Plastica. 28 (3) (pp 341–344), 1996. Date of publication: 1996	Plastics flap

(continued on next page)

Appendix 3
(continued)

Article Title	First Author	Reference	Reason Article Rejected
Closed rupture of the tibialis anterior tendon: a report of 2 cases	Neumayer F[76]	Journal of Foot & Ankle Surgery. 48(4):457–461, 2009 Jul-Aug	NA: tibialis tendon rupture
The posterolateral malleolar flap of the ankle: A distally based sural neurocutaneous flap: Report of 14 cases	Oberlin C[77]	Plastic and Reconstructive Surgery. 96 (2) (pp 400—407), 1995. Date of publication: 1995	Plastics flap
An easy and versatile method of coverage for distal tibial soft tissue defects	Ogun TC[78]	Journal of Trauma-Injury Infection & Critical Care. 50(1):53–59, 2001 Jan	Plastics flap
Congenital pseudarthrosis of the tibia	Pannier S[79]	Orthopaedics and Traumatology: Surgery and Research. 97 (7) (pp 750–761), 2011. Date of publication: November 2011	Review article
Effectiveness analysis of induced membrane technique in the treatment of infectious bone defect [Chinese]	Qiu X[80]	Chung-Kuo Hsiu Fu Chung Chien Wai Ko Tsa Chih/Chinese Journal of Reparative & Reconstructive Surgery. 31(9):1064–1068, 2017 09 15	Chinese
Dislocation and necrosis of the first, second and third wedges. Management with the Masquelet technique. A case report [Spanish]	Rincon-Cardozo DF[81]	Acta Ortopedica Mexicana. 27(1):55–59, 2013 Jan-Feb	In Spanish. Also unable to obtain online
Soft tissue preservation and reconstruction in nonsupporting foot parts [German]	Romana MC[82]	Therapeutische Umschau. 48(12):836–841, 1991 Dec	Plastics flap
Reconstruction of osseous defects using the Masquelet technique [Review] [German]	Saxer F[83]	Orthopade. 46(8):665–672, 2017 Aug	RV

Reconstruction of septic diaphyseal bone defects with the induced membrane technique	Scholz AO[84]	Injury. 46 Suppl 4:S121–124, 2015 Oct	Excluded. Did not give outcomes of MT, nor did it specify which tibias were distal
Bone propeller flap: a staged procedure	Tremp M[85]	Journal of Foot & Ankle Surgery. 53(2):226–231, 2014 Mar-Apr	Plastics flap
Technical refinement of the lateral supramalleolar flap	Valenti P[86]	British Journal of Plastic Surgery. 44(6):459–462, 1991 Aug-Sep	Plastics flap
Reconstruction of soft tissue defects of lower leg, ankle and foot using sural flap [Czech]	Vesely R[87]	Rozhledy V Chirurgii. 86(3):134–138, 2007 Mar	Plastics flap
Induction of a barrier membrane to facilitate reconstruction of massive segmental diaphyseal bone defects: an ovine model	Viateau V[88]	Veterinary Surgery. 35(5):445–452, 2006 Jul	OVINE model
The supramalleolar flap. Our experience in 35 cases [French]	Voche P[89]	Annales de Chirurgie Plastique et Esthetique. 46(2):112–124, 2001 Apr	Plastics flap
Induced membrane technique for the treatment of bone defects due to post-traumatic osteomyelitis	Wang X[90]	Bone and Joint Research. 5 (3) (pp 101–105), 2016. Date of publication: March 2016	Article did not specify distal tibia results, or even which were tibias of femurs. Tibias and femurs only
The Masquelet procedure gone awry	Assal M[91]	Orthopedics. 37 (11) (pp e1045–e1048), 2014. Date of publication: 01 Nov 2014	NA: editorial

(continued on next page)

Appendix 3
(continued)

Article Title	First Author	Reference	Reason Article Rejected
Two-stage reconstruction of post-traumatic segmental tibia bone loss with nailing	Apard T[92]	Orthop Traumatol Surg Res, 2010. 96(5): p. 549–553	Not specific
Salvage of an osteocutaneous thermonecrosis secondary to tibial reaming by the induced membrane procedure	Cambon-Binder A[93]	Clin Case Rep, 2017. 5(9): p. 1471–1476	Midshaft not distal third
Circumferential bone grafting around an absorbable gelatin sponge core reduced the amount of grafted bone in the induced membrane technique for critical-size defects of long bones	Cho JW[94]	Injury, 2017. 48(10): p. 2292–2305	Not specific enough
Reconstruction of traumatic bone loss using the induced membrane technique: preliminary results about 11 cases	Kombate NK[95]	J Orthop, 2017. 14(4): p. 489–494	No distal tibia specific
Segmental bone defect treated with the induced membrane technique	Konda SR	J Orthop Trauma, 2017. 31 Suppl 3: p. S21–S22	Femoral defect
The Masquelet technique of induced membrane for healing of bone defects. A review of 8 cases	Olesen UK[96]	Injury, 2015. 46 Suppl 8: p. S44–S47	Not clear which were distal tibia
Reconstruction of the long bones by the induced membrane and spongy autograft	Masquelet AC[97]	Ann Chir Plast Esthet. 2000 Jun 45(3):346–353. French	No specific information on location
Muscle reconstruction in reconstructive surgery: soft tissue repair and long bone reconstruction	Masquelet AC[98]	Langenbecks Arch Surg. 2003 Oct;388(5):344–346. Epub 2003 Sep 11	No specific information on location

Reamer-irrigator-aspirator bone graft and bi Masquelet technique for segmental bone defect nonunions: a review of 25 cases	Stafford PR[99]	Injury, 2010. 41 Suppl 2: p. S72–S77	Unclear whether distal tibia
Patient specific 3D printed titanium truss strut implants combined with the Masquelet technique: A novel strategy to reconstruct massive segmental bone loss	Tetsworth K[100]	Journal of Orthopaedic Research. Conference: 2017 Annual Meeting of the Orthopaedic Research Society. United States. 35 (Supplement 1) (no pagination), 2017. Date of publication: March 2017	Conference abstract only
Management of traumatic tibial diaphyseal bone defect by "induced-membrane technique"	Gupta G[101]	Indian J Orthop, 2016. 50(3): p. 290–296	Not specific
Effect of induced membrane formation followed by polymethylmethacrylate implantation on diabetic foot ulcer healing when revascularization is not feasible	Liu CY[102]	Journal of Diabetes Research. 2019:2429136, 2019	No bone grafting. PMMA cement only used for antimicrobial effect
Mixed results with the Masquelet technique: A fact or a myth?	Mi M[2]	Injury. 51 (2) (pp 132–135), 2020. Date of publication: February 2020	Review article
Infected tibia defect fractures treated with the Masquelet technique	Muhlhausser J[103]	Medicine (Baltimore), 2017. 96(20): p. e6948	Not specific
Treatment of bone loss with the induced membrane technique: techniques and outcomes	Taylor BC[104]	Journal of Orthopaedic Trauma. 29 (12) (pp 554–557), 2015. Date of publication: 01 Dec 2015	Not specific
Short-term outcomes of induced membrane technique in treatment of long bone defects in Iran	Yeganeh AM	Medicinski Arhiv. 70(4):284–287, 2016 Jul 27	Not specific

(continued on next page)

Appendix 3
(continued)

Article Title	First Author	Reference	Reason Article Rejected
Masquelet technique for treatment of posttraumatic bone defects	Wong TM[105]	ScientificWorldJournal, 2014. 2014: p. 710302	Not specific
Management of infected bone defects of the lower extremities by three-stage induced membrane technique	Zhang C[106]	Medical Science Monitor. 26:e919925, 2020 Feb 12	Not specific

Data from Refs.[12,20,35–44,46–76,77–106]

Complex Ankle Fractures
Practical Approach for Surgical Treatment

Guillermo Martin Arrondo, MD[a], German Joannas, MD[a,b,c],*

KEYWORDS

- Posterior tibial malleolus • Pilon • Tibial plafond • Posterior surgical approach
- Posteromedial approach • Modified posteromedial approach • Trimalleolar fractures
- Cuadrimalleolar fractures

KEY POINTS

- Complex ankle fractures are challenging, especially the surgical planning.
- Preoperative planning with a computed tomography axial view is mandatory to decide the surgical approach and patient positioning.
- Of the posterior tibial plafond, 40%, 64%, and 91% are visualized with the posterolateral, posteromedial, and modified posteromedial approaches, respectively.
- For decision making process, we suggest dividing the ankle into 4 areas: posterior malleolus, medial malleolus, lateral malleolus, and Chaput and/or Wagstafe fragments (supine position).
- Depending on the fracture location we suggest the following surgical approaches: posterolateral approach (posterolateral malleolus and fibula), posteromedial approach (posteromedial malleolus, medial malleolus), modified posteromedial approach (posteromedial and posterolateral malleolus, medial malleolus), medial approach (medial malleolus fracture), and anterolateral approach (Chaput tubercle and anteromedial aspect of the fibula (Wagstaffe fragment).

INTRODUCTION

Since Coppers in 1822 first described trimalleolar fractures, many articles have been published.[1–3] Anatomic reduction in complex ankle fractures is a demanding challenge. High risk of post-traumatic arthritis was observed in complex trimalleolar fractures compared with unimalleolar fractures.[4–6] Lower functional outcome was found in trimalleolar fractures when compared with unilateral

[a] Foot and Ankle Division "CEPP", Instituto Dupuytren, Av. Belgrano 3402, Ciudad Autónoma de Buenos Aires CP 1078, Argentina; [b] Foot and Ankle Division, Orthopaedics Department, Centro Artroscópico Jorge Batista SA, Pueyrredón 2446 1 Er Piso, Ciudad Autónoma de Buenos Aires (CABA) CP 1119, Argentina; [c] Instituto Barrancas, Hipolito Yrigoyen 902, QUILMES, CP 1878, Buenos Aires, Argentina
* Corresponding author.
E-mail addresses: germanjoannas@icloud.com; german_joannas@cepp.org.ar

Foot Ankle Clin N Am 25 (2020) 587–595
https://doi.org/10.1016/j.fcl.2020.08.002
1083-7515/20/© 2020 Elsevier Inc. All rights reserved.
foot.theclinics.com

or bilateral.[3] Patient positioning (supine or prone) and the surgical approach depend on the compromise of anterolateral Chaput tubercle or anterior fibular Wagstaffe fragment.

Compromise of the posterior column in ankle fractures rates are from 7% to 44%.[4] Major concerns about the importance of anatomic reduction of the posterior pilon in complex ankle fractures are increasing in literature. Anatomic reduction of the posterior malleolus is very important to stabilize the inferior tibiofibular syndesmotic complex.[3]

Computed tomography (CT) scanning is mandatory to classify and define the most useful access to the posterior plafond.[7] Bartonicek and colleagues,[8] Mason and colleagues,[9] and Haraguchi and colleagues[10] have described and classified posterior malleolar fractures. Axial CT scans allows us to determine not only the size and number of fragments, but also to define the most useful approach and patient positioning.

PLANNING

Correct preoperative planning is necessary for a good result. AP and lateral views of the ankle mortise are always indicated, but a CT scan (axial view) is mandatory because some posterior fractures may be overlooked.[4,7,11–14] Donohoe and colleagues[7] demonstrated that the use of a preoperative CT scan changed 52% of fracture identifications and in 44%, the surgical approach and patient positioning. Palmanovich and colleagues[15] found that primarily indication change after reviewing previous radiographs with CT scans.

Simple posterior malleolar fractures can be reduced with ligamentotaxis and fixed with anteroposterior screws; however, this method has some limitations. It is technically challenging to achieve anatomic reduction by fluoroscopy, and screw fixation may be difficult in small posterolateral fragments.[16] A large number of publications support direct visualization and anatomic reduction of the posterior malleolus through a posterior approach to obtain a good functional outcome.[4,17]

The posterolateral approach is useful in most cases showing posterior compromise.[18,19] However, when there is a large and split fracture of the posterior fragment, the medial aspect of the fragment is very difficult to access from this incision.[20,21] In this case, the combination of a posterolateral and a posteromedial approach is required. The modified posteromedial (MPM) approach was described to decrease the risk of complications and facilitate the reduction of the posterior malleolus.[4]

Assal and Dalmau Pastor[22] compared the percentage of exposure of the posterior plafond using 3 different approaches: posterolateral, posteromedial, and MPM. With the posterolateral approach, 40% of the surface could be visualized. From a posteromedial approach, 64% could be seen, and 91% of the plafond can be visualized from an MPM approach. Meulenkamp and colleagues[12] demonstrated that 99% of posterior plafond could be exposed using the MPM approach.

Some surgeons preferred to combined different approaches changing patient position because there are fewer anesthesia complications,[23] a decreased fluoroscopic exposure, and better visualization of the medial malleolus. However, recent anatomic publications allow the combination of posterolateral and MPM approaches with the patient in prone position to reduce and fixed most of the malleolar fractures diminishing soft tissue complications. In certain cases, when there is an anterolateral Chaput fragment or anteromedial fibula Wagstafe fragment, the patient should be changed to a supine position.

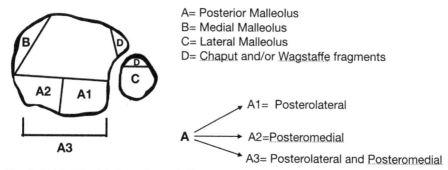

A= Posterior Malleolus
B= Medial Malleolus
C= Lateral Malleolus
D= Chaput and/or Wagstaffe fragments

A1= Posterolateral
A2=Posteromedial
A3= Posterolateral and Posteromedial

Fig. 1. Ankle CT axial view schematic illustration. Fragments are organized, as shown in the diagram.

In our experience, the ankle is divided into 4 areas on a CT axial view (**Fig. 1**):

A. Posterior malleolus (A1-A2-A3)
B. Medial malleolus
C. Lateral malleolus
D. Chaput and/or Wagstafe fragments (supine position)

Fractures line splits the posterior malleolus (A) into 3 types: A1 posterolateral, A2 posteromedial, and A3, both posterolateral and posteromedial.

SURGICAL TECHNIQUE

Different approaches are indicated depending on the fracture pattern. The posterior malleolus has to be approached first. If there is a split fracture, the posteromedial fragment has to be debrided and freed of periosteum and fixed in the first place, followed by the posterolateral fragment from a single MPM approach. When the compromise is posterolateral, the fibula can be fixed from the same posterolateral approach. If a medial approach is necessary, it could be done in the same prone position.

We suggest operating in a supine position when there is an anterior component that cannot be addressed from posterior as in Wagstaffe or Chaput type of fractures. As a helpful guideline, we suggest different approaches depending on the fracture pattern (**Fig. 2**).

Posterolateral Approach

The patient is placed in a prone position, with a bump under the ipsilateral hip, under combined lumbar plexus–sciatic nerve block anesthesia. A pneumatic tourniquet is applied to prevent bleeding. The skin incision is made between the lateral malleolus's posterior edge and the lateral aspect of the Achilles tendon. The sural nerve runs from medial to lateral and crosses the lateral aspect of the Achilles tendon, on average, 9.83 cm proximal to its insertion in the calcaneus.[24] The anatomy of the sural nerve is variable. To avoid nerve injuries, the nerve must be identified and protected throughout the procedure. After fasciotomy, dissection is performed between the peroneal tendons and the flexor hallucis longus. Now, the lateral aspect of the posterior plafond is exposed. When fixing posterolateral malleolus, the peroneal tendons are retracted laterally and flexor hallucis longus muscle medially. When fixing the fibula, the peroneal tendons are retracted medially (**Fig. 3**).

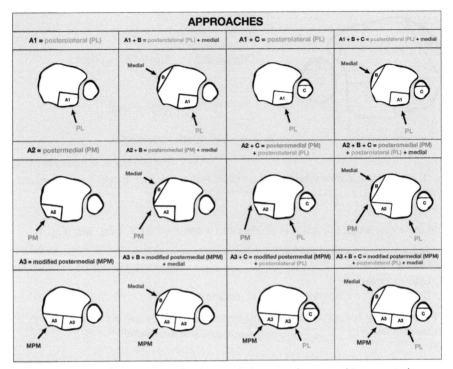

Fig. 2. Based on the fragments involved, a surgical approach proposal is presented.

Posteromedial Approach

With the patient in the prone position, under combined lumbar plexus–sciatic nerve block anesthesia, the incision is made along the posterior tibialis tendon. After the tendon sheaths are incised, the flexor digitorum longus is retracted laterally, protecting the neurovascular bundle, and the posterior tibialis tendon is mobilized and subluxated medially, allowing the visualization of 64% of the posterior plafond.[22] If a medial malleolus fracture is associated, the skin incision is extended distally, the posterior tibial tendon (TP) and flexor hallucis longus are retracted laterally. The fracture is exposed, debrided, and fixed (**Fig. 4**).

Modified Posteromedial Approach

With the patient in a prone position, under combined lumbar plexus-sciatic nerve block anesthesia, the skin incision is made 1 cm medially to the Achilles tendon, approximately 10 cm in length. The Achilles tendon, flexor hallucis longus, tendon and muscle belly are retracted laterally. The neurovascular bundle is dissected and moved medially, allowing exposure of 91% of the posterior tibial plafond.[22] From this side, platting of the posteromedial and posterolateral fractures is performed. If a medial malleolus fracture is associated, the skin incision is extended distally, and the TP, flexor digitorum longus, neurovascular bundle, and flexor hallucis longus are retracted laterally, allowing good visualization of the medial malleolus (**Fig. 5**).

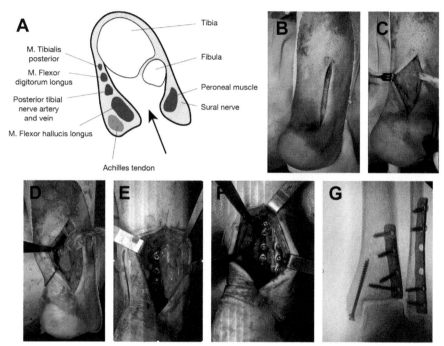

Fig. 3. Posterolateral approach: anatomic considerations. (*A*) A skin incision is made between the posterior edge of the lateral malleolus and the lateral aspect of the Achilles tendon. (*B*) Identify the peroneal tendons fascia and sural nerve. (*C*) Dissection is performed: the flexor hallucis longus medially, Peroneal tendons, and sural nerve laterally. Temporary fixation of the posterolateral fragment. (*D*) The posterolateral malleolar fragment is fixed using screws and buttress plate. (*E*) The posterolateral malleolar fragment and fibula are fixed. (*F*) Postoperative radiographs after open reduction and internal fixation of the posterolateral malleolar fragment and lateral malleolus. In the same patient from a medial approach, we made an open reduction and internal fixation of the medial malleolus with 2 screws (*G*).

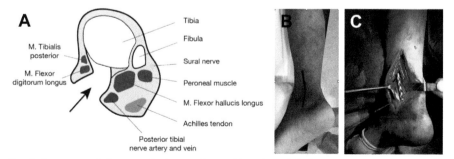

Fig. 4. Posteromedial approach. Anatomic considerations. (*A*) The incision is made along the posterior tibialis tendon. (*B*) The flexor digitorum longus is retracted laterally protecting the neurovascular bundle. Open reduction and internal fixation of the posteromedial malleolar fragment with buttress plate and lag screws (*C*).

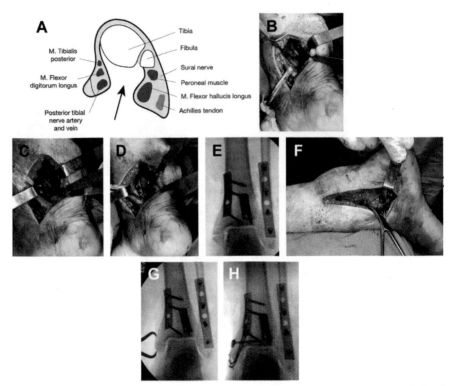

Fig. 5. MPM approach. Anatomic considerations. (*A*) Skin incision between the medial malleolus and the Achilles tendon. The neurovascular bundle is moved medially and the flexor hallucis longus laterally. (*B*) Open reduction and internal fixation of the posteromedial malleolar fragment and visualization of the posterolateral malleolar fragment. (*C*) After fixing the posteromedial malleolar fragment, we fixed the posterolateral malleolar fragment. (*D*) Fluoroscopy showing an accurate reduction of the posteromedial malleolar fragment, posterolateral malleolar fragment, and fibula. Associated medial malleolus fracture. (*E*) Same approach (MPM approach); the TP, flexor digitorum longus, neurovascular bundle, and flexor hallucis longus are retracted laterally. Reduction of the medial malleolus with a clamp (*F*). Fluoroscopy showing reduction of medial malleolus (*G*). Fluoroscopy showing a tension band for medial malleolus fracture (*H*).

Medial Approach

The patient is placed in the prone position. Although the prone position can make open reduction and internal fixation of the medial malleolus more challenging, the medial malleolus is generally the easier of the malleoli to reduce and fix.

A 4- to 5-cm long skin incision is made. Care should be taken not to damage the saphenous vein, which is retracted anteriorly. Periosteum and hematoma should be removed from the fracture site. Internal fixation of the medial malleolus is made after anatomic reduction of the articular surface is obtained (**Fig. 6**).

Anterolateral Approach

The patient is placed in a supine position. An anterolateral incision is made following the anterior border of the fibula. The superficial peroneal nerve is dissected and retracted laterally and peroneus tertius tendon medially. This incision allows excellent

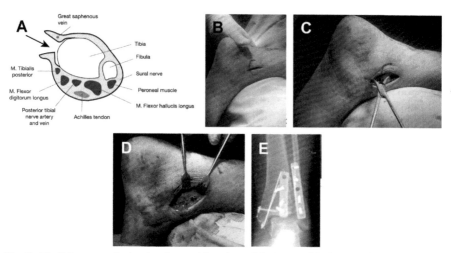

Fig. 6. Medial approach. Anatomic considerations. (*A*) A 5-cm skin incision (prone position) is made. (*B*) Reduction of the medial malleolus with a clamp. (*C*) Tension band for medial malleolus fracture. (*D*) Postoperative radiographs after open reduction and internal fixation of the posterior and lateral malleolus (*E*).

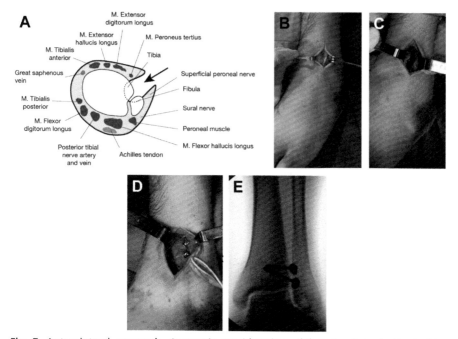

Fig. 7. Anterolateral approach. Anatomic considerations. (*A*) Anterolateral skin incision following the anterior border of the fibula. Retracted superficial peroneal nerve laterally. (*B*) Identification of a Chaput fracture. (*C*) Anatomic reduction with anteroposterior screws fixation (*D*). Postoperative mortise radiographs (*E*).

visualization of either the Chaput tubercle and anteromedial aspect of the fibula (Wagstaffe fragment) (**Fig. 7**).

Postoperative Care

It is important to protect the fracture with a nonweightbearing splint for 2 weeks owing to tendon retraction in plantar flexion. Patients are encouraged for early mobilization, and partial weightbearing is authorized at 6 weeks. Full weightbearing is allowed at 8 weeks.

SUMMARY

Anatomic reduction of the posterior malleolus is mandatory for a good functional outcome. Preoperative planning with a CT scan's axial view helps to decide which approach and surgical position we should choose. Based on posterior malleolus fracture anatomy, a guideline is suggested to facilitate decision making on which approach seems to provide the best exposure with the fewest complications.

CLINICS CARE POINTS

- The posterolateral approach is useful when there is a posterolateral compromise of the tibia and most of the fibula fractures.
- An MPM approach allows the visualization of more than 90% of the posterior malleolus.
- The supine position is indicated when there is an anterior compromise of the tibia or fibula.

DISCLOSURE

The authors do not have any relationship with a commercial company that has a direct financial interest in subject matter or materials discussed in this article or with a company making a competing product.

REFERENCES

1. McDaniel Wj, Wilson FC. Trimalleolar fractures of the ankle. An end result study. Clin Orthop Relat Res 1977;122:37–45.
2. De Vries JS, Wijgman Aj, Sierevelt IN, et al. Long-term results of ankle fractures with a posterior malleolar fragment. J Foot Ankle Surg 2005;44(3):211–7.
3. Verhage S, Hoogendoorn J, Krijen P. When and how to operate the posterior malleolus fragment in trimalleolar fractures: a systematic literature review. Arch Orthop Trauma Surg 2018;138(9):1213–22.
4. Zhong S, Shen L, Zhao JG, et al. Comparison of Posteromedial Versus Posterolateral Approach for Posterior Malleolus Fixation in Trimalleolar Ankle Fractures. Orthop Surg 2017;9(1):69–76.
5. Evers J, Fischer M, Zderic I, et al. The role of a small posterior malleolar fragment in trimalleolar fractures. Bone Joint J 2018;100-B(1):95–100.
6. Lindsijö U. Operative treatment of ankle fracture-dislocations. A follow-up study of 306/321 consecutive cases. Clin Orthop Relat Res 1985;199:28–38.
7. Donohoe S, Alluri RK, Hill JR, et al. Impact of Computed Tomography on Operative Planning for Ankle Fractures Involving the Posterior Malleolus. Foot Ankle Int 2017;38(12):1337–42.
8. Bartonicek J, Rammelt S, Tucek M. Posterior malleolar fractures: changing concepts and recent developments. Foot Ankle Clin 2017;22(1):125–45.

9. Mason LW, Marlow WJ, Widnall J, et al. Pathoanatomy and associated injuries of posterior malleolus fracture of the ankle. Foot Ankle Int 2017;38(11):1229–35.
10. Haraguchi N, Haruyama H, Toga H, et al. Pathoanatomy of posterior malleolar fractures of the ankle. J Bone Joint Surg Am 2006;88(5):1085–92.
11. Ferries JS, Decoster TA, Firoozbakhsh KK, et al. Plain radiographic interpretation in trimalleolar ankle fractures poorly assesses posterior fragment size. J Orthop Trauma 1994;8(4):328–31.
12. Meulenkamp B, Louati H, Morellato J. Posterior malleolus exposure. Orthopedic Trauma Association; 2019. p. e021.
13. Gardner MJ, Streubel PN, McCormick JJ, et al. Surgeon Practices regarding operative treatment of posterior malleolus fractures. Foot Ankle Int 2011;32(4): 385–93.
14. Macko VW, Matthews LS, Zwirkoski P, et al. The joint-contact area of the ankle. The contribution of the posterior malleolus. J Bone Joint Surg Am 1991;73(3): 347–51.
15. Palmanovich E, Brin YS, Kish B, et al. The effect of minimally displaced posterior malleolar fractures on decision making in minimally displaced lateral malleolus fractures. Int Orthop 2014;38(5):1051–6.
16. Lee Hj, Kang Ks, Kang Sy, et al. Percutaneous reduction technique using a Kirschner wire for displaced posterior malleolar fractures. Foot Ankle Int 2009; 30(2):157–9.
17. Bartonicek J, Rammelt S, Tucek M, et al. Posterior Malleolar Fractures of the ankle. Eur J Trauma Emerg Surg 2015;41:587–600b.
18. Amorosa Lf, Brown GD, Greisberg J. A surgical approach to posterior pilon fractures. J Orthop Trauma 2010;24(3):188–93.
19. Erdem MN, Erken HY, Burc H, et al. Comparison of lag screw versus buttress plate fixation of posterior malleolar fractures. Foot Ankle Int 2014;35(10):1022–30.
20. Weber M. Trimalleolar fractures with impaction of the posteromedial tibial plafond: implications for talar stability. Foot Ankle Int 2004;25(10):716–27.
21. Ogilvie-Harris DJ, Reed SC, Hedman TP. Disruption of the ankle syndesmosis: biomechanical study of the ligamentous restraints. Arthroscopy 1994;10(5): 558–60.
22. Assal M, Dalmau-Pastor M, Ray A, et al. How to Get to the Distal Posterior Tibial Malleolus? A Cadaveric Anatomic Study Defining the Access Corridors Through 3 Different Approaches. J Orthop Trauma 2017;31(4):e127–9.
23. Edgcombe H, Carter K, Yarrow S. Anaesthesia in the prone position. Br J Anaesth 2008;100(2):165–83.
24. Webb J, Moorjani N, Radford M. Anatomy of the sural nerve and its relation to the Achilles Tendon. Foot Ankle Int 2000;21(6):475–7.

Acute Deltoid Ligament Repair in Ankle Fractures

Gonzalo F. Bastias, MD[a,b,c], Jorge Filippi, MD, MBA[a,b],*

KEYWORDS

- Ankle fracture • Deltoid ligament repair • Medial clear space
- bimalleolar equivalent fracture

KEY POINTS

- The deltoid ligament complex stabilizes the ankle joint against eversion, external rotation, and plantar flexion forces.
- There is no consensus on whether deltoid ligament must be repaired in bimalleolar equivalent ankle fractures.
- Patients with extensive capsuloligamentous damage and multidirectional instability may benefit from repair to improve reduction quality, avoid loss of reduction, and regain medial/syndesmotic stability.
- Most deltoid ligament repair techniques involve direct repair or reattachment using suture anchors for augmentation. There is no evidence of the superiority of any technique in the literature.
- The authors recommend repairing the deltoid ligament complex in the setting of bimalleolar equivalent fractures associated with syndesmotic or multiligamentous instability as well as in heavier patients with greater mechanical requirements.

INTRODUCTION

There is no consensus on whether the deltoid ligament (DL) should be repaired in the setting of ankle fractures.[1–6] One of the main drawbacks is the wide spectrum of ankle fractures presenting with DL injuries ranging from the low-energy bimalleolar equivalent to complex high-energy fractures with multiligamentous and osseous involvement. Recent systematic reviews have shown better results in early stages in terms of radiologic reduction and decreased pain when the DL is repaired. Patients with high fibular

[a] Department of Orthopedic Surgery, Foot and Ankle Unit, Clinica Las Condes, Estoril 450, Las Condes, Santiago 7591047, Chile; [b] Department of Orthopedic Surgery, Foot and Ankle Unit, Hospital del Trabajador, Ramon Carnicer 185, Providencia, Santiago 7501239, Chile; [c] Department of Orthopedic Surgery, Universidad de Chile, Complejo Hospitalario San Jose, 1027 Independencia, Santiago 8380453, Chile
* Corresponding author. Estoril 450, Las Condes, Santiago 7591047, Chile.
E-mail address: jfilippi@clinicalascondes.cl

Foot Ankle Clin N Am 25 (2020) 597–612
https://doi.org/10.1016/j.fcl.2020.08.009
1083-7515/20/© 2020 Elsevier Inc. All rights reserved.

foot.theclinics.com

fractures or injuries with concomitant syndesmotic instability may benefit from DL repair.[7-9] The long-term benefits on surgical repair of the DL have not been fully demonstrated, prolonging the debate on which is the best clinical choice.[7,8,10]

This article reviews the current evidence in diagnosis, trends, and surgical techniques for repairing the DL in the acute setting and presents the authors' practical approach.

HISTORICAL PERSPECTIVE

Forty years ago, repairing the DL complex in the setting of an acute ankle fracture was the standard of practice.[1,11,12] After the results of several case series published during the 1980s and early 1990s, this trend changed, allowing the DL to heal without direct surgical repair unless reduction of the lateral malleolus or medial gutter was not obtained.[2,5,13,14]

This early body of evidence, criticized for being methodologically insufficient and low powered, modeled the widely spread conduct of not repairing the medial ligamentous complex.[1] However, in the last 2 decades, a renewed interest in optimizing the results of patients sustaining ankle fractures has resulted in revisiting this indication with a growing body of evidence supporting swinging the pendulum once again toward DL repair.[3,6,15,16]

RELEVANT ANATOMY AND BIOMECHANICS

The anatomic description of the DL and its structures has been widely studied through the years.[17-20] Even though a full understanding of its characteristics and variability is an evolving matter, there is consensus in dividing this structure into 2 main components: the superficial and deep DLs.[19,21]

Superficial Deltoid Ligament

The superficial DL spans the tibiotalar and subtalar joints coursing from the medial malleolus to the navicular and the calcaneus (**Fig. 1**).[22,23] This layer has been classically described to be constantly conformed by the tibionavicular ligament and the tibiospring ligament. In addition, there are 2 bands with variable presence: the

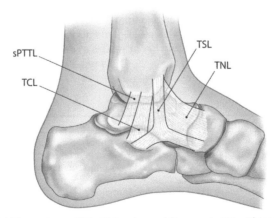

Fig. 1. Superficial DL anatomy. TCL, tibiocalcaneal ligament; TNL, tibionavicular ligament; TSL, tibiospring ligament; sPTTL, superficial posterior tibiotalar ligament. (*Courtesy of* I. Guerrero Schiappacasse, Valdivia, Chile.)

tibiocalcaneal ligament and the superficial posterior tibiotalar ligament.[23,24] Both bands have been reported to be present in as many as 94% and 97%, respectively, in different cadaveric studies.[25–27]

The tibiospring ligament also has fibers to the sustentaculum tali and merges with the calcaneonavicular portion of the spring ligament. These anatomic details, recently described, show the close relationship between DL and spring ligament as one integrated and functional entity.[25,28,29]

Deep Deltoid Ligament

The deep portion of the DL has a major constant component denominated deep posterior tibiotalar ligament usually accompanied to the anterior tibiotalar ligament (**Fig. 2**).[23,24] Panchani and colleagues[25] also described an additional deep tibiocalcaneal ligament running between both the anterior tibiotalar ligament and deep posterior tibiotalar ligament in around 12% of the ankles analyzed in their cadaveric study.

Biomechanics

The DL is the primary stabilizer of the ankle joint, restraining against valgus tilting and anterior and lateral translation of the talus.[21] The superficial and deep layers of the DL have different roles in ankle biomechanics.

The superficial DL resists eversion forces of the hindfoot[30] and plays a significant role in rotational ankle stability, resisting external rotation of the talus to the tibia, and valgus stress.[21] The specific role of its components has been further studied, showing that loss of both tibionavicular ligament and tibiospring ligament leads to an objective increment in eversion/pronation without talar tilt or subtalar gapping, whereas the tibiocalcaneal ligament specifically limits talar pronation.[23]

The principal function of the deep DL is to prevent lateral displacement and external rotation of the talus, also being the primary stabilizer against plantarflexion.[21,31] Earll and colleagues[30] established that sectioning the deep DL results in lateral talar shift only if the fibula is removed. However, sectioning of the entire deltoid complex is required to create significant medial talar tilt in otherwise intact ankles, decreasing the total tibiotalar contact by 15% to 20%.

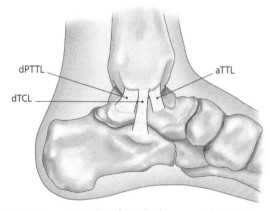

Fig. 2. Deep DL anatomy. aTTL, anterior tibiotalar ligament; dPTTL, deep posterior tibiotalar ligament; dTCL, deep tibiocalcaneal ligament. (*Courtesy of* I. Guerrero Schiappacasse, Valdivia, Chile.)

DOES THE DELTOID LIGAMENT NEED TO BE REPAIRED?
Studies Supporting Not Repairing the Deltoid Ligament

de Souza and colleagues[13] analyzed 150 external rotation–abduction ankle fractures, including 24 patients with DL disruption diagnosed radiologically. Twenty-two of these patients were treated without medial repair and were followed for 3.5 years on average. Functional results were reported as satisfactory in all patients, without clinical medial instability. The authors concluded that the ruptured DL probably does not need to be repaired as long as the lateral fracture is anatomically and rigidly fixed, and an intraoperative radiograph reveals a restored medial joint space. In 1988, similar findings were reported on another study by Harper,[2] in a retrospective study following 36 patients with ankle fractures and closed treatment of a DL injury. This study indicates that the DL heals sufficiently without repair and positive outcomes seemed to be related to maintaining the initial surgical reduction of the lateral malleolus and medial joint space until bone repair was completed.

Zeegers and van der Werken[14] reported on 28 patients presenting with lateral malleolar fractures and DL rupture treated only with open reduction and internal fixation (ORIF) of the fibula with an average follow-up of 18 months. Twenty-three patients had a perfect anatomic reduction with 5 patients presenting a slight widening of the medial joint space. Twenty patients had excellent and good results after clinical and radiologic evaluation. Eight patients were reported having poor functional outcomes correlating with radiologic findings of osteoarthritis. No medial instability was reported in any patient, and it was concluded that DL reconstruction was not necessary if an anatomic reduction is achieved.

A randomized study of 50 patients was published by Strömsöe and colleagues.[5] One group (25 patients) underwent direct DL repair and the other group only fibular stabilization with no exploration of the medial side. In both groups, syndesmotic fixation with a screw was performed when needed. No differences were found except for a longer duration of surgery in the repair group. The mean follow-up was 17 months, and the clinical evaluation was based on pain, swelling, range of motion, and whether prior work or sports activities changed or not. No clinical score was used, nor was the statistical significance for any of the results reported.

A systematic review by Chen and colleagues,[32] reported 520 ankle fractures treated with arthroscopy assisted techniques informing concomitant ligament injuries. Six studies included 322 patients (60.9%) with arthroscopically diagnosed DL injuries. Among all of the studies involved in this systematic review, none repaired the DL and no case of chronic instability was reported.

Comparative Studies

Nonrandomized controlled trials

Recent studies have tried to establish the outcomes of ankle fractures with and without DL repair in terms of functional and radiologic outcomes.[7,9,33,34] A retrospective study by Zhao and colleagues[33] compared the results of 74 patients with ankle fractures associated with DL ruptures with a mean follow-up of 53 months. Twenty patients underwent surgical repair of the DL and 54 were left unrepaired. The American Orthopaedic Foot and Ankle Society (AOFAS) score and visual analog scale (VAS) was comparable among both groups and revealed no statistical differences. The postoperative medial clear space (MCS) was significantly smaller in the DL repair group and also at latest follow-up. No malreduction (MCS of ≥5 mm) occurred at the DL repair group, however, the rate was 20.4% in the nonrepaired group. Interestingly, AO/OTA type C fractures showed a positive correlation with malreduction.

Woo and colleagues[9] retrospectively evaluated 78 consecutive cases of a ruptured DL in association with ankle fractures with an average of 17 months of follow-up. Outcomes were evaluated using the AOFAS, VAS, and fraction of failures isolated, with outcomes being comparable in both groups. Radiologic findings at final follow-up showed that MCS was significantly smaller on the DL repair group. A comparison was made between patients requiring syndesmotic fixation between both groups. The DL repair group attained better clinical outcomes and showed significantly smaller MCS values. According to these results, these investigators concluded that at final follow-up MCS had a significant influence on clinical outcomes. In addition, patients with high-grade unstable fractures and syndesmotic instability may benefit from DL repair for restoring medial stability.

Other studies have advocated for DL repair as an augmentation for syndesmosis stability proposing that anatomic reconstruction of the DL could even avoid the need for syndesmotic screws. Jones and Nunley,[4] in a retrospective series, compared 15 patients with lateral ORIF and syndesmotic fixation and 12 patients treated with DL repair for bimalleolar equivalent fractures. No statistical differences were demonstrated between the groups in functional, radiologic, or subjective outcomes. Little and collaborators[35] compared radiographic and clinical outcomes on patients with supination external rotation type IV fractures at 12 months of follow-up. Eighteen patients were treated with syndesmotic screws and 27 were treated using DL and posterior inferior tibiofibular ligament repair. The DL–posterior inferior tibiofibular ligament group had significantly better syndesmotic reduction compared with the contralateral extremity on a postoperative computed tomography scan and maintenance of MCS based on final postoperative radiographs had no significant differences. The authors' opinion is that a higher quality of evidence is needed to recommend not to stabilize the syndesmosis and to rely only on DL repair when associated syndesmotic instability is present.

Randomized controlled trials and meta-analysis

Prospective randomized studies comparing outcomes of ankle fractures in patients with and without repair of DL injuries are scarce. A prospective comparative study of 41 patients with Weber type B fractures was conducted by Sun and colleagues.[7] Patients were allocated (not randomized) upon arrival in 3 groups: augmentation of the deep DL with anchors on the talar insertion (16 patients), superficial deltoid repair with anchors on the anterior border of the medial malleolus (12 patients) and a group of patients without repair of the DL (13 patients). At 3 years of follow-up there were no statistical differences between groups in terms of AOFAS scores and MCS results. According to this study, routinely repairing DL injuries in ankle fractures does not affect long-term functional and radiologic outcomes.

Gu and colleagues[34] recently published a prospective randomized controlled study comparing 40 patients enrolled in 2 groups of 20 patients. The control group was treated only with ORIF, whereas the treatment group was treated with ORIF and DL repair. The patients were followed for at least 12 months. At 3 months postoperative, the VAS values were significantly lower in the treatment group. Radiologic results at 12 months of follow-up presented a significant difference in the MCS width between the groups in favor of the treatment group. Patients with DL repair had considerably significantly higher AOFAS scores at the latest follow-up. However, the authors divided the results into 4 categorical groups: excellent (100–90 points), good (75–89 points), fair (50–74 points), and poor (<50 points). Numerical values of the AOFAS were not reported, which makes it difficult to compare the results with other similar studies.

A systematic review comparing ORIF treatment for ankle fractures with versus without DL repair was conducted by Dabash and colleagues.[8] Four studies were eligible with a total of 281 patients; 137 of these patients underwent DL repair and 144 were left unrepaired. The conclusion was that the current evidence does not provide a clear indication for the repair of the DL at the time of ankle fracture fixation. Some advantages regarding maintenance of reduction and stability may be found in adding DL repair on high fibular fractures and in patients requiring syndesmotic fixation.

A meta-analysis by Salameh and colleagues[10] reported the outcome of DL repair in ankle fractures in terms of maintenance of MCS reduction, functional outcomes, and complication rates. Three comparative studies met the inclusion criteria for the meta-analysis with a total of 192 patients, 81 in the DL repair group and 111 in the nonrepair group. The MCS correction was superior in the DL repair group with statistical significance, although maintenance of the MCS correction at the final follow-up was also significantly better in the repair group. Although the VAS score was lower in the repair group at final follow-up, AOFAS scores did not show any difference between the 2 groups, with equal total complication rates. Even though the number of studies included in this study was small, this is the first meta-analysis to pool data from comparative studies regarding the effect of DL repair in ankle fractures with widened MCS.

Described Techniques for Deltoid Ligament Repair

Early techniques popularized before the wave for conservative treatment of DL injuries included direct suture end-to-end repair, posterior tibial tendon weave reconstruction, and allograft augmentation techniques.[1,36] Lack and colleagues[36] described an anatomic reconstruction of both superficial and deep components of the DL using an anchor-to-post reinforcement of the primary ligamentous repair using a tibial screw. Current trends for repairing DL injuries are to use anchors on the tibia or the talus to obtain osseous reattachment of the complex. Multiple anchor insertion points have been described on the medial malleolus anatomy to reproduce both superficial and deep attachments.[6,16] Yu and colleagues[37] describe the use of suture anchors inserted into the anterior margin of the medial malleolus for reattaching the superficial DL components. In cases where a distal deep DL avulsion is found, these authors used 2 anchors inserted into the medial aspect of the talus for reattaching the medial complex. Hsu and colleagues[38] in their series of 14 football players with high-energy rotational ankle fractures, recommend performing arthroscopy for removal of loose bodies, evaluation of osteochondral lesions, syndesmosis, and DL components. After the fibula and syndesmosis reduction and fixation are completed, superficial DL repair was performed by means of inserting 1 or 2 anchors 5 mm proximal to the tip of the medial malleolus directed proximal and away from the ankle joint. No direct repair was performed for the deep layer of the DL. In contrast, Woo and colleagues[9] described a reattachment technique that reconstructs both the superficial and deep portions of the DL. In their study, DL rupture after acute trauma was common in both the superficial and deep ligaments. Using the proximal avulsion of the rupture site as a reference, 1 or 2 suture anchors are placed on the medial malleolus. If both components were avulsed from the medial malleolus, an anterior suture anchor was placed for the superficial DL and a posterior suture anchor was placed for the deep DL.

Arthroscopic and endoscopic techniques for repairing the superficial DL complex have been described in the context of chronic medial insufficiency, but their role in the management of DL injuries in the context of ankle trauma is yet to be determined.[39,40]

Because most of the repair techniques described involve direct suturing or reinsertion with anchors, we can consider that there is a certain agreement that the DL has healing potential. Theoretic benefits of repairing the DL in the acute setting are a contribution to achieving anatomic joint reduction and maintaining ankle stability.[4,15] To our knowledge, the superiority of any surgical technique over another for DL repair has not been studied.

INTRAOPERATIVE EVALUATION

Although the choice to repair or not the DL can be made preoperatively, based on available imaging studies, there are strategies that allow a sequential decision making process to evaluate this determination intraoperatively.

Fluoroscopy

Intraoperative dynamic fluoroscopy is performed after fibular and syndesmotic fixation with the objective of identifying residual medial instability. The external eversion test, consisting of applying a valgus hindfoot force to quantify talar tilt, has been widely used to confirm the need for DL repair.[6] Even though, in practice, DL repair is indicated when a subjective significant opening is found, it has been proposed that a talar tilt of more than 7° is consistent with medial residual instability.[6] A comparison with the uninjured ankle may be useful for ruling out physiologic hyperlaxity. Currently, there are no studies that validate normative data on talar tilt angles, and caution should be paid to the routine use of this parameter.

A fluoroscopic external rotation test has been also described on the mortise view to assess the need for DL repair.[9] An MCS widening of more than 4 mm and 1 mm greater than the superior tibiotalar clear space was considered positive for medial residual instability.

Arthroscopy

Arthroscopic identification of intra-articular ligament injuries in the setting of ankle fractures has been studied widely.[41,42] Syndesmotic and medial injuries have been a matter of debate concerning the absence of objective criteria to determine arthroscopic instability.[43] Moreover, intra-articular tears may be unnoticed during arthroscopy.[44] Hintermann and colleagues[45] described that only 84% of the DL can be seen after ankle fractures and superficial components cannot be visualized at all. However, there is evidence sustaining an intra-articular diagnosis of DL injury in the setting of ankle fractures. Schuberth and collaborators[42] evaluated DL integrity with direct arthroscopic visualization and correlated it with widening of the MCS on standard radiographs. Arthroscopic evaluation of the DL was performed under manual stress before fracture reduction. Four of 13 arthroscopically diagnosed DL ruptures (30%) had an MCS of 4.5 mm or less. They concluded that the integrity of the DL cannot be ruled out in patients with an MCS of between 4 and 6 mm. Motley and colleagues[46] evaluated arthroscopically 19 patients with isolated fibular fractures with an MCS value of more than 4 mm on a gravity stress view. Intraoperative findings included 15 patients with a complete rupture of the DL, 2 patients with partial ruptures, and 2 patients with an intact DL. All patients with complete ruptures had MCS values of greater than 5 mm. The authors suggested conservative treatment of patients with an MCS of less than 5 mm because it could be representative of a partial rupture of the DL.

Schairer and colleagues[47] described the arthroscopic ankle drive-thru sign, consisting of the passing of a 2.9-mm shaver through the medial portal onto the medial gutter.

In the normal setting, the shaver is not able to pass through the medial space. According to the authors, the sign remaining positive after adequate syndesmotic stabilization may be related to residual medial instability.

AUTHORS' RATIONALE AND METHOD OF TREATMENT
Indications for Deltoid Ligament Repair

In accordance with current evidence, we do not perform routine DL reconstruction in all bimalleolar equivalent fractures. Even in cases with a preoperative MCS of greater than 5 mm on stress or weight-bearing radiographs, anatomic fixation of the fibula, in most cases, reduces the medial ankle joint satisfactorily, especially in low-energy injuries (**Fig. 3**). Syndesmotic evaluation by means of an external rotation stress test or the Cotton test is recommended after fixation of the fibula in all of these patients. In cases with positive instability findings, flexible or rigid syndesmotic fixation must be performed and stress maneuvers should be repeated. A persistent widened MCS can be indicative of interposition either of the DL, posterior tibial tendon or loose bodies, and medial exploration is indicated.

Nonetheless, there are some circumstances in which we recommend to proceed with DL repair:

- The authors are cautious when performing fluoroscopic external eversion tests to assess medial instability because we consider it to be unreliable and talar tilt has not been validated as a diagnostic criterion. However, in cases where gross talar

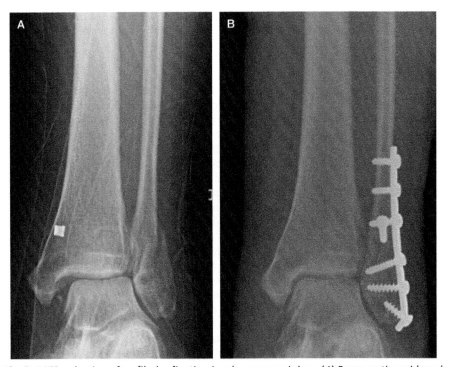

Fig. 3. MCS reduction after fibular fixation in a low energy injury. (*A*) Preoperative widened MCS. (*B*) Postoperative radiograph demonstrating adequate MCS reduction and tibiotalar congruity.

tilting is found in comparison with the uninjured side (a difference of >15°–20°), we proceed with DL repair (**Fig. 4**).

- Bimalleolar equivalent fractures associated with gross syndesmotic instability, both in the coronal and sagittal planes, are candidates for DL repair. Commonly, syndesmosis stability is tested on the coronal plane while instability on the sagittal plane is rarely assessed.[48] New trends in the intraoperative assessment of syndesmosis instability and reduction include the lateral relationship of the tibia and the fibula, which may be more sensitive for detecting sagittal plane syndesmotic instability.[49] Medial instability correction will contribute to reestablishing ankle stability.

- DL injuries can coexist with medial malleolar fractures. This combination has been previously described by Tornetta[50] and Kusnezov and associates,[51] and it can be explained mainly because the medial injury occurs partly through the bone, anteriorly, and continuing through the deep portion of the DL, posteriorly. Because the deep portion of the DL is torn, the fixation of the anterior fragment does not restore medial stability. In our experience, the competence of the DL after medial malleolar fixation can be at high risk, especially in heavier or obese patients. Accordingly, we suggest being aware of potential failures in the form of medial insufficiency after medial malleolar fixation owing to this cause and consider repairing the DL in this group of patients.

- An important component of multiplanar instability is the presence of concomitant lateral ligamentous injuries. Usually, the commonly accepted ring theory establishes that an ankle fracture is unstable if 2 or more parts of the ring are disrupted.[52] Most of the current knowledge supports the fact that, in ankle fractures, lateral stability is regained once fibular fixation is achieved. However, concomitant lateral ligament injuries have been reported to be present as many as 65% of patients with fibular fractures.[53] The exact clinical implications of these injuries are unclear and yet to be determined.[53,54] In high-energy fractures, concomitant soft tissue injuries may explain why certain patients maintain disruption of the ring after fibular fixation and also explain the proximal migration of the fibula in certain patterns

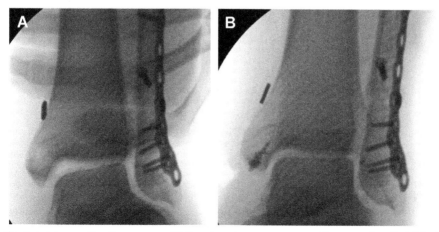

Fig. 4. Intraoperative fluoroscopy. (*A*) Eversion stress maneuver with gross talar tilt (16°) after fibular fixation and syndesmosis repair. (*B*) Eversion stress maneuver after DL repair was performed.

of ankle fractures. We have coined the concept of a lateral equivalent type of injury in cases where fibular fracture and severe lateral ligament rupture coexist (**Fig. 5**). These combined injuries may also benefit from augmented stability given by DL repair (**Fig. 6**).

Authors' Technique for Deltoid Ligament Repair

We perform standard fixation of the fibular fractures using a 3.5-mm lateral or postero-lateral plate with screws through a conventional lateral approach. Even though we do

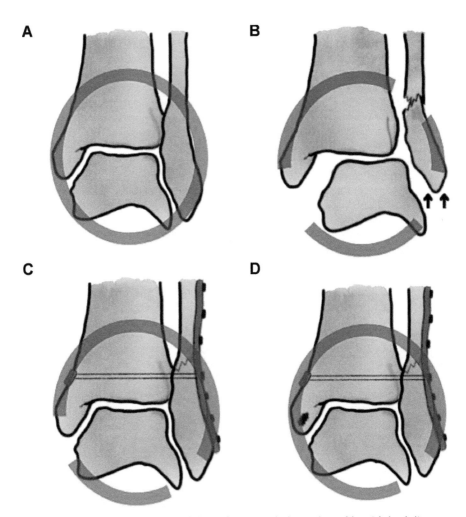

Fig. 5. Lateral equivalent concept. (*A*) On the coronal plane, the ankle with both ligament and bony stabilizers acts as a stable ring. The ring is considered unstable if it has more than 2 points of failure. (*B*) A lateral malleolar fracture with both severe deltoid and lateral complex injuries "breaks" the ring in 3 parts with subsequent instability. (*C*) Fibular and syndesmotic fixation changes the injury into a 2-part lesion of the ring but still unstable. (*D*) After the repair of the DL the stability of the ring is reestablished. (*Courtesy of* J. Jofre, MD, Santiago, Chile.)

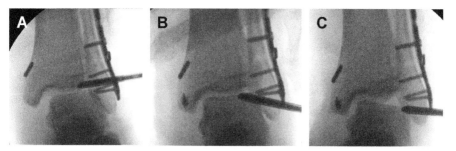

Fig. 6. Intraoperative fluoroscopy. Patient with high energy AO/OTA type C fibular fracture with multiligamentous instability. (*A*) Eversion stress maneuver after syndesmosis fixation showing persistent MCS widening. (*B*) Eversion stress maneuver after DL repair with normalization of the MCS. (*C*) Inversion stress maneuver compatible with persistent lateral equivalent instability.

not perform routine preoperative MRI or intraoperative arthroscopy, syndesmotic and medial instability can be suspected preoperatively based on radiographs and computed tomography scan findings.

Once the fracture is fixed, we proceed to assess MCS normalization and perform a syndesmotic stress test. If necessary, the syndesmosis is stabilized, and then if there are any of the previously aforementioned indications, we proceed with the DL repair. There is debate about whether to fixate the syndesmosis before fixing the deltoid or vice versa. In our opinion, there is no high-quality evidence that an unstable syndesmosis should be left unrepaired relying only on DL fixation. Considering that flexible fixation has been related to improved syndesmosis reduction we prefer to go first with syndesmotic fixation and then proceed to DL repair. Caution must be taken during syndesmosis reduction not to forcefully reduce the MCS at expense of overcompressing the mortise, resulting in sagittal malreduction. In this context, an initial medial exploration may be indicated to allow an effortless mortise reduction.

An arciform approach 5 mm distal to the tip of the medial malleolus is used (**Fig. 7**A) and proceeding with blunt dissection until the identification of the more anterior

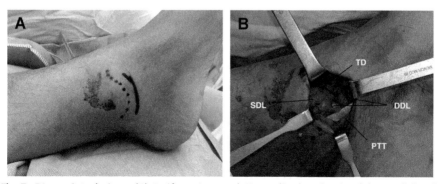

Fig. 7. DL repair technique. (*A*) Arciform Approach 5 mm distal to the tip of the medial malleolus. (*B*) Identification of the superficial DL (SDL), deep DL (DDL), Talus dome (TD), and the posterior tibial tendon (PTT).

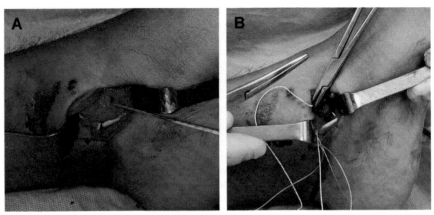

Fig. 8. DL repair technique. (*A*) Insertion of a 5.0-mm anchor in the most posterior part of the anterior colliculus following the midline of the medial malleolus and avoiding the sulcus. (*B*) Repair of the deep DL with a full-thickness, horizontal mattress suture pattern using 2 strands.

superficial component and the posterior deep portion are identified. This approach has proven useful for allowing wide visualization and permitting identification of both fascicles of the DL as well as the complete visualization of the posterior tibial tendon, which is retracted posteroinferiorly throughout the procedure (**Fig. 7**B). A rongeur is used to create bleeding on the cancellous aspect of the medial malleolus allowing soft tissue healing. One 5.0-mm or two 3.5-mm anchors with 4 high-resistance suture strands are inserted in the most posterior part of the anterior colliculus following the midline of the medial malleolus and avoiding the sulcus (**Fig. 8**A). Before knotting, a varus and inversion maneuver should be performed. Two of the strands are used to repair and advance the deep DL creating a full-thickness, horizontal mattress suture pattern (**Fig. 8**B). The remaining strands are left for similarly repairing the superficial portion forming a double row configuration (**Fig. 9**). This type of repair can be considered anatomic for the superficial DL and nonanatomic for the deep DL. In cases where there is evidence that the deep DL has been avulsed from its insertion on the talus, we use a longitudinal medial approach to allow placement of 1 or 2 anchors on the medial aspect of the talus.

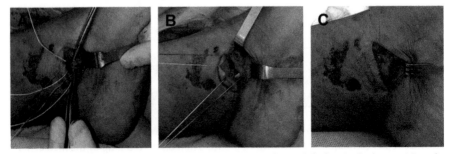

Fig. 9. DL repair technique. (*A*) The 2 remaining strands are left for similarly repairing the superficial portion. (*B*) A double row configuration. (*C*) Final appearance after repair.

SUMMARY

The long-term clinical benefits of repairing the DL have yet to be proven and further high-quality randomized controlled studies are necessary considering the characteristics of the current body of evidence. Patients with extensive capsuloligamentous damage and multidirectional instability may benefit from DL repair to improve MCS reduction quality, avoid loss of reduction, and regain medial and syndesmotic stability. Most DL repair techniques involve direct repair or reattachment using suture anchors for augmentation, but there is no evidence of the superiority of any technique in the literature. The authors recommend repairing the DL complex in the setting of bimalleolar equivalent fractures associated with syndesmotic or multiligamentous instability as well as in heavier patients with greater mechanical requirements.

CLINICS CARE POINTS

- There is no consensus on whether the DL must be repaired in bimalleolar equivalent ankle fractures. The long-term clinical benefits have yet to be proven considering the current body of evidence.
- DL repair can improve MCS reduction quality, avoid loss of reduction, and regain medial and syndesmotic stability, especially in patients with extensive capsuloligamentous damage and multidirectional instability.
- DL repair is recommended in the setting of bimalleolar equivalent fractures associated with syndesmotic or multiligamentous instability as well as in heavier patients with greater mechanical requirements.

ACKNOWLEDGMENTS

The authors acknowledge Javiera Jofre and Isabel Guerrero for their help on the preparation of the illustrations appearing in this publication.

DISCLOSURE

The authors have no disclosures.

REFERENCES

1. Bluman EM. Deltoid ligament injuries in ankle fractures: should I leave it or fix it? Foot Ankle Int 2012;33(3):236–8.
2. Harper MC. The deltoid ligament. An evaluation of need for surgical repair. Clin Orthop Relat Res 1988;226:156–68.
3. Hintermann B, Knupp M, Pagenstert GI. Deltoid ligament injuries: diagnosis and management. Foot Ankle Clin 2006;11(3):625–37.
4. Jones CR, Nunley JA 2nd. Deltoid ligament repair versus syndesmotic fixation in bimalleolar equivalent ankle fractures. J Orthop Trauma 2015;29(5):245–9.
5. Strömsöe K, Höqevold HE, Skjeldal S, et al. The repair of a ruptured deltoid ligament is not necessary in ankle fractures. J Bone Joint Surg Br 1995;77(6):920–1.
6. Lee S, Lin J, Hamid KS, et al. Deltoid ligament rupture in ankle fracture: diagnosis and management. J Am Acad Orthop Surg 2019;27(14):e648–58.
7. Sun X, Li T, Sun Z, et al. Does routinely repairing deltoid ligament injuries in type B ankle joint fractures influence long term outcomes? Injury 2018;49(12):2312–7.
8. Dabash S, Elabd A, Potter E, et al. Adding deltoid ligament repair in ankle fracture treatment: is it necessary? A systematic review. Foot Ankle Surg 2019;25(6):714–20.

9. Woo SH, Bae S-Y, Chung H-J. Short-term results of a ruptured deltoid ligament repair during an acute ankle fracture fixation. Foot Ankle Int 2018;39(1):35–45.

10. Salameh M, Alhammoud A, Alkhatib N, et al. Outcome of primary deltoid ligament repair in acute ankle fractures: a meta-analysis of comparative studies. Int Orthop 2019. https://doi.org/10.1007/s00264-019-04416-9.

11. Lindsjö U. Operative treatment of ankle fractures. Acta Orthop Scand Suppl 1981;189:1–131.

12. Hughes J. The medial malleolus in ankle fractures. Orthop Clin North Am 1980; 11(3):649–60.

13. de Souza LJ, Gustilo RB, Meyer TJ. Results of operative treatment of displaced external rotation-abduction fractures of the ankle. J Bone Joint Surg Am 1985; 67(7):1066–74.

14. Zeegers AV, van der Werken C. Rupture of the deltoid ligament in ankle fractures: should it be repaired? Injury 1989;20(1):39–41.

15. Butler BA, Hempen EC, Barbosa M, et al. Deltoid ligament repair reduces and stabilizes the talus in unstable ankle fractures. J Orthop 2020;17:87–90.

16. Rigby RB, Scott RT. Role for Primary Repair of Deltoid Ligament Complex in Ankle Fractures. Clin Podiatr Med Surg 2018;35(2):183–97.

17. Milner CE, Soames RW. Anatomy of the collateral ligaments of the human ankle joint. Foot Ankle Int 1998;19(11):757–60.

18. Pankovich AM, Shivaram MS. Anatomical basis of variability in injuries of the medial malleolus and the deltoid ligament. I. Anatomical studies. Acta Orthop Scand 1979;50(2):217–23.

19. Kelikian AS, Sarrafian SK. Sarrafian's anatomy of the foot and ankle: descriptive, topographic, functional. Lippincott Williams & Wilkins; 2011.

20. Siegler S, Block J, Schneck CD. The mechanical characteristics of the collateral ligaments of the human ankle joint. Foot Ankle 1988;8(5):234–42.

21. Savage-Elliott I, Murawski CD, Smyth NA, et al. The deltoid ligament: an in-depth review of anatomy, function, and treatment strategies. Knee Surg Sports Traumatol Arthrosc 2013;21(6):1316–27.

22. Jeong MS, Choi YS, Kim YJ, et al. Deltoid ligament in acute ankle injury: MR imaging analysis. Skeletal Radiol 2014;43(5):655–63.

23. Hintermann B, Golanó P. The Anatomy and Function of the Deltoid Ligament. Tech Foot Ankle Surg 2014;13(2):67–72.

24. Campbell KJ, Michalski MP, Wilson KJ, et al. The ligament anatomy of the deltoid complex of the ankle: a qualitative and quantitative anatomical study. J Bone Joint Surg Am 2014;96(8):e62.

25. Panchani PN, Chappell TM, Moore GD, et al. Anatomic study of the deltoid ligament of the ankle. Foot Ankle Int 2014;35(9):916–21.

26. Won H-J, Koh IJ, Won H-S. Morphological variations of the deltoid ligament of the medial ankle. Clin Anat 2016;29(8):1059–65.

27. Yammine K. The Morphology and Prevalence of the Deltoid Complex Ligament of the Ankle. Foot Ankle Spec 2017;10(1):55–62.

28. Cromeens BP, Kirchhoff CA, Patterson RM, et al. An attachment-based description of the medial collateral and spring ligament complexes. Foot Ankle Int 2015; 36(6):710–21.

29. Bastias GF, Dalmau-Pastor M, Astudillo C, et al. Spring Ligament Instability. Foot Ankle Clin 2018;23(4):659–78.

30. Earll M, Wayne J, Brodrick C, et al. Contribution of the deltoid ligament to ankle joint contact characteristics: a cadaver study. Foot Ankle Int 1996;17(6):317–24.

31. Michelsen JD, Ahn UM, Helgemo SL. Motion of the ankle in a simulated supination-external rotation fracture model. J Bone Joint Surg Am 1996;78(7): 1024–31.

32. Chen X-Z, Chen Y, Liu C-G, et al. Arthroscopy-assisted surgery for acute ankle fractures: a systematic review. Arthroscopy 2015;31(11):2224–31.

33. Zhao H-M, Lu J, Zhang F, et al. Surgical treatment of ankle fracture with or without deltoid ligament repair: a comparative study. BMC Musculoskelet Disord 2017; 18(1):543.

34. Gu G, Yu J, Huo Y, et al. Efficacy of deltoid ligament reconstruction on the curative effect, complication and long-term prognosis in ankle fracture-dislocation with deltoid ligament injury. Int J Clin Exp Med 2017;10(9):13778–83.

35. Little MMT, Berkes MB, Schottel PC, et al. Anatomic fixation of supination external rotation type IV equivalent ankle fractures. J Orthop Trauma 2015;29(5):250–5.

36. Lack W, Phisitkul P, Femino JE. Anatomic deltoid ligament repair with anchor-to-post suture reinforcement: technique tip. Iowa Orthop J 2012;32:227–30.

37. Yu G-R, Zhang M-Z, Aiyer A, et al. Repair of the acute deltoid ligament complex rupture associated with ankle fractures: a multicenter clinical study. J Foot Ankle Surg 2015;54(2):198–202.

38. Hsu AR, Lareau CR, Anderson RB. Repair of acute superficial deltoid complex avulsion during ankle fracture fixation in National Football League players. Foot Ankle Int 2015;36(11):1272–8.

39. Lui TH. Endoscopic repair of the superficial deltoid ligament and spring ligament. Arthrosc Tech 2016;5(3):e621–5.

40. Acevedo JI, Kreulen C, Cedeno AA, et al. Technique for arthroscopic deltoid ligament repair with description of safe zones. Foot Ankle Int 2020;41(5):605–11.

41. Chiang C-C, Tzeng Y-H, Jeff Lin C-F, et al. Arthroscopic reduction and minimally invasive surgery in supination-external rotation ankle fractures: a comparative study with open reduction. Arthroscopy 2019;35(9):2671–83.

42. Schuberth JM, Collman DR, Rush SM, et al. Deltoid ligament integrity in lateral malleolar fractures: a comparative analysis of arthroscopic and radiographic assessments. J Foot Ankle Surg 2004;43(1):20–9.

43. Guyton GP, DeFontes K 3rd, Barr CR, et al. Arthroscopic Correlates of Subtle Syndesmotic Injury. Foot Ankle Int 2017;38(5):502–6.

44. Stufkens SAS, van den Bekerom MPJ, Knupp M, et al. The diagnosis and treatment of deltoid ligament lesions in supination-external rotation ankle fractures: a review. Strategies Trauma Limb Reconstr 2012;7(2):73–85.

45. Hintermann B, Regazzoni P, Lampert C, et al. Arthroscopic findings in acute fractures of the ankle. J Bone Joint Surg Br 2000;82(3):345–51.

46. Motley T, Carpenter B, Clements JR, et al. Evaluation of the Deltoid Complex in Supination External Rotation Ankle Fractures. Foot Ankle Online J 2010;3(4). https://doi.org/10.3827/faoj.2010.0304.0001.

47. Schairer WW, Nwachukwu BU, Dare DM, et al. Arthroscopically assisted open reduction-internal fixation of ankle fractures: significance of the arthroscopic ankle drive-through sign. Arthrosc Tech 2016;5(2):e407–12.

48. Candal-Couto JJ, Burrow D, Bromage S, et al. Instability of the tibio-fibular syndesmosis: have we been pulling in the wrong direction? Injury 2004;35(8):814–8.

49. Abarca M, Besa P, Palma J, et al. A new intraoperative measurement that predicts ankle syndesmotic joint malreduction. Foot Ankle Orthop 2019;4(4). 2473011419S00079.

50. Tornetta P 3rd. Competence of the deltoid ligament in bimalleolar ankle fractures after medial malleolar fixation. J Bone Joint Surg Am 2000;82(6):843–8.

51. Kusnezov NA, Eisenstein ED, Diab N, et al. Medial malleolar fractures and associated deltoid ligament disruptions: current management controversies. Orthopedics 2017;40(2):e216–22.
52. Wailing A, Sanders RW, Behboudi A, et al. Chapter 37: ankle fractures. In: Coughlin MJ, Saltzman CL, editors. Mann's surgery of the foot and ankle. Elsevier; 2014. p. 2003–40.
53. Gardner MJ, Demetrakopoulos D, Briggs SM, et al. The ability of the Lauge-Hansen classification to predict ligament injury and mechanism in ankle fractures: an MRI study. J Orthop Trauma 2006;20(4):267–72.
54. Faqi MK, AlJawder A, Alkhalifa F, et al. Weber B fracture of the lateral malleolus with concomitant anterior talofibular ligament injury following an ankle supination injury. Case Rep Orthop 2016;2016:8035029.

Strategies to Avoid Syndesmosis Malreduction in Ankle Fractures

Derek S. Stenquist, MD[a],*, John Y. Kwon, MD[b]

KEYWORDS

- Syndesmosis • Ankle fracture • Instability • Malreduction

KEY POINTS

- Up to 45% of surgically treated ankle fractures have associated syndesmotic disruption. Quality of syndesmotic reduction appears to affect functional outcomes.
- Syndesmotic malreduction ranges from 15% to 50% in the literature, and achieving anatomic reduction remains a significant challenge.
- Certain ankle fractures are more prone to malreduction: pronation injuries, fracture-dislocations, comminuted fibula fractures, and trimalleolar ankle fractures.
- Preoperative computed tomography scan can identify a posterior malleolus fracture or syndesmotic anatomy that may predispose to malreduction.
- It is essential to have a stepwise plan and an understanding of reliable fluoroscopic parameters for evaluating the reduction in both coronal and sagittal planes intraoperatively.

INTRODUCTION

Ankle fractures are among the most common injuries treated by orthopedic surgeons,[1] and achieving anatomic reduction of the syndesmosis remains a significant challenge. Ankle fractures account for more than 50% of lower extremity fractures and 14% of fracture-related hospital admissions,[1,2] and a significant number have concomitant syndesmotic disruption.[3,4] Syndesmotic malreduction has been associated with poor functional outcomes[5–11] and the development of osteoarthritis.[12] Although achieving accurate reduction is recognized as a critical component of treating ankle fractures with syndesmotic instability,[11] the most reliable method for doing so continues to be debated.[13] This article focuses on strategies to avoid malreduction of the syndesmosis during surgical fixation of ankle fractures.

[a] Harvard Combined Orthopaedic Residency Program, Massachusetts General Hospital, 55 Fruit Street, Boston, MA 02114, USA; [b] Orthopaedic Foot & Ankle Service, 330 Brookline Avenue, Boston, MA 02215, USA
* Corresponding author.
E-mail address: derek.s.stenquist@gmail.com

Foot Ankle Clin N Am 25 (2020) 613–630
https://doi.org/10.1016/j.fcl.2020.08.001
1083-7515/20/© 2020 Elsevier Inc. All rights reserved.

MECHANISM AND BIOMECHANICS OF SYNDESMOTIC INJURY

Lauge-Hansen's mechanistic theory of supination-external rotation (SER) ankle fractures states that as an external rotation (ER) force is applied to a supinated foot, the fibula externally rotates and first disrupts the anterior inferior tibiofibular ligament (AITFL) and/or creates an avulsion fragment. As rotation continues, an oblique fibula fracture occurs followed by injury to the posterior malleolus or posterior syndesmotic ligaments. In addition, the deforming force results in a medial osseoligamentous injury.[3,14] Although syndesmotic injury occurs in approximately 20% of SER injuries, there is an even higher incidence with pronation-type injuries.[15]

Syndesmotic injuries produce instability, which alters ankle kinematics and may lead to altered contact areas and abnormal contact pressures.[16–21] These alterations in joint loading have been posited to cause long-term loss of function and the development of arthritis.[7,11,12] Based on the classic experiments of Ramsey and Hamilton,[18] which were corroborated by subsequent investigations, 1 to 2 mm of loss of mortise congruency constitutes an indication for surgical fixation to prevent abnormal ankle kinematics and poor outcomes.[17,18,22–24] Biomechanical studies indicate that fibular rotation as well as sagittal reduction influences ankle kinematics.[17,21]

OUTCOMES AFTER SYNDESMOTIC INJURY AND FIXATION

Ankle fractures with syndesmotic injury seem to be associated with worse functional outcomes than those without,[25] although evidence is limited to retrospective and observational studies. Weening and Bhandari[5] found that syndesmotic malreduction was the only significant predictor of functional outcomes in a retrospective cohort of 51 patients. Sagi and colleagues[7] documented significantly worse outcomes with minimum 2-year follow-up in patients with syndesmotic malreduction, independent of injury severity.[26] In a retrospective series of 120 patients, Ray and colleagues[12] found that malreduction was an independent predictor for the development of arthrosis.

Other investigators have refuted the association between syndesmotic malreduction and poor outcomes.[27,28] Cherney and colleagues[27] found no difference in functional outcomes using thresholds of 3 mm and 10° to 15° of malreduction at 1 year. However, a recent study by Andersen and colleagues[11] of 87 patients with minimum 2-year clinical follow-up found that a threshold of 2 mm for malreduction was a predictor of poor outcomes. Given the biomechanical evidence for altered tibiotalar joint mechanics and the clinical association between functional outcome and quality of reduction, it is essential to strive for anatomic reduction during surgical treatment.[29]

PREVALENCE OF AND RISK FACTORS FOR MALREDUCTION

Achieving anatomic syndesmotic reduction remains a significant technical challenge because reported rates of malreduction after surgery range from 16% to 52%.[11,30–32] Reduction technique, parameters used for intraoperative evaluation of reduction, and choice of implants are variable and may influence the quality of reduction.[29,32] Although many studies have failed to find definitive predictors of malreduction,[33] an understanding of pitfalls and predisposing factors can help surgeons optimize outcomes.

Rates of syndesmotic malreduction have been shown to be higher in Weber C ankle fractures compared with Weber B patterns (**Fig. 1**).[28,34] Schottel and colleagues[35] found twice the rate of malreduction when comparing a cohort of pronation-ER (PER) injuries with SER injuries. They suggested heightened scrutiny of the reduction

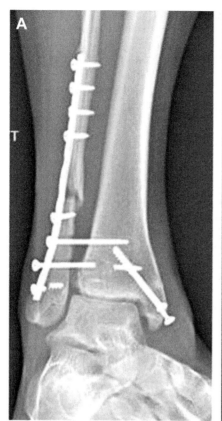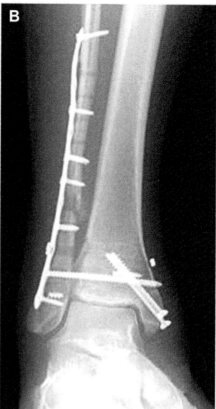

Fig. 1. A 30-year-old woman presented with fibular nonunion and syndesmotic diastasis after open reduction with internal fixation of a Weber C ankle fracture (A). This fracture was revised with fibular bone grafting and revision plating, arthroscopic ankle debridement, syndesmotic reduction and revision fixation, deltoid ligament repair, and suture-tape augmentation of the anterior syndesmotic ligaments (B).

when treating fractures with pronation injuries. In their comparative cohort study of PER fractures, Warner and colleagues[36] found similarly high rates of syndesmotic malreduction regardless of dislocation status, but fracture-dislocation was associated with worse functional outcomes postoperatively.

The osseous morphology of the incisura varies between individuals and certain shapes are predisposed to specific patterns of malreduction.[37] Using axial computed tomography (CT) scan with the uninjured extremity as a control, Cherney and colleagues[38] showed that shallow incisura correlated with anterior fibular malreduction but were less likely to have rotational malreduction, whereas patients with a deep concave incisura were more likely to be posteriorly and rotationally malreduced. Boszczyk and colleagues[39] found that incisural anteversion or retroversion predisposed to anterior and posterior fibular translation respectively, and patients with deep incisura were at higher risk for overcompression

The posterior malleolus and the posterior inferior tibiofibular ligament (PITFL) play an important role in stability[40,41] and syndesmotic reduction,[42] and may influence functional outcomes after rotational ankle fractures.[43] In a small series, Cherney and colleagues[34] found that the absence of a posterior malleolar injury was protective against rotational malreduction but not overcompression. A recent cadaver study by Fitzpatrick and colleagues[42] evaluated the impact of a malreduced posterior malleolus fragment on the quality of syndesmotic reduction and found that malreduction of a large posterior malleolus fracture involving the incisura can affect syndesmotic reduction in both sagittal and coronal planes. When a posterior malleolus fracture is appreciated on plain films, a preoperative CT scan may be useful given the potential impact of both syndesmotic anatomy and posterior malleolus fragment morphology on quality of syndesmotic reduction.[44]

ACHIEVING SYNDESMOTIC REDUCTION
Intraoperative Radiographic Stress Testing

Intraoperative stress testing after fibular fixation should always be performed to assess syndesmotic integrity.[45,46] In cases of significant disruption, instability is occasionally detected on preoperative stress radiography, especially in the setting of a Maisonneuve or ligamentous-equivalent injury (**Fig. 2**). Intraoperative assessment is most commonly performed using a lateral fibular stress test (Cotton test) or the ER stress test,[47] although biomechanical studies suggest the ER stress test may overestimate syndesmotic instability because it can result in an abnormal medial clear space (MCS) with isolated deltoid ligament disruption.[48] The Cotton test is performed by applying a lateral distraction force using a surgical clamp applied to the distal fibula approximately 1 to 2 cm proximal to the plafond (**Fig. 3**). Radiographs are then evaluated using previously defined parameters for normal alignment on anteroposterior (AP) radiographs, including tibiofibular clear space (TFCS), tibiofibular overlap (TFO), and MCS.[8,49–52] However, asymptomatic patients may meet traditional thresholds for syndesmotic injury (**Fig. 4**), so contralateral radiographs should be obtained before prepping and draping to allow for intraoperative comparison.[53,54] Many factors influence the accuracy of stress radiography, including ankle position and force

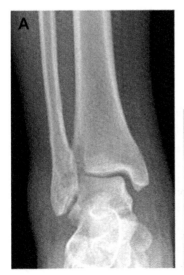
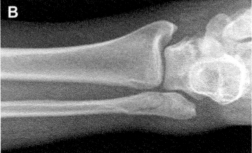

Fig. 2. A 39-year-old woman with a bimalleolar-equivalent ankle fracture (A). Gravity stress view shows not only mortise instability but also syndesmotic ligament disruption (B).

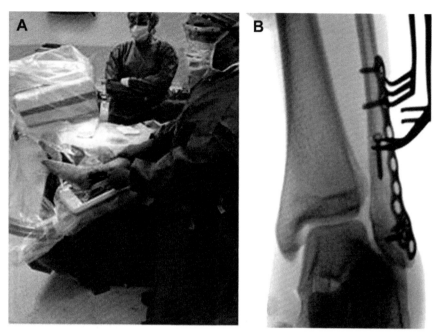

Fig. 3. The Cotton test. A point-to-point reduction clamp is placed on or around the fibula. A mortise view is obtained. It is our preference to use live fluoroscopy when applying a posterolateral distraction force. Counter pressure is applied proximally (as opposed to on the foot) to prevent a false-negative test (*A*). The mortise view is scrutinized for any pathologic changes to the tibiofibular overlap, clear space, and/or medial clear space (*B*).

applied.[55,56] Once syndesmotic instability is confirmed by intraoperative Cotton test, reduction and fixation are performed.

Patient Positioning

Several investigators have suggested the potential for foot position at the time of fixation to influence syndesmotic reduction.[57,58] In a cadaver study, Boszczyk and

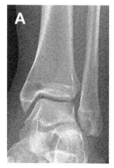
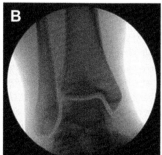
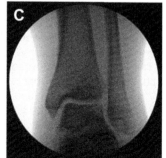

Fig. 4. A 47-year-old woman who sustained a twisting injury to the ankle with anterolateral pain. Lack of tibiofibular overlap on mortise radiograph was suspicious for syndesmotic injury (*A*). Fluoroscopy confirmed normal anatomic variation with similar appearance to the uninjured contralateral ankle (*B, C*).

colleagues[58] confirmed their clinical suspicion that supporting the foot beneath the heel during syndesmotic reduction could predispose to anterior fibular subluxation. Plantarflexion during syndesmotic fixation has long been thought to predispose to overcompression because of the narrower posterior aspect of the talus.[59] However, multiple studies have failed to show any effect of ankle position during fixation on maximal dorsiflexion.[60,61] To our knowledge, no study has investigated the relative risk of malreduction depending on supine versus prone positioning, but most techniques for achieving and evaluating syndesmotic reduction have been described for use in the supine position.

Screw Trajectory

The AO (Arbeitsgemeinschaft für Osteosynthesefragen) Foundation has traditionally recommended that screws be placed parallel and 2 cm proximal to the plafond and inserted obliquely posterior to anterior at an angle of approximately 30°.[62] However, studies have increasingly shown that individual anatomic variation makes finding the ideal screw trajectory challenging.[39,63] In addition, intraoperative perception of trajectory is influenced by the position of the ankle at the time of screw insertion. For example, the ankle will already be internally rotated approximately 15° if the screw is being inserted under fluoroscopic guidance on a mortise view.

Mendelsohn and colleagues[64] reported that the distal tibiofibular axis is $32° \pm 6°$ externally rotated from the transepicondylar femoral axis. Putnam and colleagues[65] correlated CT to radiograph and found the trans-syndesmotic angle (TSA) was aimed 21.5° anterior to the plane of a lateral radiograph. In a CT study of 200 normal ankles, Kennedy and colleagues[66] calculated that the optimal force vector for anatomic reduction passed through the fibula within 2.5 mm of the lateral cortical apex and the anterior half of the medial malleolus in 100% of the ankles studied. They suggested that, with a start point on the lateral cortical ridge of the fibula, the anterior half of the medial malleolus can be used as a reliable target.

Regarding screw position relative to the plafond, screws are traditionally placed parallel to avoid theoretic iatrogenic lengthening or shortening of the fibula.[66] Several investigators have found no difference in clinical or radiological outcomes between trans-syndesmotic and suprasyndesmotic screw placement.[67–70] At present, it seems that acceptable outcomes can be achieved by placing syndesmotic fixation between 2 and 5 cm proximal to the plafond.

Indirect Reduction

Various methods of indirect reduction have been described. Clamp reduction before implant placement is a well-described technique,[34,71] although some investigators argue that this may predispose to malreduction.[57] In a cadaver study, Miller and colleagues[72] showed that clamp angles of 0°, 15°, and 30° from the posterolateral corner of the fibula resulted in predictable patterns of syndesmotic malreduction on CT scan[71] and concluded that accurate reduction cannot be reliably achieved with a clamp alone.[72] Cosgrove and colleagues[71] determined that placement of the medial tine in the anterior third of the tibia on a lateral radiograph was associated with the lowest risk of malreduction. They concluded that sagittal plane reduction is highly sensitive to clamp obliquity, and off-axis clamping is likely a major culprit in iatrogenic malreduction.[71]

Putnam and colleagues[65] attempted to define the optimal position of a clamp along the TSA to facilitate anatomic reduction using CT scans of 45 normal patients. They determined that the average TSA was 21.5° anterior to a lateral view of the ankle. Using three-dimensional reconstructions, they then simulated clamp placement in the optimal average trajectory. With the lateral tine assumed to be placed on the fibular ridge, the optimal medial tine placement was approximately 23% of the distance from the anterior to the posterior tibial cortex on a simulated lateral radiograph view.[65] In a cadaver study, Cosgrove and colleagues[63] used specimen-specific CT scans to plan clamp placement. Although they were able to accurately achieve clamp placement along the TSA using CT planning, clamp use increased the risk of malreduction and overcompression compared with manual digital reduction under direct visualization.[63] In addition, Hoshino and colleagues[73] noted a specific pattern of malreduction resulting in anterior subluxation of the talus. They reported on 3 patients with anterior translation and ER of the fibula causing talar subluxation after screw fixation and hypothesized that the malreduction resulted from posterior placement of the fibular clamp tine.[73] These studies show the pitfalls of indirect reduction with a clamp, including malreduction rates up to 50% and the potential for overcompression.[31]

Direct Open Reduction

Methods of direct open reduction involve direct palpation or visualization of the fibula within the incisura to confirm reduction. Described techniques have focused on palpation or visualization of the anterior syndesmosis. Although a direct approach to the fibula can be used, access is facilitated by slightly curving the distal incision anteriorly. In a cadaver study, LaMothe and colleagues[74] compared tibial plafond contact area, contact force, and peak contact pressure after 3 different reduction techniques: indirect clamp and screw reduction, indirect reduction using a suture button (SB) implant, and thumb reduction (manual palpation) followed by screw placement. None of the reduction techniques restored ankle loading mechanics to the intact state, but thumb reduction performed significantly better than the 2 indirect reduction techniques.[74] Miller and colleagues[30] compared the quality of reduction on CT for a large cohort treated with open reduction under direct visualization compared with 25 historical controls treated with indirect fluoroscopic reduction. They found a 50% malreduction rate in the indirect group compared with 16% in the direct visualization group.[30]

Open reduction under direct visualization has traditionally been performed by attempting to center the fibula within the tibial incisura, judging the articulation at the anterior aspect of the tibiofibular joint, approximately at the level of the ankle joint.[30] Pang and colleagues[75] recently found no difference between direct visualization and blind palpation of the reduction at this location in a cadaver study. In another cadaver study, Tornetta and colleagues[76] suggested that the anterior articular surface visualized through a separate incision may be a more accurate visual reference than the incisura for direct open reduction. Reb and colleagues[77] attempted to establish the tibiofibular line as a method to objectively judge the quality of direct open syndesmotic reduction. However, intraobserver and interobserver reliability were poor for this technique, showing the continued subjective nature of judging reduction despite direct visualization and palpation. Although overall conclusions are limited by the variation in methods between these studies, direct open reduction does seem to result in lower rates of malreduction compared with indirect reduction.[30,63]

Overcompression

Another potential mode of malreduction involves overmedialization of the fibula within the incisura. Clamp reduction has been associated with overcompression in several studies.[4,34] In their series of 27 patients treated with clamp reduction, Cherney and colleagues[34] found a 44% rate of overcompression, defined as 1 mm of overmedialization of the fibula on CT compared with the contralateral normal ankle.

A cadaveric study of SB fixation showed that this device commonly causes over-compression, defined as lower syndesmotic volume on CT compared with the intact state.[78] However, according to another cadaver study by Morellato and colleagues,[79] adequate SB tension resulting in overcompression was required in order to maintain reduction and reapproximate the degree of physiologic motion at the distal tibiofibular joint. They showed excessive motion on stress CT when the SB was not adequately tensioned.[79]

Severe overcompression has been documented to cause anteromedial or inferior talar subluxation requiring revision.[59,60,80,81] The syndesmosis is known to widen slightly over time regardless of whether the syndesmotic hardware is intact, broken, or removed,[82] but the clinical significance of overcompression continues to be debated. Although severe overcompression causing talar subluxation is to be avoided, the optimal degree of initial compression and subsequent widening to restore physiologic motion remains unknown because studies correlating compression with functional outcomes are lacking.[82,83]

EVALUATING THE REDUCTION: INTRAOPERATIVE IMAGING

Imaging parameters used for intraoperative evaluation of reduction may influence the quality of reduction, and many fluoroscopic techniques to assess reduction have been described. Surgeons should assess the position of the fibula within the incisura as well as fibular rotation and length. There is no agreement on the optimal parameters or threshold measurements, but it is suggested that they should equal or at least approach values for the same parameters for the contralateral uninjured side.[84]

Fluoroscopy

The utility of traditional parameters has been investigated both for detecting syndesmotic injury[85] and for evaluating reduction intraoperatively.[86,87] Marmor and colleagues[87] showed the limitations of plain radiographs for detecting malreduction after fixation in a cadaver model. When assessing various degrees of intentional malalignment, they showed that up to 30° of ER malreduction can go undetected when using TFCS and TFO.[87] Fig. 5 provides a clinical example of these limitations. Chang and colleagues[88] suggested 2 new parameters for judging fibular rotation on AP radiograph based on the contour of the distal fibula and the appearance of the lateral malleolar fossa. Futamura found high sensitivity and specificity of 3 indices for detecting malreduction, including TFCS, anterior tibiofibular interval, and fibular rotation compared with contralateral AP radiographs. They did not describe parameters for assessing sagittal plane reduction.[89]

Several techniques for assessing sagittal plane reduction on fluoroscopy have been described.[90–92] Loizou and colleagues[91] showed excellent agreement using the anterior fibular line ratio and posterior fibular line distance to assess sagittal reduction according to the relationship of the posterior fibular cortex to the posterior tibial articular margin on lateral views. Similarly, Grenier and colleagues[92] described the anteroposterior tibiofibular ratio, which assesses where the anterior fibular cortex intersects the tibial physeal scar. As discussed previously, Cosgrove and colleagues[71] found a relationship between quality of reduction and location of the medial reduction clamp tine on a lateral radiograph.

Many recent techniques for fluoroscopic evaluation of reduction rely on comparison with contralateral fluoroscopic views obtained at the time of surgery. In a cadaver study, Koenig and colleagues[86] simulated malreduction on lateral ankle radiographs and asked fellowship-trained trauma surgeons to detect varying amounts of malalignment

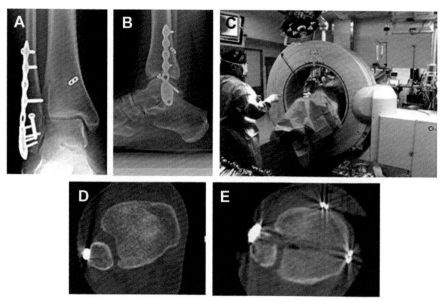

Fig. 5. A 32-year-old woman with continued anterolateral pain approximately 1 year after lateral malleolar and syndesmotic fixation. The suture button was misdirected posteriorly resulting in an externally rotated and posteriorly translated syndesmotic malreduction (*D*). Note how radiographic parameters such as tibiofibular overlap, TFCS, MCS, and sagittal plane tibiofibular alignment appear grossly normal (*A, B*). Use of intraoperative CT allowed confirmation of anatomic syndesmotic alignment during revision surgery (*C, E*).

compared with a normal contralateral radiograph. Anterior translation and greater magnitudes of displacement in general were most easily diagnosed to a threshold of 2.5 mm. All reviewers had the most difficulty detecting 2.5 mm of posterior displacement. Surgeons who routinely used comparison views of the contralateral lateral radiograph in clinical practice were more accurate.[86] Summers and colleagues[93] described a technique for obtaining accurate syndesmotic reduction by comparison with mortise and lateral fluoroscopic views of the uninjured ankle. They obtained provisional fixation and then used intraoperative CT to confirm reduction. CT changed their reduction in only 1 out of 18 patients, indicating their technique may obviate the need for intraoperative CT.[93] Baek and colleagues[94] found that measurement of TFCS and TFO can fail to detect sagittal malreduction diagnosed on CT, indicating the importance of scrutinizing intraoperative lateral radiograph views (**Fig. 6**).

Computed Tomography

CT is more sensitive than plain radiography for detecting malalignment.[53,95–97] Multiple investigators have described means of measuring syndesmotic alignment using CT,[95,96,98–101] and the contralateral normal ankle seems to be the best control for assessing reduction. Investigations to determine the most accurate, reliable, and practical CT parameters are ongoing.[102,103] Some centers have advocated the use of intraoperative CT to minimize malreduction, but this resource is not widely available. In a retrospective study of 251 patients, Franke and colleagues[104] found that the use of intraoperative CT altered surgical outcomes in approximately one-third of patients. However, in a smaller study comparing 2 centers using intraoperative fluoroscopy versus CT, Davidovitch and colleagues[105] found no significant difference in malreduction rates. Although the

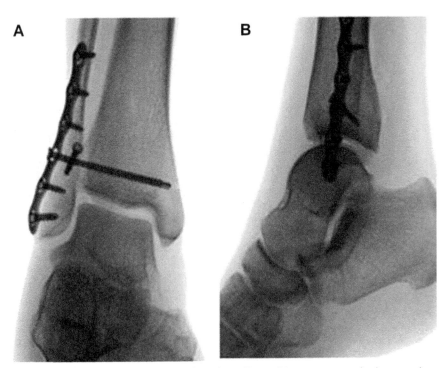

Fig. 6. Syndesmotic malreduction. Although radiographic parameters look normal on mortise radiograph (*A*), lateral view shows anterior subluxation of the talus within the plafond and anterior positioning of the fibula in relation to the tibia, both consistent with syndesmotic malreduction (*B*). The screw was removed and revised to obtain an anatomic reduction.

use of intraoperative three-dimensional CT may decrease malreduction rates, it may not be feasible in settings with limited resources. Furthermore, increased operative times and radiation exposure are of concern. Therefore, it is important to develop reliable and practical methods for reduction under fluoroscopic guidance.

The utility of routine postoperative CT continues to be debated. In a prospective study, Kotwal and colleagues[106] evaluated the utility of a low-dose postoperative CT protocol and found more than 40% of patients were malreduced using a threshold of 2 mm. However, they concluded that there is no role for routine postoperative CT because 84% of malreduced patients who provided functional outcomes had good to excellent results. These conclusions are limited by significant loss to follow-up in the study.[106] Increased availability and use of intraoperative CT may further enhance the ability to assess anatomic reduction or perform revision fixation (**Fig. 5**). Bilateral CT imaging is the modality of choice before revision surgery for suspected syndesmotic malreduction, especially in the setting of metal implants.[29]

CHOICE OF IMPLANT

Syndesmotic screws (SSs) and SB devices are the mainstay for surgical treatment. Systematic reviews have concluded that, in general, the number of screws, screw diameter, and number of cortices engaged have no effect on clinical outcomes and no definitive correlation with loss of syndesmotic reduction.[70,107] Screws may be superior to SBs for certain injury patterns that require enhanced stability, especially in the setting of axially unstable fractures.[108,109] If axial length is not restored by internal fixation, SB devices may be inadequate to prevent fibular shortening resulting in talar tilt and lateral talar displacement.[110] Screws have also been shown to have better torsional resistance to sagittal fibular translation.[108,109] Disadvantages of screws include higher rates of reoperation and implant breakage,[111,112] although some new implants, such as the R3lease screw (Paragon 28, Englewood, CO), are designed with a controlled break point to allow a return to physiologic motion and prevent the need for implant removal.[113]

Multiple randomized controlled trials (RCTs) have compared reduction and clinical outcomes after SS versus SB fixation for syndesmotic injury. The SB device has been found to provide improved functional outcomes with lower rates of malreduction.[112] In a recent prospective multicenter RCT, Sanders and colleagues[32] found lower malreduction rates with SB (15%) versus SS fixation (39%). There were no significant differences in functional scores but the study was underpowered for this outcome. The choice of clamp or thumb technique for open reduction in the SS fixation group was at the surgeons' discretion.[32] In a retrospective series by Miller and colleagues,[30] the investigators found an 18% malreduction rate with SS fixation under direct visualization, similar to the rate reported for SB in the RCT by Sanders and colleagues.[32] Although a direct comparison between the studies cannot be made, experienced surgeons may be able to achieve similarly low malreduction rates with screws under direct visualization.

Several investigators have suggested a rationale for the lower observed malreduction rates with the SB construct. Westermann and colleagues[114] showed the ability of the SB to mitigate deliberate clamp malreduction in a cadaveric model. In a similar study also in cadavers, Honeycutt and Riehl[115] concluded that the size difference between the suture diameter and drill hole effectively allows the fibula to be pulled and seated into the tibial incisura fibularis in spite of a potentially incorrect drill path. Peterson and colleagues[116] noted some loss of coronal reduction as measured by TFO and TFCS at short-term follow-up after SB fixation, indicating mild creep. This widening did not correlate with adverse patient outcomes.

CLINICS CARE POINTS

Although patient-specific and fracture-specific characteristics may influence treatment algorithms, choice of implants, and order of fixation, the authors generally prefer the following techniques for the diagnosis and management of patients with known or suspected syndesmotic injuries:

- Preoperative imaging: we obtain bilateral preoperative ankle CT scans for patients with trimalleolar ankle fractures, fracture-dislocations, Weber C fractures, and those with radiographs only obtained in splint/cast material. We do so given (1) the high rate of change in operative plans based on CT imaging as shown by Black and colleagues,[44] and (2) the higher incidence of potential syndesmotic disruption in these cohorts.
- Intraoperative contralateral fluoroscopy: intraoperative CT scan is not widely available. We obtain a perfect mortise and lateral fluoroscopic image of the contralateral uninjured ankle in the operating room as a template per the work of Summers and colleagues.[93] This imaging is most easily obtained before prepping and draping, and the use of fluoroscopy allows manipulation of the uninjured ankle to ensure perfect contralateral imaging. Contralateral fluoroscopy provides an understanding of normal fibular length, rotation, radiographic overlaps, and sagittal plane alignment. Images are saved for later comparison during the procedure.

- Fibular reduction: if an associated lateral malleolus fracture is present, we first obtain length and correct rotation by direct fracture reduction or indirect reduction if comminution exists. Appropriate length is confirmed by examining the relative distance from the tip of the fibula to the lateral talar process with the ankle in neutral position compared with the contralateral ankle.[117] Rotation is confirmed by examination of the lateral malleolar fossa compared with the contralateral ankle.[88,118]
- Syndesmotic reduction and fixation: if syndesmotic instability is confirmed by intraoperative Cotton test (see **Fig. 3**), reduction and fixation are pursued. A bolster under the heel is avoided to prevent an anterior drawer effect.[58] Gentle thumb pressure is applied to the distal fibula while the foot is slightly supinated and medialized. As the surgical assistant drills for placement of the syndesmotic device, counterpressure is applied to the medial tibia while the mortise is held reduced. If counterpressure is applied solely on the medial foot without maintaining reduction, a distraction force can be inadvertently created, resulting in a fixed malreduction once the implant is placed. Appropriate alignment is confirmed using fluoroscopy as stabilization proceeds.
- Assessing the reduction: at the conclusion of the procedure, perfect AP, mortise, and lateral views are obtained and radiographic parameters compared with contralateral fluoroscopy to mitigate limitations of traditional measurements, as previously discussed. The lateral radiograph is initially obtained holding only the leg in order to elevate the extremity off the table without any pressure or force applied to the foot. Pressure on the foot and/or manual dorsiflexion can artificially reduce the talus posteriorly and hide subtle sagittal plane malreduction such as that shown in **Fig. 6**. The contralateral lateral fluoroscans are scrutinized for symmetry, considering the parameters described by Loizou and colleagues[91] and Grenier and colleagues.[92] If the talus is subluxated within the mortise and/or sagittal plane tibiofibular overlap appears incorrect, malreduction is possible and fixation is revised.

DISCLOSURE

J.Y. Kwon receives intellectual property royalties from, and is a paid consultant for, Paragon 28. D.S. Stenquist has nothing to disclose.

REFERENCES

1. Shibuya N, Davis ML, Jupiter DC. Epidemiology of foot and ankle fractures in the United States: an analysis of the National Trauma Data Bank (2007 to 2011). J Foot Ankle Surg 2014;53(5):606–8.
2. Jennison T, Brinsden M. Fracture admission trends in England over a ten-year period. Ann R Coll Surg Engl 2019;101(3):208–14.
3. Dattani R, Patnaik S, Kantak A, et al. Injuries to the tibiofibular syndesmosis. J Bone Joint Surg Br 2008;90(4):405–10.
4. Haynes J, Cherney S, Spraggs-Hughes A, et al. Increased reduction clamp force associated with syndesmotic overcompression. Foot Ankle Int 2016; 37(7):722–9.
5. Weening B, Bhandari M. Predictors of functional outcome following transsyndesmotic screw fixation of ankle fractures. J Orthop Trauma 2005;19(2):102–8.
6. Kennedy JG, Soffe KE, Vedova PD, et al. Evaluation of the syndesmotic screw in low weber C ankle fractures. J Orthop Trauma 2000. https://doi.org/10.1097/00005131-200006000-00010.

7. Sagi HC, Shah AR, Sanders RW. The functional consequence of syndesmotic joint malreduction at a minimum 2-year follow-up. J Orthop Trauma 2012; 26(7):439–43.
8. Roberts RS. Surgical treatment of displaced ankle fractures. Clin Orthop Relat Res 1983;172:164–70.
9. Reckling FW, McNamara GRDA. Problems in the diagnosis and treatment of ankle fractures. J Trauma 1981;21(11):943–50.
10. Leeds HCEM. Instability of the distal tibiofibular syndesmosis after bimalleolar and trimalleolar ankle fractures. J Bone Joint Surg Am 1984;66(4):490–503.
11. Andersen MR, Diep LM, Frihagen F, et al. Importance of syndesmotic reduction on clinical outcome after syndesmosis injuries. J Orthop Trauma 2019;33(8): 397–403.
12. Ray R, Koohnejad N, Clement ND, et al. Ankle fractures with syndesmotic stabilisation are associated with a high rate of secondary osteoarthritis. Foot Ankle Surg 2019;25(2):180–5.
13. Hak DJ, Egol KA, Gardner MJ, et al. The "not so simple" ankle fracture: avoiding problems and pitfalls to improve patient outcomes. Instr Course Lect 2011;60: 73–88. Available at: http://www.ncbi.nlm.nih.gov/pubmed/21553763.
14. Massri-Pugin J, Lubberts B, Vopat BG, et al. Role of the Deltoid Ligament in Syndesmotic Instability. Foot Ankle Int 2018;39(5):598–603.
15. Ebraheim NA, Elgafy H, Padanilam T. Syndesmotic disruption in low fibular fractures associated with deltoid ligament injury. Clin Orthop Relat Res 2003. https://doi.org/10.1097/01.blo.0000052935.71325.30.
16. Fitzpatrick DC, Otto JK, McKinley TO, et al. Kinematic and contact stress analysis of posterior malleolus fractures of the ankle. J Orthop Trauma 2004;18(5): 271–8. Available at: http://www.ncbi.nlm.nih.gov/pubmed/15105748.
17. Lloyd J, Elsayed S, Hariharan K, et al. Revisiting the concept of talar shift in ankle fractures. Foot Ankle Int 2006;27(10):793–6.
18. Ramsey PL, Hamilton W. Changes in tibiotalar area of contact caused by lateral talar shift. J Bone Joint Surg Am 1976;58(3):356–7. Available at: http://www.ncbi.nlm.nih.gov/pubmed/1262367.
19. Kelly M, Vasconcellos D, Osman WS, et al. Alterations in tibiotalar joint reaction force following syndesmotic injury are restored with static syndesmotic fixation. Clin Biomech (Bristol) 2019;69:156–63.
20. Hunt KJ, Goeb Y, Behn AW, et al. Ankle joint contact loads and displacement with progressive syndesmotic injury. Foot Ankle Int 2015;36(9):1095–103.
21. Stroh DA, DeFontes K, Paez A, et al. Distal fibular malrotation and lateral ankle contact characteristics. Foot Ankle Surg 2019;25(1):90–3.
22. Macko VW, Matthews LS, Zwirkoski P, et al. The joint-contact area of the ankle. The contribution of the posterior malleolus. J Bone Joint Surg Am 1991;73(3): 347–51. Available at: http://www.ncbi.nlm.nih.gov/pubmed/2002072.
23. Vrahas M, Fu F, Veenis B. Intraarticular contact stresses with simulated ankle malunions. J Orthop Trauma 1994;8(2):159–66. Available at: http://www.ncbi.nlm.nih.gov/pubmed/8207574.
24. Kimizuka M, Kurosawa H, Fukubayashi T. Load-bearing pattern of the ankle joint. Contact area and pressure distribution. Arch Orthop Trauma Surg 1980; 96(1):45–9.
25. Egol KA, Pahk B, Walsh M, et al. Outcome after unstable ankle fracture: effect of syndesmotic stabilization. J Orthop Trauma 2010;24(1):7–11.
26. Sagi C, Shah A. In response. J Orthop Trauma 2013;27(10):e247–8.

27. Cherney SM, Cosgrove CT, Spraggs-Hughes AG, et al. Functional outcomes of syndesmotic injuries based on objective reduction accuracy at a minimum 1-year follow-up. J Orthop Trauma 2018;32(1):43–51.

28. Ntalos D, Rupprecht M, Grossterlinden LG, et al. Incidence and severity of malreduction of the tibiofibular syndesmosis following surgical treatement of displaced ankle fractures and impact on the function -Clinical study and MRI evaluation. Injury 2018;49(6):1220–7.

29. Scolaro JA, Marecek G, Barei DP. Management of syndesmotic disruption in ankle fractures. JBJS Rev 2014;2(12):1.

30. Miller AN, Carroll EA, Parker RJ, et al. Direct visualization for syndesmotic stabilization of ankle fractures. Foot Ankle Int 2009;30(5):419–26.

31. Gardner MJ, Demetrakopoulos D, Briggs SM, et al. Malreduction of the tibiofibular syndesmosis in ankle fractures. Foot Ankle Int 2006;27(10):788–92.

32. Sanders D, Schneider P, Taylor M, et al, Canadian Orthopaedic Trauma Society. Improved reduction of the tibiofibular syndesmosis with tightrope compared with screw fixation: results of a randomized controlled study. J Orthop Trauma 2019;33(11):531–7.

33. Franke J, von Recum J, Suda AJ, et al. Predictors of a persistent dislocation after reduction of syndesmotic injuries detected with intraoperative three-dimensional imaging. Foot Ankle Int 2014;35(12):1323–8.

34. Cherney SM, Haynes JA, Spraggs-Hughes AG, et al. In vivo syndesmotic overcompression after fixation of ankle fractures with a syndesmotic injury. J Orthop Trauma 2015;29(9):414–9.

35. Schottel PC, Berkes MB, Little MTM, et al. Comparison of clinical outcome of pronation external rotation versus supination external rotation ankle fractures. Foot Ankle Int 2014;35(4):353–9.

36. Warner SJ, Schottel PC, Hinds RM, et al. Fracture-dislocations demonstrate poorer postoperative functional outcomes among pronation external rotation IV ankle fractures. Foot Ankle Int 2015;36(6):641–7.

37. Ebraheim NA, Lu J, Yang H, et al. The fibular incisure of the tibia on CT scan: a cadaver study. Foot Ankle Int 1998;19(5):318–21.

38. Cherney SM, Spraggs-Hughes AG, McAndrew CM, et al. Incisura morphology as a risk factor for syndesmotic malreduction. Foot Ankle Int 2016;37(7):748–54.

39. Boszczyk A, Kwapisz S, Krümmel M, et al. Correlation of Incisura anatomy with syndesmotic malreduction. Foot Ankle Int 2018;39(3):369–75.

40. Miller AN, Carroll EA, Parker RJ, et al. Posterior malleolar stabilization of syndesmotic injuries is equivalent to screw fixation. Clin Orthop Relat Res 2010;468(4):1129–35.

41. Gardner MJ, Brodsky A, Briggs SM, et al. Fixation of posterior malleolar fractures provides greater syndesmotic stability. Clin Orthop Relat Res 2006;447:165–71.

42. Fitzpatrick E, Goetz JE, Sittapairoj T, et al. Effect of posterior malleolus fracture on syndesmotic reduction: a cadaveric study. J Bone Joint Surg Am 2018;100(3):243–8.

43. Kang C, Hwang D-S, Lee J-K, et al. Screw fixation of the posterior malleolus fragment in ankle fracture. Foot Ankle Int 2019. https://doi.org/10.1177/1071100719865895. 1071100719865895.

44. Black EM, Antoci V, Lee JT, et al. Role of preoperative computed tomography scans in operative planning for malleolar ankle fractures. Foot Ankle Int 2013; 34(5):697–704.

45. Stark E, Tornetta P, Creevy WR. Syndesmotic instability in Weber B ankle fractures: a clinical evaluation. J Orthop Trauma 2007;21(9):643–6.
46. Hunt KJ, Phisitkul P, Pirolo J, et al. High ankle sprains and syndesmotic injuries in athletes. J Am Acad Orthop Surg 2015;23(11):661–73.
47. Matuszewski PE, Dombroski D, Lawrence JTR, et al. Prospective intraoperative syndesmotic evaluation during ankle fracture fixation: stress external rotation versus lateral fibular stress. J Orthop Trauma 2015;29(4):e157–60.
48. Jiang KN, Schulz BM, Tsui YL, et al. Comparison of radiographic stress tests for syndesmotic instability of supination-external rotation ankle fractures: a cadaveric study. J Orthop Trauma 2014;28(6):e123–7.
49. Harper MC, Keller TS. A radiographic evaluation of the tibiofibular syndesmosis. Foot Ankle 1989;10(3):156–60.
50. Harper MC. An anatomic and radiographic investigation of the tibiofibular clear space. Foot Ankle 1993;14(8):455–8.
51. Ostrum RF, De Meo P, Subramanian R. A critical analysis of the anterior-posterior radiographic anatomy of the ankle syndesmosis. Foot Ankle Int 1995;16(3): 128–31.
52. DeAngelis JP, Anderson R, DeAngelis NA. Understanding the superior clear space in the adult ankle. Foot Ankle Int 2007;28(4):490–3.
53. Switaj PJ, Mendoza M, Kadakia AR. Acute and chronic injuries to the syndesmosis. Clin Sports Med 2015;34(4):643–77.
54. Shah AS, Kadakia AR, Tan GJ, et al. Radiographic evaluation of the normal distal tibiofibular syndesmosis. Foot Ankle Int 2012;33(10):870–6.
55. Saldua NS, Harris JF, LeClere LE, et al. Plantar flexion influences radiographic measurements of the ankle mortise. J Bone Joint Surg Am 2010;92(4):911–5.
56. Park SS, Kubiak EN, Egol KA, et al. Stress radiographs after ankle fracture: the effect of ankle position and deltoid ligament status on medial clear space measurements. J Orthop Trauma 2006;20(1):11–8. Available at: http://www.ncbi.nlm.nih.gov/pubmed/16424804.
57. Tornetta P. Invited commentary related to: a novel indirect reduction technique in ankle syndesmotic injuries: a cadaveric study. J Orthop Trauma 2018;32(7): 367–8.
58. Boszczyk A, Kordasiewicz B, Kiciński M, et al. Operative setup to improve sagittal syndesmotic reduction: technical tip. J Orthop Trauma 2019;33(1): e27–30.
59. Tornetta P, Spoo JE, Reynolds FA, et al. Overtightening of the ankle syndesmosis: is it really possible? J Bone Joint Surg Am 2001;83(4):489–92.
60. Gonzalez T, Egan J, Ghorbanhoseini M, et al. Overtightening of the syndesmosis revisited and the effect of syndesmotic malreduction on ankle dorsiflexion. Injury 2017;48(6):1253–7.
61. Pallis MP, Pressman DN, Heida K, et al. Effect of ankle position on tibiotalar motion with screw fixation of the distal tibiofibular syndesmosis in a fracture model. Foot Ankle Int 2018;39(6):746–50.
62. Hahn DM, Chong K. Malleoli. In: Buckley RE, Moran CG, Apivatthakakul T, editors. AO principles of fracture management. 3rd edition. Davos Platz (CH): AO Publishing; 2017. p. 933–60.
63. Cosgrove CT, Spraggs-Hughes AG, Putnam SM, et al. A novel indirect reduction technique in ankle syndesmotic injuries: a cadaveric study. J Orthop Trauma 2018;32(7):361–7.
64. Mendelsohn ES, Hoshino CM, Harris TG, et al. CT characterizing the anatomy of uninjured ankle syndesmosis. Orthopedics 2014;37(2):157–61.

65. Putnam SM, Linn MS, Spraggs-Hughes A, et al. Simulating clamp placement across the trans-syndesmotic angle of the ankle to minimize malreduction: a radiological study. Injury 2017;48(3):770–5.

66. Kennedy MT, Carmody O, Leong S, et al. A computed tomography evaluation of two hundred normal ankles, to ascertain what anatomical landmarks to use when compressing or placing an ankle syndesmosis screw. Foot (Edinb) 2014;24(4):157–60.

67. Stuart K, Panchbhavi VK. The fate of syndesmotic screws. Foot Ankle Int 2011; 32(5):S519–25.

68. Kukreti S, Faraj A, Miles JNV. Does position of syndesmotic screw affect functional and radiological outcome in ankle fractures? Injury 2005;36(9):1121–4.

69. McBryde A, Chiasson B, Wilhelm A, et al. Syndesmotic screw placement: a biomechanical analysis. Foot Ankle Int 1997;18(5):262–6.

70. Peek AC, Fitzgerald CE, Charalambides C. Syndesmosis screws: how many, what diameter, where and should they be removed? a literature review. Injury 2014;45(8):1262–7.

71. Cosgrove CT, Putnam SM, Cherney SM, et al. Medial clamp tine positioning affects ankle syndesmosis malreduction. J Orthop Trauma 2017;31(8):440–6.

72. Miller AN, Barei DP, Iaquinto JM, Ledoux WR, Beingessner DM. Iatrogenic Syndesmosis Malreduction via Clamp and Screw Placement. J Orthop Trauma 2013;27(2):100–6. Available at: www.jorthotrauma.com.

73. Hoshino CM, Mendelsohn ES, Zinar DM, et al. Anterior subluxation of the talus: a complication of malreduction of the ankle syndesmosis: a report of three cases. JBJS Case Connect 2012;2(4):e78.

74. LaMothe J, Baxter JR, Gilbert S, et al. Effect of complete syndesmotic disruption and deltoid injuries and different reduction methods on ankle joint contact mechanics. Foot Ankle Int 2017;38(6):694–700.

75. Pang EQ, Coughlan M, Bonaretti S, et al. Assessment of open syndesmosis reduction techniques in an unbroken fibula model: visualization versus palpation. J Orthop Trauma 2019;33(1):e14–8.

76. Tornetta P, Yakavonis M, Veltre D, et al. Reducing the syndesmosis under direct vision: where should i look? J Orthop Trauma 2019;33(9):450–4.

77. Reb CW, Hyer CF, Collins CL, et al. Clinical adaptation of the "tibiofibular line" for intraoperative evaluation of open syndesmosis reduction accuracy: a cadaveric study. Foot Ankle Int 2016;37(11):1243–8.

78. Schon JM, Mikula JD, Backus JD, et al. 3D model analysis of ankle flexion on anatomic reduction of a syndesmotic injury. Foot Ankle Int 2017;38(4):436–42.

79. Morellato J, Louati H, Bodrogi A, et al. The effect of varying tension of a suture button construct in fixation of the tibiofibular syndesmosis-evaluation using stress computed tomography. J Orthop Trauma 2017;31(2):103–10.

80. Mahapatra P, Rudge B, Whittingham-Jones P. Is it possible to overcompress the syndesmosis? J Foot Ankle Surg 2018;57(5):1005–9.

81. Gesink DS, Anderson JG. Over-tightening of the syndesmosis after ankle fracture: a case report. JBJS Case Connect 2015;5(4):e85.

82. Gennis E, Koenig S, Rodericks D, et al. The fate of the fixed syndesmosis over time. Foot Ankle Int 2015;36(10):1202–8.

83. Jordan TH, Talarico RH, Schuberth JM. The radiographic fate of the syndesmosis after trans-syndesmotic screw removal in displaced ankle fractures. J Foot Ankle Surg 2011;50(4):407–12.

84. van den Heuvel SB, Dingemans SA, Gardenbroek TJ, et al. Assessing quality of syndesmotic reduction in surgically treated acute syndesmotic injuries: a systematic review. J Foot Ankle Surg 2019;58(1):144–50.

85. Nielson JH, Gardner MJ, Peterson MGE, et al. Radiographic measurements do not predict syndesmotic injury in ankle fractures: an MRI study. Clin Orthop Relat Res 2005;(436):216–21.

86. Koenig SJ, Tornetta P, Merlin G, et al. Can we tell if the syndesmosis is reduced using fluoroscopy? J Orthop Trauma 2015;29(9):e326–30.

87. Marmor M, Hansen E, Han HK, et al. Limitations of standard fluoroscopy in detecting rotational malreduction of the syndesmosis in an ankle fracture model. Foot Ankle Int 2011;32(6):616–22.

88. Chang S-M, Li H-F, Hu S-J, et al. A reliable method for intraoperative detection of lateral malleolar malrotation using conventional fluoroscopy. Injury 2019;50(11): 2108–12.

89. Futamura K, Baba T, Mogami A, et al. Malreduction of syndesmosis injury associated with malleolar ankle fracture can be avoided using Weber's three indexes in the mortise view. Injury 2017;48(4):954–9.

90. Schreiber JJ, McLawhorn AS, Dy CJGE. Intraoperative contralateral view for assessing accurate syndesmosis reduction. Orthopedics 2013;36(5):360–1.

91. Loizou CL, Sudlow A, Collins R, et al. Radiological assessment of ankle syndesmotic reduction. Foot (Edinb) 2017;32:39–43.

92. Grenier S, Benoit B, Rouleau DM, et al. APTF: anteroposterior tibiofibular ratio, a new reliable measure to assess syndesmotic reduction. J Orthop Trauma 2013; 27(4):207–11.

93. Summers HD, Sinclair MK, Stover MD. A reliable method for intraoperative evaluation of syndesmotic reduction. J Orthop Trauma 2013;27(4):196–200.

94. Baek JH, Kim TY, Kwon YB, et al. Radiographic change of the distal tibiofibular joint following removal of transfixing screw fixation. Foot Ankle Int 2018;39(3): 318–25.

95. Nault ML, Hébert-Davies J, Laflamme GY, et al. CT scan assessment of the syndesmosis: a new reproducible method. J Orthop Trauma 2013;27(11):638–41.

96. Ebraheim NA, Lu J, Yang H, et al. Radiographic and CT evaluation of tibiofibular syndesmotic diastasis: a cadaver study. Foot Ankle Int 1997;18(11):693–8.

97. Dikos GD, Heisler J, Choplin RH, et al. Normal tibiofibular relationships at the syndesmosis on axial CT imaging. J Orthop Trauma 2012;26(7):433–8. Available at: www.jorthotrauma.com.

98. Malhotra G, Cameron J, Toolan BC. Diagnosing chronic diastasis of the syndesmosis: a novel measurement using computed tomography. Foot Ankle Int 2014; 35(5):483–8.

99. Lepojärvi S, Pakarinen H, Savola O, et al. Posterior translation of the fibula may indicate malreduction: CT study of normal variation in uninjured ankles. J Orthop Trauma 2014;28(4):205–9.

100. Abdelaziz ME, Hagemeijer N, Guss D, et al. Evaluation of Syndesmosis reduction on CT scan. Foot Ankle Int 2019;40(9):1087–93.

101. Patel S, Malhotra K, Cullen NP, et al. Defining reference values for the normal tibiofibular syndesmosis in adults using weight-bearing CT. Bone Joint J 2019; 101-B(3):348–52.

102. Yeung TW, Chan CYG, Chan WCS, et al. Can pre-operative axial CT imaging predict syndesmosis instability in patients sustaining ankle fractures? seven years' experience in a tertiary trauma center. Skeletal Radiol 2015;44(6):823–9.

103. Schon JM, Brady AW, Krob JJ, et al. Defining the three most responsive and specific CT measurements of ankle syndesmotic malreduction. Knee Surg Sports Traumatol Arthrosc 2019;27(9):2863–76.

104. Franke J, Von Recum J, Suda AJ, et al. Intraoperative three-dimensional imaging in the treatment of acute unstable syndesmotic injuries. J Bone Joint Surg Am 2012;94(15):1386–90.

105. Davidovitch RI, Weil Y, Karia R, et al. Intraoperative syndesmotic reduction: three-dimensional versus standard fluoroscopic imaging. J Bone Joint Surg Am 2013;95(20):1838–43.

106. Kotwal R, Rath N, Paringe V, et al. Targeted computerised tomography scanning of the ankle syndesmosis with low dose radiation exposure. Skeletal Radiol 2016;45(3):333–8.

107. Michelson JD, Wright M, Blankstein M. Syndesmotic ankle fractures. J Orthop Trauma 2018;32(1):10–4.

108. Clanton TO, Whitlow SR, Williams BT, et al. Biomechanical comparison of 3 current ankle syndesmosis repair techniques. Foot Ankle Int 2017;38(2):200–7.

109. Ebramzadeh E, Knutsen AR, Sangiorgio SN, et al. Biomechanical comparison of syndesmotic injury fixation methods using a cadaveric model. Foot Ankle Int 2013;34(12):1710–7.

110. Riedel MD, Miller CP, Kwon JY. Augmenting suture-button fixation for maisonneuve injuries with fibular shortening: technique tip. Foot Ankle Int 2017; 38(10):1146–51.

111. Laflamme M, Belzile EL, Bédard L, et al. A prospective randomized multicenter trial comparing clinical outcomes of patients treated surgically with a static or dynamic implant for acute ankle syndesmosis rupture. J Orthop Trauma 2015; 29(5):216–23.

112. Shimozono Y, Hurley ET, Myerson CL, et al. Suture button versus syndesmotic screw for syndesmosis injuries: a meta-analysis of randomized controlled trials. Am J Sports Med 2018. https://doi.org/10.1177/0363546518804804. 363546518804804.

113. Stenquist D, Velasco BT, Cronin PK, et al. Syndesmotic fixation utilizing a novel screw: a retrospective case series reporting early clinical and radiographic outcomes. Foot Ankle Spec 2019. https://doi.org/10.1177/1938640019866322. 193864001986632.

114. Westermann RW, Rungprai C, Goetz JE, et al. The effect of suture-button fixation on simulated syndesmotic malreduction: a cadaveric study. J Bone Joint Surg Am 2014;96(20):1732–8.

115. Honeycutt MW, Riehl JT. Effect of a dynamic fixation construct on syndesmosis reduction: a cadaveric study. J Orthop Trauma 2019;33(9):460–4.

116. Peterson KS, Chapman WD, Hyer CF, et al. Maintenance of reduction with suture button fixation devices for ankle syndesmosis repair. Foot Ankle Int 2015;36(6): 679–84.

117. Panchbhavi VK, Gurbani BN, Mason CB, et al. Radiographic assessment of fibular length variance: the case for "fibula minus". J Foot Ankle Surg 2018; 57(1):91–4.

118. Fitzpatrick EP, Kwon JY. Use of a pointed reduction clamp placed on the distal fibula to ensure proper restoration of fibular length and rotation and anatomic reduction of the syndesmosis: a technique tip. Foot Ankle Int 2014;35(9): 943–8.

Chronic Syndesmotic Injuries

Arthrodesis versus Reconstruction

Stefan Rammelt, MD, PhD[a],*, Andrzej Boszczyk, MD, PhD[b]

KEYWORDS

- Ankle • Instability • Syndesmosis • Syndesmotic avulsion • Reconstruction
- Ankle malunion • Ankle arthritis

KEY POINTS

- Chronic syndesmotic injury covers a broad range of symptoms and pathologies. Antero-lateral ankle impingement from scarring after syndesmotic injury without instability is treated by arthroscopic debridement and arthrolysis.
- Subacute syndesmotic injuries are treated by arthroscopic or open debridement followed by secondary stabilization using suture button device or permanent placement of syndesmotic screws.
- Chronic syndesmotic instability is treated by a near-anatomic ligamentoplasty supplemented by screw fixation. In case of poor bone stock, failed ligament reconstruction, or comorbidities, tibiofibular fusion with bone grafting is preferred.
- Malleolar malunions and particularly anterior or posterior syndesmotic avulsions must be corrected in order to achieve a stable and congruent ankle mortise.
- In the presence of manifest tibiotalar arthritis, corrective ankle fusion or arthroplasty combined with syndesmotic fusion and deformity correction are salvage options.

INTRODUCTION

The treatment of syndesmotic injuries has been a subject of continued interest and debate for more than 100 years.[1–6] There is increasing consensus that adequate treatment of syndesmotic injuries is a key to improving overall treatment results of ankle joint injuries.[7–11]

With a more regular use of computed tomography (CT) scanning after fixation of unstable syndesmotic injuries it became clear that up to 52% of the syndesmotic injuries

[a] University Center for Orthopaedics, Trauma and Plastic Surgery, University Hospital Carl Gustav Carus at the TU Dresden, Fetscherstrasse 74, Dresden 01307, Germany; [b] Department of Traumatology and Orthopaedics, Centre of Postgraduate Medical Education, Adam Gruca Clinical Hospital, Konarskiego Str. 13, Otwock 05-400, Poland
* Corresponding author.
E-mail address: stefan.rammelt@uniklinikum-dresden.de

Foot Ankle Clin N Am 25 (2020) 631–652
https://doi.org/10.1016/j.fcl.2020.08.006
1083-7515/20/© 2020 Elsevier Inc. All rights reserved.

remain malreduced after closed reduction and 16% after open reduction of the syndesmosis.[12–15] With meticulous technique this percentage can be reduced to 15% and less[16–18] but still not close to zero. Simultaneously, it has been shown that fractures including syndesmotic injury requiring fixation[19] as well as malreduction of the distal fibula with regard to the tibial incisura[13,15,20–23] carry a worse prognosis. This is of great clinical importance, as the distal tibiofibular syndesmosis is injured in 20% to 45% of all operatively treated ankle fractures.[24,25]

Chronic syndesmotic injury is an umbrella term covering a broad range of symptoms and functional restrictions of variable severity and presentation. Consequently, there is a great variety of methods of delayed treatment and reconstruction after missed or malreduced syndesmotic injury. The reported methods range from physical therapy and arthroscopic debridement[26] to complex triligamentous ligamentoplasty and tibiofibular fusion.[27,28] Furthermore, as most of the syndesmotic injuries occurs in the wake of ankle fractures, the bony component of the injury and malunion has to be considered.[5] With an individual choice of treatment almost uniformly good results are reported.[29] This requires a thorough assessment of the individual pathology. This review, therefore, aims at giving a structured approach to the evaluation and treatment of chronic conditions following syndesmotic injury.

PATHOANATOMY OF CHRONIC SYNDESMOTIC INJURY

The detailed description of anatomy is beyond the scope of this review, and the reader is referred to texts dedicated to this topic.[30,31] A strong ligamentous tibiofibular bond exists over the full length of the fibula. The term syndesmosis is typically used for the distal portion that is crucial for stability of the ankle mortise. The distal tibiofibular syndesmosis consists of 5 ligamentous connections between distal tibia and distal fibula: anterior inferior tibiofibular ligament (AITFL), posterior inferior tibiofibular ligament (PITFL), transverse tibiofibular ligament, interosseous tibiofibular ligament (IOL), and the distal portion of the interosseous membrane. In addition, the deltoid ligament also is an important contributor to syndesmotic stability.[32,33]

Of these 5 ligaments, the AITFL and PITFL receive most attention, as they are surgically available for reconstruction. Both ligaments share similar anatomic features as consisting of 2 parallel parts, being flat, wide, and relatively short, giving them an appearance more of a ribbon than a rope. The injury of these ligaments can take a form of pure ligamentous injury as well as avulsion injuries of their bony attachments. These avulsions have been long recognized as a part of malleolar fractures and are sources of chronic pain and instability if not addressed properly.[34,35] However, clinical and biomechanical studies have also highlighted the importance of the strong tibiofibular interosseous ligament that is not amenable to direct suture or reconstruction but may as well contribute to chronic instability of the ankle mortise.[32,33,36]

The avulsion of the tibial attachment of the AITFL, the anterior tibial tubercle, is known under the eponym of Tillaux-Chaput.[2] The avulsion of the fibular attachment of the AITFL carries the eponym Le Fort-Wagstaffe.[37] An avulsion of PITFL at the posterior tibial tubercle was first described by Earle but is widely referred to as posterior Volkmann triangle or posterior malleolus.[38] Recent studies using CT imaging revealed that besides a basic triangular pattern, anatomy of the posterior malleolar fracture may be more complex including intercalary fragments, joint impaction ("posterior pilon"), and extension into the medial malleolus.[34,39–42] In the classification system by Bartoníček and colleagues[40] the typical avulsion of PITFL is mostly found in type 2 fractures corresponding to a small posterolateral fragment. However, it is conceivable that with increasing size the posterior tibial fragment carries a larger portion of the PITFL and

IOL, resulting in a more unstable injury pattern. Injuries to the distal tibiofibular syndesmosis typically result from forced external rotation of the foot with respect to the tibia or internal rotation of the lower leg with the foot fixed. The talus rotates in the ankle mortise forcing the malleoli apart.[43] With the foot in dorsiflexion, the broader posterior part of the talus is forced into the ankle mortise, thus putting an additional strain on the syndesmotic ligaments.[44,45] Relevant syndesmotic instability therefore has to be expected in but is not limited to pronation injuries.[5,25,46,47]

The ruptures typically start anteriorly with ATFL and continue through the IOL and finally the PTFL, which results in variable malposition of the fibula in cases of late diastasis. Primary displacement may be rotation and posterior translation—in case of ATFL insufficiency and retained PTFL acting as a pivot (**Fig. 1**A). Primary displacement may also be diastasis—in cases where all 3 ligaments are insufficiently healed (**Fig. 1**B).

Definition of chronicity varies, but typically a 6 to 8 weeks postinjury cutoff is used for an acute injury because this is the time that ligaments typically take to heal. Injuries may be considered subacute after a lapse of 6 weeks to 6 months.[48] The time from injury to reconstruction does not seem to be crucial for the functional results. Successful reconstructions have been reported from 2[49] to 120 months[50] after initial injury.

Chronic syndesmotic instability and diastasis results from failure to detect and treat instability of the ankle mortise in case of acute syndesmotic rupture.[5] As most syndesmotic injuries occur in the wake of malleolar fractures, chronic syndesmotic insufficiency is frequently accompanied by bony malunion.[51,52] In particular, failure to address bony syndesmotic avulsions at the time of injury will lead to incongruity of

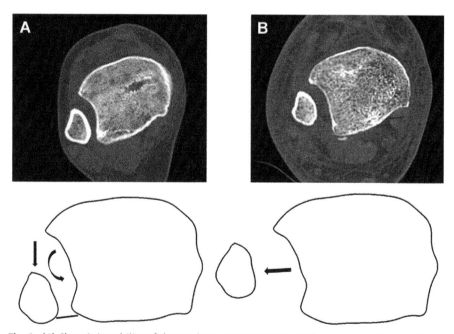

Fig. 1. (*A*) Chronic instability of the syndesmosis can present with rotation and translation of the distal fibula if either the anterior or posterior tibiofibular ligament is still intact and acts as a hinge. (*B*) If the anterior, interosseous, and posterior ligaments are disrupted, a diastasis results.

the tibial incisura and tibiofibular malalignment.[5,34,35,53,54] Apart from inadequate treatment of acute syndesmotic injuries, chronic syndesmotic instability may also result from relevant comorbidities such as obesity, complicated diabetes and osteoporosis, or patient incompliance with the postoperative protocol. In a clinical study by Mendelsohn and collaborators, obese patients were 12 times more likely to sustain early failure of syndesmotic stabilization than nonobese controls.[55] Diabetes mellitus, especially when complicated by neuropathy, impairs healing of bone and ligaments by several mechanisms.[56]

CLINICAL ASSESSMENT

The major symptoms of chronic injury include diffuse pain on weight bearing, a subjective feeling of instability (giving way) on uneven grounds, reduced range of motion, and persistent swelling of the ankle region.[27,57] Tenderness may be aggravated by forced dorsiflexion at the ankle. The symptoms tend to be uncharacteristic, and delayed diagnosis is not uncommon. With chronic diastasis there is a valgus deformity of the ankle that may be accentuated with any bony malunion, most commonly shortening and valgus of the fibula.[51] The clinical tests for chronic syndesmotic instability mimic those for acute injuries but may be less specific with chronic conditions. Pain over the syndesmosis and anterolateral aspect of the ankle can be elicited with dorsiflexion and forced external rotation of the foot against the fixed lower leg.[44] Further clinical tests include the calf squeeze test, the cross-legged test, and a functional stabilization test mainly used in athletes with suspected syndesmosis sprains.[58,59] In a study by Han and colleagues[60] palpation of the anterior syndesmosis evoked dull tenderness in 18 of 20 confirmed chronic injuries, 3/20 patients had positive external rotation test, and 2/20 had positive squeeze test translating to 90%, 15%, and 10% specificity, respectively. Symptoms related to syndesmotic instability may overlap with those resulting from posttraumatic ankle arthritis, particularly in long-standing deformities.

IMAGING STUDIES
Plain Radiographs

Standing radiographs of both ankles in standardized projections (lateral and anteroposterior views with the foot in 20° of internal rotation, "mortise view") remains the first-line standard for assessing posttraumatic ankle deformities including chronic syndesmotic instability (**Fig. 2**). The "ligne claire" (tibiofibular clear space [TCS]), as described by Chaput,[2] is the radiographic measure for syndesmotic integrity. Other radiographic landmarks include the tibiofibular overlap (TFO) and the medial clear space (MCS). Weight bearing mimics the physiologic loading of the ankle and uncovers ligamentous mortise instability that remains unnoticed in non–weight-bearing radiographs.

The establishment of normal values for radiographic anatomic measurements is hampered by the great variability of the anatomy of the distal fibula and tibial incisura.[61,62] Generally, a TCS of less than 6 mm and a TFO greater than 1 mm in the mortise view are considered to be normal.[63] Both are larger in men than in women.[13,64] Shah and colleagues,[65] in an analysis of 392 ankle radiographs, found a mean tibiofibular overlap of 8.3 mm in the true anteroposterior view and 3.5 mm in the mortise view. The mean TCS was 4.6 mm and 4.3 mm, respectively. Interestingly, the investigators found a subset of patients with a complete lack of tibiofibular overlap in the mortise view as a normal variant underlining the necessity for bilateral radiographs.[65,66] Widening of the TCS and MCS of 2 mm and more compared with the unaffected side is considered to be pathologic.[45]

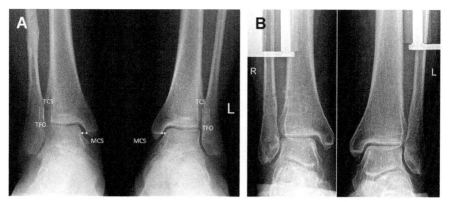

Fig. 2. (A) Standing anteroposterior radiographs 17 months after pronation eversion stage 3 (Weber C) fracture and 8 months after hardware removal for residual pain in the right ankle. Note the increased ligne claire (tibiofibular clear space [TCS]), reduced tibiofibular overlap (TFO), and increased medial clear space (MCS) on the right side as compared with the unaffected left ankle. (B) In the absence of a frank diastasis, stress radiographs can reveal chronic syndesmotic insufficiency (latent diastasis).[32]

For detecting subtle syndesmotic injury, analysis of the lateral view is mandatory,[67] as posterior migration of the fibula precedes widening of the mortise.[68] However, plain radiography is insensitive to rotational deformity, prompting a generous use of CT scanning in suspected chronic syndesmotic injury.[54]

Computed Tomography

Bilateral CT imaging is the gold standard for assessment of syndesmosis instability.[32,54] The standard plane of assessment is a coronal scan located 10 mm proximal to the plafond in most studies,[17] but a lower level close to the tibial plafond has been suggested.[69] Numerous measurements have been proposed[12,18,70–74] (**Fig. 3**), but still no gold standard of measurement exists. Because of the high interindividual variability,[61,75] but low intraindividual variation[67,76] of important radiographic parameters of syndesmotic anatomy such as the tibiofibular interval, position, and rotation of the distal fibula, the patients' contralateral, uninjured ankle, rather than a population norm, should be used for assessment of syndesmotic reduction.[54,77,78] A side-to-side difference in fibular translation or tibiofibular diastasis exceeding 2 mm is considered abnormal. With respect to fibular malrotation, 5° lead to a significant load shift in cadaveric ankles,[79] whereas 15° and more seem to be clinically relevant.[13]

Recent studies suggest a role of standing CT for assessment of subtle syndesmotic injuries combining the benefits of 3-dimensional imaging and physiologic loading.[80–82] It still remains unclear if it is superior to conventional CT in detecting acute or chronic instability.[81,83]

MRI

MRI has a high specificity and sensitivity for acute injuries of the AITFL and PITFL with a high interobserver agreement. It is less useful in chronic conditions but may reveal additional lesions such as chronic injuries to the tendons and chondral damage.[57,84] However, MRI findings may not correlate with the clinical symptoms and lead to overestimation or underestimation of the severity of the lesion.[85]

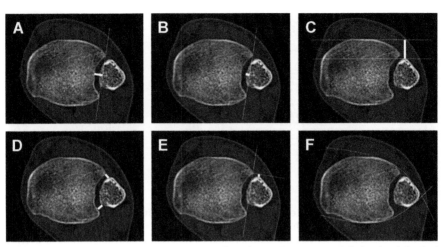

Fig. 3. Examples of linear CT measurements of syndesmotic anatomy: (*A*) depth of the incisura,[75] (*B*) engagement of the fibula into the incisura,[18] (*C*) anterior tibiofibular distance,[78] (*D*) anterior and posterior distance,[71] (*E*) fibular translation,[74] (*F*) anterior and posterior tibiofibular alignment on an elliptical line.[69].

Ultrasound

The anterior syndesmotic ligaments are accessible to ultrasound imaging, and dynamic testing can be performed to detect tibiofibular instability. Additional pathologies and instability of the lateral ankle ligaments and the tendons may also be assessed dynamically. The use of ultrasound examination is limited by high intraobserver variability and subjectivity of assessment.

Arthroscopy

The instability of the syndesmosis is easily visualized under arthroscopy, but this invasive method is not without limitations. Firstly, no standard definition of instability exists: stressed diastasis of 1 mm,[57] 2 mm,[26,60] 3 mm,[86] and 4 mm[87] have all been used as cutoff value. Secondly, standard ankle arthroscopy allows for assessment of the anterior part of the syndesmosis, with the interosseous and posterior part being less accessible for anterior ankle arthroscopy. Still, arthroscopy may be useful if apart from syndesmotic instability further pathologies are suspected that may be detected and treated arthroscopically as intraarticular adhesions[26] or osteochondral lesions that occur frequently in rotational ankle fractures with syndesmotic injury.[88]

TREATMENT OF CHRONIC SYNDESMOTIC INJURY

The term "chronic syndesmotic instability" covers injuries of highly variable pathoanatomy and severity. In the following section, treatment options are discussed according to the 5 most commonly seen clinical presentations of the problem.

Ligamentous Injury Without Static Diastasis

In this clinical scenario the most commonly seen mode of injury is sporting injury involving the AITFL, also referred to as "high ankle sprain." High ankle sprains are known for prolonged healing and propensity for long-term disability.[89] However, with a 3-staged protocol of immobilization, physical therapy, and rehabilitation including neuromuscular control and sport-specific tasks, the results of nonoperative management of syndesmosis sprains are favorable with good to excellent outcomes in 86% to 100% and full return to sports in almost all cases.[59,90]

Chronic pain after syndesmotic injury without instability typically results from impingement of scar tissue and hypertrophic synovium between tibia and fibula. Treatment consists of arthroscopic debridement of the syndesmotic scars (**Fig. 4**) and is typically effective.[26,60,91] In a first series by Ogilvie-Harris and Reed, arthroscopic resection of the torn interosseous ligament and chondroplasty relieved symptoms in all 19 patients after an average of 2 years of symptoms in the short term.[26,91] Han and colleagues reported significant functional improvement with improved range of motion at the ankle from arthroscopic marginal resection of chronically injured syndesmosis ligaments.[60] Additional prophylactic syndesmotic stabilization with screws[92] or suture button[87] does not lead to better outcome.[60]

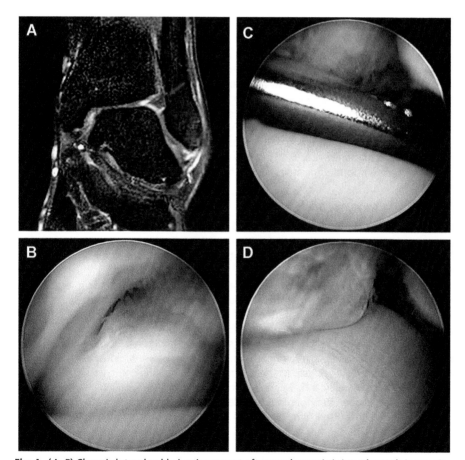

Fig. 4. (*A, B*) Chronic lateral ankle impingement after syndesmotic injury through ingrowing fibrous tissue from the syndesmosis without instability. (*C, D*) Treatment consists of arthroscopic debridement.

Tibiofibular Ossifications and Synostosis

Heterotopic ossifications at the distal tibiofibular joint have been observed in up to 50% of patients with radiographic follow-up after syndesmotic injury.[93] The majority seems to be asymptomatic and the functional impact remains unclear.[94] On CT examination these patients typically display an incomplete synostosis at the level of the syndesmosis and distal IOM and require no further treatment.[32]

The prevalence of a complete tibiofibular synostosis has been reported in 1.7% to 18.2%.[5] Hinds and colleagues,[95] in a study of 564 ankle fractures, identified male sex, syndesmotic screw fixation, and initial tibiofibular dislocation as independent risk factors for the development of a complete synostosis (as seen in 16.1% of all patients) and incomplete bony bridging (seen in 8.2%). Plantarflexion, dorsiflexion, and inversion were significantly reduced by 11%, 6%, and 20%, respectively, in patients with radiographic tibiofibular synostosis. No significant differences in functional outcome were detected between the groups. Karapinar and colleagues[96] noted a higher rate of tibiofibular synostosis but similar functional outcomes at 2 years after quadricortical screw fixation compared with tricortical screw fixation. Similarly, Marvan and colleagues[97] observed similar function in patients with and without complete synostosis, which was observed in 11% of 269 cases. Still, sagittal motion was restricted in 61% of these patients. Albers and colleagues[98] followed 9 patients on average for 14 years after synostosis development. They observed reduced range of motion in 2 patients who developed complications, whereas in 7 uncomplicated patients the dorsiflexion remained equal to the contralateral side. Droog and colleagues[99] observed reduction in dorsiflexion among all patients at an average of 10 years after sustaining an ankle fracture. The reduction was not significantly higher in patients with a complete tibiofibular synostosis (5%), averaging 2.7° in this group. Again, no functional differences were found between patients with and without synostosis.

Painful, complete synostosis should be resected and the debrided areas sealed with bone wax to avoid recurrence.[32,100] In a few reported cases, all patients returned to full activity including sports after resection of the synostosis.[100]

Ligamentous Injury with Static Diastasis

Mechanically relevant ligamentous injury to the syndesmosis will lead to static, frank diastasis of the ankle mortise. Such patients would typically present with more severe symptoms than patients with dynamic diastasis only. The chances for progressing to arthritis are also increased.

Most investigators agree that some form of reduction and fixation is mandatory.[27,50,87,92] The methods, however, vary considerably and range from repeat screw fixation to tibiofibular fusion. Regardless of the method of fixation, a congruent ankle mortise must be restored before fixation, and this typically requires debridement of the syndesmotic area from debris, intervening soft tissue and pannus. If the medial clear space remains wide after syndesmotic reduction, it must be explored and any intervening tissue removed.[5] Repair of the deltoid ligament is only indicated in rare cases of gross medial instability with valgus tilt of the talus.[32]

Arthroscopic or open debridement followed by secondary fixation with syndesmotic screws or suture-button implants has been successfully used by several investigators.[57,87,92,101]

Because the syndesmosis physiologically provides a dynamic stability to the ankle mortise, many investigators have propagated a dynamic ligament reconstruction. Beumer and colleagues[102] reported favorable outcomes in 9 patients treated with medial and proximal advancement of a bone block at the anterior tibial tubercle, thus stretching out the AITFL. A positioning screw was added. These results were confirmed by Wagener and colleagues[86] in another small series of 12 patients. Colcuc and collaborators[57] used one screw and one suture-button for fixation, and Ryan and Rodriguez[87] used 2 to 3 suture buttons. Implants are only removed if symptomatic.

If there is insufficient scar tissue, a graft may be used to replace the syndesmotic ligaments. Options include the peroneus brevis tendon,[103] split peroneus longus tendon,[27] a free hamstring allograft,[104] free semitendinosus tendon autograft,[50] free gracilis autograft,[105] periosteal flap, and plantaris tendon.[57]

The investigators prefer to use a split peroneus longus tendon graft for a near-anatomic reconstruction of the AITFL, IOL, and PITFL at the level of the chronically unstable syndesmosis (**Fig. 5**) in order to reconstruct the 3-point fixation of the distal fibula.[27] Because the peroneus longus tendon contributes less to eversion of the foot than the peroneus brevis tendon and half of the tendon remains in continuity, no functional deficits such as loss of eversion strength or lateral ankle instability have to be expected. The peroneus longus tendon is split from the distal tip of the fibula upwards at a length of 18 cm. The anterior part of the split tendon is guided through 3 bony channels in the distal tibia and fibula mimicking the anatomic conditions of the

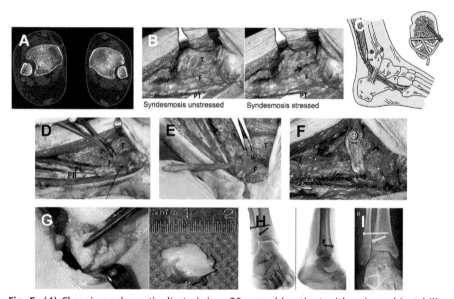

Fig. 5. (A) Chronic syndesmotic diastasis in a 36-year-old patient with pain and instability (same patient as in **Fig. 2**). (B) Intraoperative appearance of the syndesmotic region with external rotation (intraoperative Frick test). (C) Treatment consists of a ligamentoplasty with a split peroneus longus tendon graft. (D) The graft is guided through the oblique fibular tunnel and the tibial tunnel from posterior, replacing the PITFL. (E) The graft is pulled through the straight fibular hole from the tibial canal, thus replacing the interosseous ligament. (F) The graft is then fixed with a screw and washer to the anterior tibial tubercle, replacing the AITFL and resulting in a 3-ligament reconstruction. (G) If the medial clear space remains wide after syndesmosis reduction, it is cleared from debris. (H, I) A syndesmotic screw is placed that may be removed after 8 weeks. F, Fibula; PB, peroneus brevis tendon; PL, peroneus longus tendon; PT, peroneal tendons; T, Tibia. [C] From Rammelt S, Zwipp H, Hansen ST. Posttraumatic reconstruction of the foot and ankle. In: Browner BD, Jupiter JB, Krettek C, Anderson PA (eds.): Skeletal Trauma, 6th Edition, Philadelphia, Elsevier Saunders, 2019, pp 2650; with permission.

syndesmotic complex. The free end of the tendon is then secured with a 3.5-mm cancellous screw and washer inserted obliquely to the tibial canal. The ligamento-plasty is protected by a syndesmosis screw for 8 weeks postoperatively. The results from a first series of 16 patients followed for an average of 18 months were encouraging with 15 out of 16 being relieved of pain and instability.[27] The investigators have meanwhile treated more than 150 patients with that method. Failures were seen in the presence of symptomatic arthritis or bony defects at the distal tibia or fibula at the time of revision surgery. No secondary lateral ankle instability has been noted.

Several investigators have advocated tibiofibular fusion with bone grafting for chronic syndesmotic insufficiency[4,106,107] but only few results have been reported. Katznelson and collaborators[49] saw no recurrences at short-term follow-up in a small series of 5 patients. Olson and colleagues[28] reported favorable results of tibiofibular arthrodesis in 10 patients at a minimum follow-up of 2 years. Three patients required reoperation but no secondary ankle fusion became necessary.

Syndesmotic fusion requires a thorough debridement of the distal tibiofibular syndesmosis from insufficient scar tissue, anatomic reduction of the ankle mortise, and introduction of a bicortical bone block in the clear space between the distal tibia and fibula (**Fig. 6**). The fusion is typically completed with tibiofibular screws that may be connected via a small plate in order to enhance overall stability of the construct.

It should be borne in mind that a tibiofibular synostosis results in a nonphysiological stiffness of the ankle mortise by eliminating the 3-dimensional fibular motion with tibiotalar motion. There is concern that this may lead to subsequent tibiotalar arthritis.[108,109] The scarce clinical data on tibiofibular fusion do not support this notion, showing no progression of arthritis in the medium term.[28,49] In addition, as discussed earlier, spontaneous posttraumatic tibiofibular synostosis rarely becomes symptomatic and typically does not result in significant functional restrictions.[95–97,99]

It also needs to be considered that a limited range of motion is typically present in patients with chronic syndesmotic injury as a result of scarring, altered joint mechanics, and ongoing arthritic changes. In the investigators' experience, successful reconstruction improves function by providing painless and stable joint, but restoration of a full range of motion is not regularly experienced. The authors prefer tibiofibular fusion as a valid salvage option in cases of failed ligamentoplasty or in cases where a ligamentous reconstruction as described earlier is not feasible because of avascular necrosis of the lateral tibial plafond, poor overall bone quality, or severe scarring of the peroneal tendons.

Malunited Avulsions after Malleolar Fracture

The increasing use of CT imaging in the assessment of ankle fractures has increased awareness and understanding of bony syndesmotic avulsions.[54,110,111] These avulsion fractures have been observed since the nineteenth century[2,37] and reproduced experimentally by Lauge-Hansen.[112]

Most of the posterior malleolar fractures, in particular Bartoníček & Rammelt types 2 to 4, can be considered avulsion fractures of the PITFL and therefore destabilize the syndesmosis.[5,53,113] The same is true for the anterior avulsion fragments of the AITFL from the distal tibia or fibula.[35,114]

Reduction and internal fixation of these avulsion fragments is in fact reconstruction of the integrity of the syndesmosis.[5,53] In addition, anatomic reduction of both the anterior and posterior tibial tubercle restores the bony contour of the tibial incisura, thus facilitating fibular reduction at the time of the initial injury. Failure to address these injuries, in turn, frequently leads to fibular and syndesmotic malreduction, potentially resulting in chronic syndesmotic instability.[35,54]

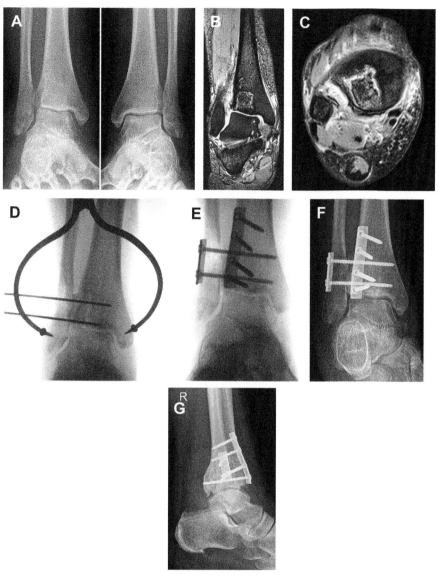

Fig. 6. (*A–C*) Chronic syndesmotic insufficiency in the presence of avascular necrosis of the distal tibia preventing ligamentoplasty in a 76-year-old woman 5 years after pronation abduction stage 3 trimalleolar fracture. (*D, E*) Treatment consists of syndesmosis debridement, curettage of the lateral tibial metaphysis, and tibiofibular fusion with an autologous bone block from the iliac crest. (*F, G*) Radiographs at 12 weeks demonstrate solid fusion and a congruent ankle mortise.

Therefore, the presence of malunited syndesmotic avulsions may be even considered a positive prognostic factor in patients with chronic syndesmotic instability. First, debridement followed by anatomic reduction of the avulsed fragments will result in recreation of the incisura and therefore also anatomic reduction of syndesmosis in most cases (**Fig. 7**). Second, bone-to-bone healing is more reliable than healing of

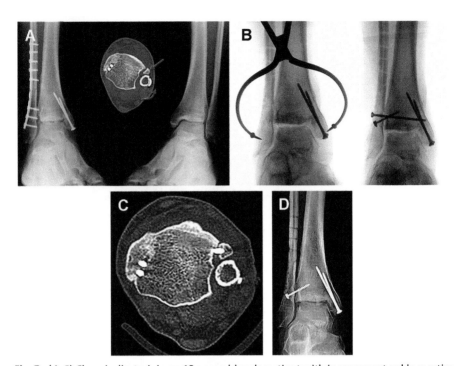

Fig. 7. (*A*, *B*) Chronic diastasis in an 18-year-old male patient with incongruent ankle mortise and first signs of posttraumatic arthritis 1 year after a pronation eternal rotation stage 3 malleolar fracture. CT imaging (insert) shows internal rotation and anterior translation of the distal fibula due to a displaced syndesmotic avulsion from the anterior tibial (Chaput) tubercle. (*B*) Treatment consists of debridement, reduction, and fixation of the anterior tibial tubercle and ankle mortise followed by syndesmotic screw fixation. (*C*) CT imaging after reduction showing correct placement of the fibula within the tibial incisura (notch). (*D*) The syndesmotic screw was removed at 8 weeks postoperatively.

ligamentous tissue. Still, additional placement of either syndesmotic screws or suture button implants is advisable to increase stability in chronic conditions. Both are only removed if symptomatic.

Syndesmotic Insufficiency with Fibular Malunion/Nonunion

As most of the acute syndesmotic injuries occur in the wake of ankle fractures, a substantial number of cases with chronic syndesmotic instability will be accompanied by osseous malunion. Many of these patients underwent operative treatment and have had the implants already removed, as the symptoms were often attributed to their presence.

The prerequisite for successful restitution of the syndesmosis is the ability to restore osseous anatomy and relationship between distal tibia and fibula by the means of a corrective osteotomy. The most common fibular malunion is shortening with external rotation and valgus deformity.[46,52,115,116]

Fibular malunion and nonunion combined with syndesmosis diastasis requires restoration of fibular anatomy as the first step of reconstruction. Yasui and colleagues[105] when performing anatomic syndesmosis reconstruction with a free gracilis autograft performed an additional fibular osteotomy in 3 of 6 cases. Fibular correction follows the principles of corrective osteotomy as laid out in the classic works by Weber[116] and Marti.[52] Lengthening, derotation, and varization of the distal fibula recreates the ankle mortise and adds a lateral restraint against a talar shift.[46,117] Frequently, a lengthening osteotomy of the distal fibula above the syndesmosis will stretch out the scar tissue at the level of the syndesmosis and thus obviate the need of an additional ligamentous reconstruction even in cases of a chronic

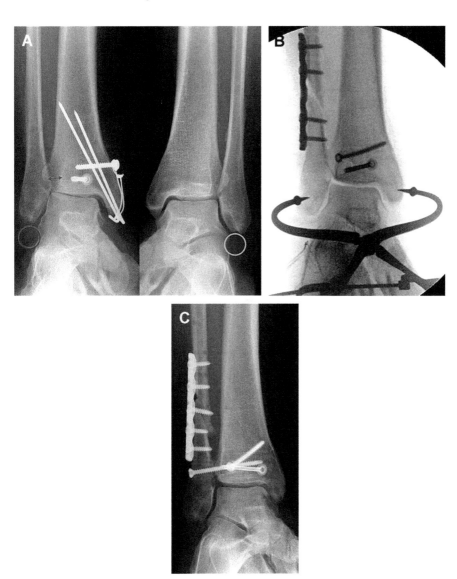

Fig. 8. (*A*) Fibular malunion combined with chronic diastasis of the ligne claire (*double arrow*) in a 44-year-old woman 6 months after internal fixation of a pronation external rotation stage 3 malleolar fracture. Note the Weber circle[4] (dime sign) as a token of fibular shortening. (*B, C*) Both fibular malunion and chronic syndesmotic diastasis need to be addressed. In this case, an oblique lengthening osteotomy of the fibula was combined with a peroneus longus ligamentoplasty[27] as described earlier.

ligamentous instability of the ankle mortise.[51] If widening of the ankle mortise prevails after fibular correction, a syndesmosis ligamentoplasty is added (**Fig. 8**).

Syndesmotic Insufficiency with Ankle Arthritis

Diastasis of the syndesmosis is accompanied by lateral translation of the talus underneath the tibia, which in turn leads to significant reduction in contact area and increase in contact stresses across the ankle joint.[45,79,118,119] This forms a background for rapid onset of posttraumatic ankle arthritis. In an analysis of 735 tibial plafond fractures, failure to detect syndesmosis injuries and syndesmotic avulsions at the distal tibia and fibula was associated with a 95% rate of posttraumatic arthritis, which was significantly higher than that after early detection and treatment after controlling for malreduction.[120] Besides malunion and instability the cartilage damage at the time of the injury and inflammatory mediators play a role in the development of posttraumatic ankle arthritis.[121,122]

If manifest tibiotalar arthritis is present, joint-preserving reconstructions will not lead to substantial improvement of pain and function. When considering the data from studies on malleolar and supramalleolar osteotomies, results are inferior with preexisting Kellgren & Lawrence grade III arthritis at the ankle.[117,123] Therefore, in these cases, fusion or arthroplasty should be considered. The same is true for failed joint-preserving reconstruction of chronic syndesmotic injury.

Comparing the benefits of ankle fusion versus ankle replacement is beyond the scope of this review.[124] In the presence of chronic syndesmotic instability and ankle arthritis, ankle fusion has the potential to correct residual deformity, restore stability, and reduce pain by the time of union in a single procedure.[125,126] If ankle arthroplasty is considered,

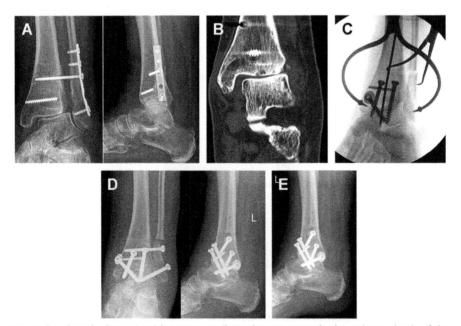

Fig. 9. (*A, B*) Wide diastasis with severe cartilage damage over the lateral two-thirds of the tibial plafond. (*C–E*) Ankle fusion with syndesmotic stabilization remains a valid salvage option in these cases. For that purpose, the original 4-screw technique[125] is modified with addition of a fibular osteotomy and a fifth, tibiofibular screw.

ligamentous stability and ankle and hindfoot alignment have to be restored in either the same surgery or as a staged procedure.[127,128] Because these procedures may be time consuming, staging seems to be a reasonable option. As with purely ligamentous reconstruction, important parameters such as deltoid ligament instability, bone defect, or avascular necrosis of the lateral tibial plafond and any residual fibular deformity must be considered during reconstruction.[126] In the investigators' experience, ankle fusion provides a safe and reliable salvage option for achieving a stable, functional foot and substantial pain relief (**Fig. 9**). It should be particularly considered in patient with significant risk factors such as diabetes and obesity.

SUMMARY

Chronic syndesmotic injury covers a broad range of symptoms and pathologies. The choice of reconstructive procedures for these conditions depends on several factors:

- Pathoanatomy (ligamentous, bony, combined)
- Observation of static/dynamic diastasis
- Presence of symptomatic synostosis
- Presence of syndesmotic avulsions
- Malleolar malunion
- Posttraumatic arthritis
- Comorbidities (diabetes mellitus with complications, obesity, substance abuse/noncompliance)

There is a wide array of treatment options, and treatment must be tailored to the individual pathology and patient characteristics.

Overall, in the current literature, favorable results are reported for the treatment of chronic syndesmotic injury.[29,32,48] However, the evidence is based on retrospective cases series, and comparison between the studies is difficult because of the great variety of pathologies and treatment modalities. In the following section, the investigators' preferred treatment algorithm is provided.

CLINICS CARE POINTS

- *Anterolateral ankle impingement* from scarring after syndesmotic injury in the absence of instability is treated by arthroscopic debridement and arthrolysis. Rarely, takedown of a symptomatic tibiofibular synostosis is warranted.
- *Subacute syndesmotic injuries* are treated by arthroscopic or open debridement followed by secondary stabilization using suture button device or permanent placement of syndesmotic screws.
- *Chronic syndesmotic instability* is treated by a near-anatomic ligamentoplasty supplemented by screw fixation. In case of poor bone stock, failed ligament reconstruction, or comorbidities, tibiofibular fusion with bone grafting is preferred.
- *Malleolar malunions* and particularly anterior or posterior *syndesmotic avulsions* must be corrected in order to achieve a stable and congruent ankle mortise.
- In the presence of *manifest tibiotalar arthritis*, corrective ankle fusion or arthroplasty combined with syndesmotic fusion and deformity correction are salvage options.

DISCLOSURE

Dr S. Rammelt is a paid consultant for KLS Martin and has received travel support by AO Trauma as a member of the AO Foot & Ankle Expert Group and AO Foot & Ankle

Education Task Force. Dr S. Rammelt has no conflict of interest resulted for the purpose of this review. Dr A. Boszczyk provided paid training for Arthrex and Stryker as well as received financial support from Johnson and Johnson devoted to continued education. Dr A. Boszczyk has no conflict of interest resulted for the purpose of this review.

REFERENCES

1. Fick R. Handbuch der Anatomie und Mechanik der Gelenke unter Berücksichtigung der bewegenden Muskeln. Teil I. Jena (DE): Gustav Fischer Verlag; 1904.
2. Chaput V. Les Fractures Malléolaires Du Cou-de-Pied et Les Accidents Du Travail. Paris (FR): Masson; 1907.
3. Quénu E. Du diastasis de l'articulation tibiopéronière inférieure. Rev Chir 1907; 35:897.
4. Weber B. Die Verletzungen des oberen Sprunggelenkes. In: Aktuelle probleme in der Chirurgie. Bern (CH): Huber; 1966. p. 102.
5. Rammelt S, Obruba P. An update on the evaluation and treatment of syndesmotic injuries. Eur J Trauma Emerg Surg 2015;41(6):601–14.
6. Swords MP, Sands A, Shank JR. Late treatment of syndesmotic injuries. Foot Ankle Clin 2017;22(1):65–75.
7. Pettrone FA, Gail M, Pee D, et al. Quantitative criteria for prediction of the results after displaced fracture of the ankle. J Bone Joint Surg Am 1983;65(5):667–77.
8. Chissell HR, Jones J. The influence of a diastasis screw on the outcome of Weber type-C ankle fractures. J Bone Joint Surg Br 1995;77(3):435–8.
9. Kennedy JG, Soffe KE, Dalla Vedova P, et al. Evaluation of the syndesmotic screw in low Weber C ankle fractures. J Orthop Trauma 2000;14(5):359–66.
10. Weening B, Bhandari M. Predictors of functional outcome following transsyndesmotic screw fixation of ankle fractures. J Orthop Trauma 2005;19(2):102–8.
11. Wikerøy AKB, Høiness PR, Andreassen GS, et al. No difference in functional and radiographic results 8.4 years after quadricortical compared with tricortical syndesmosis fixation in ankle fractures. J Orthop Trauma 2010;24(1):17–23.
12. Gardner MJ, Demetrakopoulos D, Briggs SM, et al. Malreduction of the tibiofibular syndesmosis in ankle fractures. Foot Ankle Int 2006;27(10):788–92.
13. Vasarhelyi A, Lubitz J, Gierer P, et al. Detection of fibular torsional deformities after surgery for ankle fractures with a novel CT method. Foot Ankle Int 2006; 27(12):1115–21.
14. Miller AN, Carroll EA, Parker RJ, et al. Posterior malleolar stabilization of syndesmotic injuries is equivalent to screw fixation. Clin Orthop Relat Res 2010;468(4): 1129–35.
15. Sagi HC, Shah AR, Sanders RW. The functional consequence of syndesmotic joint malreduction at a minimum 2-year follow-up. J Orthop Trauma 2012; 26(7):439–43.
16. Cherney SM, Spraggs-Hughes AG, McAndrew CM, et al. Incisura morphology as a risk factor for syndesmotic malreduction. Foot Ankle Int 2016;37(7):748–54.
17. Boszczyk A, Kwapisz S, Krümmel M, et al. Correlation of incisura anatomy with syndesmotic malreduction. Foot Ankle Int 2017;39(3). 1071100717744332.
18. Boszczyk A, Kwapisz S, Krümmel M, et al. Anatomy of the tibial incisura as a risk factor for syndesmotic injury. Foot Ankle Surg 2019;25(1):51–8.
19. Egol KA, Pahk B, Walsh M, et al. Outcome after unstable ankle fracture: effect of syndesmotic stabilization. J Orthop Trauma 2010;24(1):7–11.

20. Berkes MB, Little MTM, Lazaro LE, et al. Articular congruity is associated with short-term clinical outcomes of operatively treated SER IV ankle fractures. J Bone Joint Surg Am 2013;95(19):1769–75.
21. Warner SJ, Garner MR, Hinds RM, et al. Correlation between the Lauge-Hansen classification and ligament injuries in ankle fractures. J Orthop Trauma 2015; 29(12):574–8.
22. Andersen MR, Diep LM, Frihagen F, et al. Importance of syndesmotic reduction on clinical outcome after syndesmosis injuries. J Orthop Trauma 2019;33(8): 397–403.
23. Vetter SY, Euler J, Beisemann N, et al. Validation of radiological reduction criteria with intraoperative cone beam CT in unstable syndesmotic injuries. Eur J Trauma Emerg Surg 2020. https://doi.org/10.1007/s00068-020-01299-z.
24. Driesman AS, Egol KA. An update on the treatment of malleolar fractures. Fuss-Sprungg 2016;14(2):55–65.
25. Tornetta PIII, Axelrad TW, Sibai TA, et al. Treatment of the stress positive ligamentous se4 ankle fracture: incidence of syndesmotic injury and clinical decision making. J Orthop Trauma 2012;26(11):659–61.
26. Ogilvie-Harris DJ, Reed SC. Disruption of the ankle syndesmosis: diagnosis and treatment by arthroscopic surgery. Arthroscopy 1994;10(5):561–8.
27. Grass R, Rammelt S, Biewener A, et al. Peroneus longus ligamentoplasty for chronic instability of the distal tibiofibular syndesmosis. Foot Ankle Int 2003; 24(5):392–7.
28. Olson KM, Dairyko GH, Toolan BC. Salvage of chronic instability of the syndesmosis with distal tibiofibular arthrodesis: functional and radiographic results. J Bone Joint Surg Am 2011;93(1):66–72.
29. Krähenbühl N, Weinberg MW, Hintermann B, et al. Surgical outcome in chronic syndesmotic injury: a systematic literature review. Foot Ankle Surg 2019;25(5): 691–7.
30. Bartoníček J. Anatomy of the tibiofibular syndesmosis and its clinical relevance. Surg Radiol Anat 2003;25(5–6):379–86.
31. Lilyquist M, Shaw A, Latz K, et al. Cadaveric analysis of the distal tibiofibular syndesmosis. Foot Ankle Int 2016;37(8):882–90.
32. Rammelt S, Zwipp H, Grass R. Injuries to the distal tibiofibular syndesmosis: an evidence-based approach to acute and chronic lesions. Foot Ankle Clin 2008; 13(4):611–33.
33. Massri-Pugin J, Lubberts B, Vopat BG, et al. Role of the deltoid ligament in syndesmotic instability. Foot Ankle Int 2018;39(5):598–603.
34. Weber M. Trimalleolar fractures with impaction of the posteromedial tibial plafond: implications for talar stability. Foot Ankle Int 2004;25(10):716–27.
35. Marx C, Schaser KD, Rammelt S. Early corrections after failed ankle fracture fixation. Z Orthop Unfall 2020. https://doi.org/10.1055/a-1079-6476.
36. Hoefnagels EM, Waites MD, Wing ID, et al. Biomechanical comparison of the interosseous tibiofibular ligament and the anterior tibiofibular ligament. Foot Ankle Int 2007;28(5):602–4.
37. Le Fort L. Note on an undescribed variety of vertical fracture of the lateral malleolus by avulsion. Bull Gen Ther 1886;110:193–9.
38. Bartoníček J. Avulsed posterior edge of the tibia. Earle's or Volkmann's triangle? J Bone Joint Surg Br 2004;86(5):746–50.
39. Haraguchi N, Haruyama H, Toga H, et al. Pathoanatomy of posterior malleolar fractures of the ankle. J Bone Joint Surg Am 2006;88(5):1085–92.

40. Bartoníček J, Rammelt S, Kostlivý K, et al. Anatomy and classification of the posterior tibial fragment in ankle fractures. Arch Orthop Trauma Surg 2015;135(4): 505–16.
41. Bartoníček J, Rammelt S, Tuček M, et al. Posterior malleolar fractures of the ankle. Eur J Trauma Emerg Surg 2015;41(6):587–600.
42. Sultan F, Zheng X, Pan Z, et al. Characteristics of intercalary fragment in posterior malleolus fractures. Foot Ankle Surg 2019. [Epub ahead of print].
43. Edwards GS, DeLee JC. Ankle diastasis without fracture. Foot Ankle 1984;4(6): 305–12.
44. Frick H. Diagnosis, therapy and results of acute instability of the syndesmosis of the upper ankle joint (isolated anterior rupture of the syndesmosis) [in German]. Orthopade 1986;15(6):423–6.
45. Xenos JS, Hopkinson WJ, Mulligan ME, et al. The tibiofibular syndesmosis. Evaluation of the ligamentous structures, methods of fixation, and radiographic assessment. J Bone Joint Surg Am 1995;77(6):847–56.
46. Rammelt S, Zwipp H, Mittlmeier T. Operative treatment of pronation fracture–dislocations of the ankle [in German]. Oper Orthop Traumatol 2013;25(3):273–93.
47. Boszczyk A, Fudalej M, Kwapisz S, et al. Ankle fracture - correlation of Lauge-Hansen classification and patient reported fracture mechanism. Forensic Sci Int 2018;282:94–100.
48. van den Bekerom MPJ, de Leeuw PAJ, van Dijk CN. Delayed operative treatment of syndesmotic instability. Current concepts review. Injury 2009;40(11): 1137–42.
49. Katznelson A, Lin E, Militiano J. Ruptures of the ligaments about the tibio-fibular syndesmosis. Injury 1983;15(3):170–2.
50. Zamzami MM, Zamzam MM. Chronic isolated distal tibiofibular syndesmotic disruption: diagnosis and management. Foot Ankle Surg 2009;15(1):14–9.
51. Marti RK, Raaymakers ELFB, Rammelt S. Rekonstruktion fehlverheilter Sprunggelenkfrakturen. FussSprung 2009;7(2):78–87.
52. Marti RK, Raaymakers EL, Nolte PA. Malunited ankle fractures. The late results of reconstruction. J Bone Joint Surg Br 1990;72(4):709–13.
53. Bartoníček J, Rammelt S, Tuček M. Posterior malleolar fractures: changing concepts and recent developments. Foot Ankle Clin 2017;22(1):125–45.
54. Rammelt S, Boszczyk A. Computed tomography in the diagnosis and treatment of ankle fractures: a critical analysis review. JBJS Rev 2018;6(12):e7.
55. Mendelsohn ES, Hoshino CM, Harris TG, et al. The effect of obesity on early failure after operative syndesmosis injuries. J Orthop Trauma 2013;27(4):201–6.
56. Rammelt S. Management of ankle fractures in the elderly. EFORT Open Rev 2016;1(5):239–46.
57. Colcuc C, Fischer S, Colcuc S, et al. Treatment strategies for partial chronic instability of the distal syndesmosis: an arthroscopic grading scale and operative staging concept. Arch Orthop Trauma Surg 2016;136(2):157–63.
58. Kiter E, Bozkurt M. The crossed-leg test for examination of ankle syndesmosis injuries. Foot Ankle Int 2005;26(2):187–8.
59. Williams GN, Jones MH, Amendola A. Syndesmotic ankle sprains in athletes. Am J Sports Med 2007;35(7):1197–207.
60. Han SH, Lee JW, Kim S, et al. Chronic tibiofibular syndesmosis injury: the diagnostic efficiency of magnetic resonance imaging and comparative analysis of operative treatment. Foot Ankle Int 2007;28(3):336–42.
61. Mukhopadhyay S, Metcalfe A, Guha AR, et al. Malreduction of syndesmosis–are we considering the anatomical variation? Injury 2011;42(10):1073–6.

62. Anand Prakash A. Syndesmotic stability: is there a radiological normal?—a systematic review. Foot Ankle Surg 2018;24(3):174–84.
63. Harper MC, Keller TS. A radiographic evaluation of the tibiofibular syndesmosis. Foot Ankle 1989;10(3):156–60.
64. Ostrum RF, De Meo P, Subramanian R. A critical analysis of the anterior-posterior radiographic anatomy of the ankle syndesmosis. Foot Ankle Int 1995;16(3): 128–31.
65. Shah AS, Kadakia AR, Tan GJ, et al. Radiographic evaluation of the normal distal tibiofibular syndesmosis. Foot Ankle Int 2012;33(10):870–6.
66. Nault M, Hébert-Davies J, Laflamme G-Y, et al. CT scan assessment of the syndesmosis: a new reproducible method. J Orthop Trauma 2013;27(11):638–41.
67. Grenier S, Benoit B, Rouleau DM, et al. APTF: anteroposterior tibiofibular ratio, a new reliable measure to assess syndesmotic reduction. J Orthop Trauma 2013; 27(4):207–11.
68. Beumer A, Valstar ER, Garling EH, et al. Effects of ligament sectioning on the kinematics of the distal tibiofibular syndesmosis: a radiostereometric study of 10 cadaveric specimens based on presumed trauma mechanisms with suggestions for treatment. Acta Orthop 2006;77(3):531–40.
69. Bartoníček J, Rammelt S, Kašper Š, et al. Pathoanatomy of Maisonneuve fracture based on radiologic and CT examination. Arch Orthop Trauma Surg 2019;139(4):497–506.
70. Ebraheim NA, Lu J, Yang H, et al. The fibular incisure of the tibia on CT scan: a cadaver study. Foot Ankle Int 1998;19:318–21.
71. Elgafy H, Semaan HB, Blessinger B. Computed tomography of normal distal tibiofibular syndesmosis. Skeletal Radiol 2010;39(6):559–64.
72. Mendelsohn ES, Hoshino CM, Harris TG, et al. CT characterizing the anatomy of uninjured ankle syndesmosis. Orthopedics 2014;37(2):157–60.
73. Phisitkul P, Ebinger T, Goetz J, et al. Forceps reduction of the syndesmosis in rotational ankle fractures: a cadaveric study. J Bone Joint Surg Am 2012; 94(24):2256–61.
74. Ebinger T, Goetz J, Dolan L, et al. 3D model analysis of existing CT syndesmosis measurements. Iowa Orthop J 2013;33:40–6.
75. Höcker K, Pachucki A. The fibular incisure of the tibia. The cross-sectional position of the fibula in distal syndesmosis [in German]. Unfallchirurgie 1989;92(8): 401–6.
76. Summers HD, Sinclair MK, Stover MD. A reliable method for intraoperative evaluation of syndesmotic reduction. J Orthop Trauma 2013;27(4):196–200.
77. Franke J, von Recum J, Suda AJ, et al. Intraoperative three-dimensional imaging in the treatment of acute unstable syndesmotic injuries. J Bone Joint Surg Am 2012;94(15):1386–90.
78. Dikos GD, Heisler J, Choplin RH, et al. Normal tibiofibular relationships at the syndesmosis on axial CT imaging. J Orthop Trauma 2012;26(7):433–8.
79. Thordarson DB, Motamed S, Hedman T, et al. The effect of fibular malreduction on contact pressures in an ankle fracture malunion model. J Bone Joint Surg Am 1997;79(12):1809–15.
80. Hagemeijer NC, Chang SH, Abdelaziz ME, et al. Range of normal and abnormal syndesmotic measurements using weightbearing CT. Foot Ankle Int 2019; 40(12):1430–7.
81. Osgood GM, Shakoor D, Orapin J, et al. Reliability of distal tibio-fibular syndesmotic instability measurements using weightbearing and non-weightbearing cone-beam CT. Foot Ankle Surg 2019;25(6):771–81.

82. Malhotra K, Welck M, Cullen N, et al. The effects of weight bearing on the distal tibiofibular syndesmosis: a study comparing weight bearing-CT with conventional CT. Foot Ankle Surg 2019;25(4):511–6.

83. Krähenbühl N, Bailey TL, Weinberg MW, et al. Is load application necessary when using computed tomography scans to diagnose syndesmotic injuries? a cadaver study. Foot Ankle Surg 2020;26(2):198–204.

84. Jain SK, Kearns SR. Ligamentous advancement for the treatment of subacute syndesmotic injuries. Report of a new technique in 5 cases. Foot Ankle Surg 2014;20(4):281–4.

85. Krähenbühl N, Weinberg MW, Davidson NP, et al. Imaging in syndesmotic injury: a systematic literature review. Skeletal Radiol 2018;47(5):631–48.

86. Wagener ML, Beumer A, Swierstra BA. Chronic instability of the anterior tibiofibular syndesmosis of the ankle. Arthroscopic findings and results of anatomical reconstruction. BMC Musculoskelet Disord 2011;12(1):212.

87. Ryan PM, Rodriguez RM. Outcomes and return to activity after operative repair of chronic latent syndesmotic instability. Foot Ankle Int 2016;37(2):192–7.

88. Lambers KTA, Saarig A, Turner H, et al. Prevalence of osteochondral lesions in rotational type ankle fractures with syndesmotic injury. Foot Ankle Int 2019;40(2): 159–66.

89. Gerber JP, Williams GN, Scoville CR, et al. Persistent disability associated with ankle sprains: a prospective examination of an athletic population. Foot Ankle Int 1998;19(10):653–60.

90. Amendola A, Williams G, Foster D. Evidence-based approach to treatment of acute traumatic syndesmosis (high ankle) sprains. Sports Med Arthrosc Rev 2006;14(4):232–6.

91. Ogilvie-Harris DJ, Gilbart MK, Chorney K. Chronic pain following ankle sprains in athletes: the role of arthroscopic surgery. Arthroscopy 1997;13(5):564–74.

92. Schuberth JM, Jennings MM, Lau AC. Arthroscopy-assisted repair of latent syndesmotic instability of the ankle. Arthroscopy 2008;24(8):868–74.

93. Taylor DC, Englehardt DL, Bassett FH. Syndesmosis sprains of the ankle. The influence of heterotopic ossification. Am J Sports Med 1992;20(2):146–50.

94. Hopkinson WJ, Pierre P St, Ryan JB, et al. Syndesmosis sprains of the ankle. Foot Ankle 1990;10(6):325–30.

95. Hinds RM, Lazaro LE, Burket JC, et al. Risk factors for posttraumatic synostosis and outcomes following operative treatment of ankle fractures. Foot Ankle Int 2014;35(2):141–7.

96. Karapinar H, Kalenderer O, Karapinar L, et al. Effects of three- or four-cortex syndesmotic fixation in ankle fractures. J Am Podiatr Med Assoc 2007;97(6): 457–9.

97. Marvan J, Dzupa V, Krbec M, et al. Distal tibiofibular synostosis after surgically resolved ankle fractures: an epidemiological, clinical and morphological evaluation of a patient sample. Injury 2016;47(11):2570–4.

98. Albers GH, de Kort AF, Middendorf PR, et al. Distal tibiofibular synostosis after ankle fracture. A 14-year follow-up study. J Bone Joint Surg Br 1996;78(2): 250–2.

99. Droog R, Verhage SM, Hoogendoorn JM. Incidence and clinical relevance of tibiofibular synostosis in fractures of the ankle which have been treated surgically. Bone Joint J 2015;97-B(7):945–9.

100. Veltri DM, Pagnani MJ, O'Brien SJ, et al. Symptomatic ossification of the tibiofibular syndesmosis in professional football players: a sequela of the syndesmotic ankle sprain. Foot Ankle Int 1995;16(5):285–90.

101. Harper MC. Delayed reduction and stabilization of the tibiofibular syndesmosis. Foot Ankle Int 2001;22(1):15–8.
102. Beumer A, Heijboer RP, Fontijne WP, et al. Late reconstruction of the anterior distal tibiofibular syndesmosis: good outcome in 9 patients. Acta Orthop Scand 2000;71(5):519–21.
103. Castaing J, Le Chevallier PL, Meunier M. Repeated sprain or recurring subluxation of the tibio-tarsal joint. A simple technic of external ligamentoplasty. Rev Chir Orthop Reparatrice Appar Mot 1961;47:598–608 [in French].
104. Morris MWJ, Rice P, Schneider TE. Distal tibiofibular syndesmosis reconstruction using a free hamstring autograft. Foot Ankle Int 2009;30(6):506–11.
105. Yasui Y, Takao M, Miyamoto W, et al. Anatomical reconstruction of the anterior inferior tibiofibular ligament for chronic disruption of the distal tibiofibular syndesmosis. Knee Surg Sports Traumatol Arthrosc 2011;19(4):691–5.
106. Outland T. Sprains and separations of the inferior tibiofibular joint without important fracture. Am J Surg 1943;59(2):320–9.
107. Loder BG, Frascone ST, Wertheimer SJ. Tibiofibular arthrodesis for malunion of the talocrural joint. J Foot Ankle Surg 1995;34(3):283–8.
108. Ney R, Jend JJ, Schöntag H. Tibiofibular mobility and arthrosis in patients with postoperative ossification in the area of syndesmosis of the upper ankle joint [in German]. Unfallchirurgie 1987;13(5):274–7.
109. Peña FA, Coetzee JC. Ankle syndesmosis injuries. Foot Ankle Clin 2006;11(1): 35–50, viii.
110. Birnie MFN, van Schilt KLJ, Sanders FRK, et al. Anterior inferior tibiofibular ligament avulsion fractures in operatively treated ankle fractures: a retrospective analysis. Arch Orthop Trauma Surg 2019;139(6):787–93.
111. Rammelt S. Malleolar fractures. In: Rammelt S, Swords M, Dhillon M, et al, editors. Manual of fracture management - foot and ankle. Stuttgart (NY): Thieme; 2020. p. 115–30.
112. Lauge-Hansen N. Fractures of the ankle. II. Combined experimental-surgical and experimental-roentgenologic investigations. Arch Surg 1950;60(5):957–85.
113. Gardner MJ, Brodsky A, Briggs SM, et al. Fixation of posterior malleolar fractures provides greater syndesmotic stability. Clin Orthop Relat Res 2006;447: 165–71.
114. Kamin K, Notov D, Al-Sadi O, et al. Treatment of ankle fractures: standards, tricks and pitfalls [in German]. Unfallchirurg 2020;123(1):43–56.
115. Ovaska MT, Mäkinen TJ, Madanat R, et al. A comprehensive analysis of patients with malreduced ankle fractures undergoing re-operation. Int Orthop 2014; 38(1):83–8.
116. Weber BG. Lengthening osteotomy of the fibula to correct a widened mortice of the ankle after fracture. Int Orthop 1981;4(4):289–93.
117. Weber D, Weber M. Corrective osteotomies for malunited malleolar fractures. Foot Ankle Clin 2016;21(1):37–48.
118. Ramsey PL, Hamilton W. Changes in tibiotalar area of contact caused by lateral talar shift. J Bone Joint Surg Am 1976;58(3):356–7.
119. Leeds HC, Ehrlich MG. Instability of the distal tibiofibular syndesmosis after bimalleolar and trimalleolar ankle fractures. J Bone Joint Surg Am 1984;66(4): 490–503.
120. Haller JM, Githens M, Rothberg D, et al. Syndesmosis and syndesmotic equivalent injuries in tibial plafond fractures. J Orthop Trauma 2019;33(3):e74–8.

121. Godoy-Santos AL, Ranzoni L, Teodoro WR, et al. Increased cytokine levels and histological changes in cartilage, synovial cells and synovial fluid after malleolar fractures. Injury 2017;48:S27–33.

122. Godoy-Santos AL, Lopes D, Giarola I, et al. Changes in cartilage, synovial cells and synovial fluid after malleolar fractures: what its importance for post-traumatic ankle osteoarthitis? FussSprung 2019;17(2):68–74.

123. Reidsma II, Nolte PA, Marti RK, et al. Treatment of malunited fractures of the ankle: a long-term follow-up of reconstructive surgery. J Bone Joint Surg Br 2010;92(1):66–70.

124. Barg A, Wimmer MD, Wiewiorski M, et al. Total ankle replacement. Dtsch Arztebl Int 2015;112(11):177–84.

125. Zwipp H, Rammelt S, Endres T, et al. High union rates and function scores at midterm followup with ankle arthrodesis using a four screw technique. Clin Orthop Relat Res 2010;468(4):958–68.

126. Swords M, Brilhault J, Sands A. Acute and chronic syndesmotic injury: the authors' approach to treatment. Foot Ankle Clin 2018;23(4):625–37.

127. Hobson SA, Karantana A, Dhar S. Total ankle replacement in patients with significant pre-operative deformity of the hindfoot. J Bone Jointt Surg Br 2009; 91(4):481–6.

128. Queen RM, Adams SB, Viens NA, et al. Differences in outcomes following total ankle replacement in patients with neutral alignment compared with tibiotalar joint malalignment. J Bone Joint Surg Am 2013;95(21):1927–34.

Talar Neck Fractures: Single or Double Approach?

Florencio Pablo Segura, MD[a,b,*], Santiago Eslava, MD[c]

KEYWORDS

- Displaced talar neck fractures • Open reduction and fixation • Surgical approaches

KEY POINTS

- Correct approach selection in talar neck injuries is crucial to obtain adequate access to the entire fracture site avoiding malreduction and angular deformity.
- The major concern about a single incision technique is lack of visualization.
- Combined lateral and medial approaches are strongly recommended in complex talar neck fractures providing better control of dorsal and varus displacement of the talar head.
- The major discussion in the literature about combining double approach is preservation of talus vascularity.
- Soft tissues surrounding the talus must be preserved, in particular posteromedial vessels from posterior tibial artery at the tarsal canal that provide the majority of the blood supply.

INTRODUCTION

Surgical treatment of displaced talar neck fractures is among the most challenging procedures in foot and ankle trauma for several reasons: their relative infrequency (1%–3% of all foot and ankle fractures)[1]; high-energy mechanism usually involved; and a unique anatomic feature of the talus, including no muscle or tendon attachments, two-thirds of its surface covered by articular cartilage and a particular vascular supply.[2–4]

Approach selection is crucial as is precise planning of fracture reduction and fixation for return to optimal function. Adequate visualization may prevent articular malreduction or malalignment when certain degree of collapse is overlook and minimize complications, such as posttraumatic arthritis or malunion including rotational or varus deviation.[2–6]

[a] Department of Orthopaedics, Faculty of Medicine, Universidad Nacional de Córdoba, Nuevo Hospital San Roque, Bajada Pucará 1900, Piso 6, Ciudad de Córdoba, CP 5000, Argentina; [b] Centro Privado de Ortopedia y Traumatología, Urquiza 358, Piso 8, Ciudad de Córdoba, CP 5000, Argentina; [c] Foot and Ankle Division, Instituto Dupuytren, Av. Belgrano 3402, Ciudad Autónoma de Buenos Aires, CP 1078, Argentina
* Corresponding author.
E-mail address: fpablosegura@gmail.com

Foot Ankle Clin N Am 25 (2020) 653–665
https://doi.org/10.1016/j.fcl.2020.08.007
1083-7515/20/© 2020 Elsevier Inc. All rights reserved.
foot.theclinics.com

This article describes different surgical approaches for talar neck fractures and provides selection criteria that could help as guidelines for each fracture pattern.

ANATOMIC CONSIDERATIONS

Osteonecrosis is a devastating complication: in some recent studies using combined lateral and medial incisions, it may be expected up to 30% to 50% of talar neck fractures.[3,7,8] It is also suggested that depending on which incision is performed, it can increase the risk of diminishing blood supply to the talar body.[9]

For this reason, a thorough knowledge of talus body's extraosseous and intraosseous blood supply is necessary to not increase the risk of vascular damage.

Extraosseous Vascularity

Since the first publication by Lexer and colleagues in 1904,[10] many investigators described talar vascular supply. It is well known that the 3 major arteries that irrigate the talar body are the dorsalis pedis, the posterior tibial artery, and the perforating peroneal artery, originating a complex and rich extraosseous network. Little irrigation is provided from ligament and other soft tissue attachments. The major component of this network is the connection between the tarsal canal artery, arising from posterior tibial artery 1 cm proximal to the medial and lateral plantar arteries, and the artery of the sinus tarsi, a branch of perforating peroneal artery, providing most of blood supply to the talar body. There also is an important connection between vessels from the peroneal artery and calcaneal branches of the posterior tibial artery at the posterior tubercle of the talus (**Fig. 1**).[11–13]

With three-fifths of talar surface covered by cartilage, only a small amount of bone can be perforated by small vessels of these main arteries creating vascular foramina, small tunnels through the cortex of the nonarticular surface that provide the entrance to the medullary bone. Cadaveric studies found the highest amount and density of them in the inferior talar neck from vessels arising from the connection of tarsal canal and sinus tarsi arteries. Foramina also are described in 4 other regions: the superior neck, the transition zone of the sinus tali to the talus neck (both from branches of dorsalis pedis artery), the medial facet of the talus directly beneath the articular surface (from deltoid branch of posterior tibial artery), and the posterior process (**Fig. 2**).[14,15]

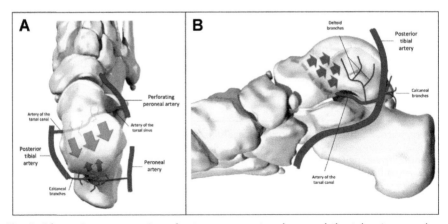

Fig. 1. Schematic representation of extraosseous network around the talus. Large red arrows show main retrograde flow to the body from connection between tarsal canal artery-artery of the tarsal sinus. (*A*) Superior view. (*B*) Medial view.

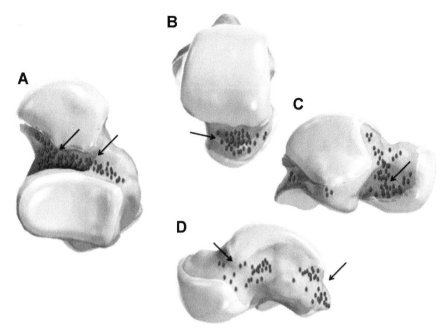

Fig. 2. Schematic representation of vascular foramina of the talus. (*A*) Vascular foramina of the sulcus tali. (*B*) Vascular foramina on the superior neck, (*C*) sinus tarsi, and (*D*) medial surface of the body: note the lower amount and density in comparison to the sulcus tali.

Intraosseous Vascularity

The tarsal canal artery is the single major source blood supply to the body of the talus, providing one-half to two-thirds of its surface. There are other minor contributions from posterior tibial artery branches: the deltoid branch—that gives the medial one-third of the body—and the posterior tubercle branches—which supplies a small region of the posterior tubercle and have communications with the tarsal canal artery determining an antegrade flow. The only area of the talus body that does not depend on posterior tibial artery is the lateral one-fifth, supplied by branches of the sinus tarsi artery (**Fig. 3**).[9,11–13]

This higher qualitative contribution of posteromedial vessels is also reflected quantitatively in the literature: in a cadaveric study using gadolinium-enhanced magnetic resonance imaging of the talus, Miller and colleagues[9] determined that, on average, the posterior tibial artery supplied 47.0%. of the total vascularity of the talus, the anterior tibial artery 36.2%, and the peroneal artery 16.9%.

In summary, much of the arterial supply of the talus body comes from posteromedial vessels, with the posterior tibial artery the main contributor, with entry points at tarsal canal, medial body's surface, and posterior tubercle. Care should be taken respect the surrounding soft tissues, particularly at the posteromedial side, where the deltoid branch and the tarsal canal artery always should be preserved.

SURGICAL TECHNIQUES AND CURRENT EVIDENCE

Although there is increasing support in literature of combining lateral and medial approaches for talar neck fractures, some controversy remains on when to use 1 or 2 incisions.

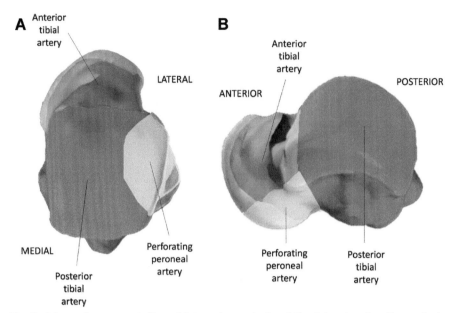

Fig. 3. Schematic representation of internal vascularity of the talus showing the posterior tibial artery and branches as the major blood source to the body of the talus. (*A*) Dorsal view. (*B*) Medial view.

Single Approach

The most frequent single approach described in literature is the anteromedial.[3,16–19] The incision is sharply made between the anterior and posterior tibial tendons behind the saphenous nerve and vein, giving access to the most inferomedial aspect of the dorsal neck. Typically, it starts over the medial malleolus, progressing slightly curved to the navicular tuberosity (**Fig. 4**). It can be extended proximally if a chevron-type malleolus osteotomy is added, allowing excellent visualization of the entire medial side of

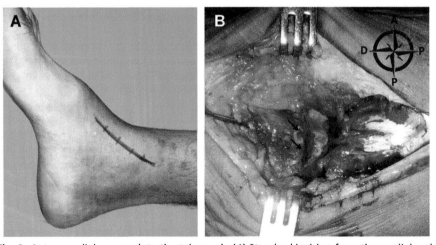

Fig. 4. Anteromedial approach to the talar neck. (*A*) Standard incision from the medial malleollus to the navicular. (*B*) Intraoperative view of the fracture line (*arrows*).

the talus. Oblique cuts are made with the tip a little above the articular line, descending posteriorly to the medial malleolus and anteriorly to the tibial plafond. Predrilling of 2 parallel holes for further fixation with two 4.0-mm cancellous screws decreases the risk of secondary displacement (**Fig. 5**).[20]

An alternative single approach described is the anterior.[17,21] Soft tissues are dissected through the interval between the anterior tibial and extensor hallucis longus tendons. The incision starts approximately 3 cm proximal to the ankle joint just lateral to the palpable tibial crest and runs straight over the ankle joint following the lateral margin of the anterior tibial tendon, allowing good exposure of the dorsal talar neck but limited of both talar sides (**Fig. 6**).

The major concern about a single approach technique is lack of visualization: full extension of the fracture site cannot be seen and checked during or after reduction maneuvers.[16–21] Even though medial or superior cortex of the talar neck may look perfectly aligned through an isolated anteromedial or anterior approach, an opening of the fracture line with loss of contact of the main fragments on the lateral side or tilting of the distal fragment in supination or pronation can occur (**Fig. 7**). This situation is more likely to happen when some comminution is present, because the talar shape is complex and difficult to reconstruct even for the most experienced surgeons and hard to evaluate with fluoroscopy during surgery. Eventual bone loss of very thin intermediate fragments and inappropriate compression results in shortening of the neck or, worse, in tilting of the cervicocephalic fragment, by opening the opposite side.[16–21]

Therefore, the single approach technique could be recommended only for simple vertical talar neck fractures with no conminution and minimum initial displacement (**Fig 8**).

Combined Lateral and Medial Approach

For the past 20 years, the literature has strongly recommended combined lateral and medial approaches for surgical treatment of talar neck fractures.[1–3,5,6,8,17–19,22–28]

Better control of fracture reduction and visualization of both sides are possible with a dual-access technique, especially in complex patterns (**Fig. 9**), avoiding residual displacement, which invariably is associated with poor functional outcome. In a cadaveric study, slight dorsal or varus 2-mm malreductions were found to alter

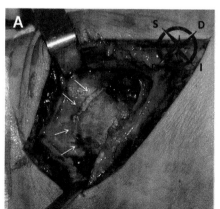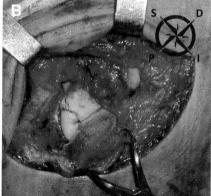

Fig. 5. Extended anteromedial approach to the talar neck with medial malleolus osteotomy. (*A*) Chevron-type cut with the tip above tibial plafond. (*B*) Distal fragment moved distally giving access to body's fracture line extension.

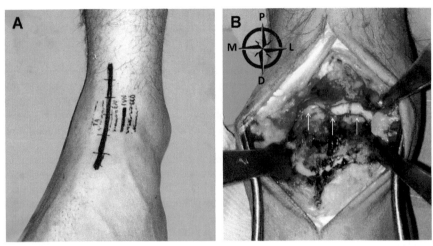

Fig. 6. Anterior approach to the talar neck. (*A*) Incision between the anterior tibial and extensor hallucis longus tendons. (*B*) Intraoperative view of the dorsal tarsal neck with the fracture line (*arrows*).

subtalar joint congruency and, therefore, joint motion, leading to arthritis in 32% of talar neck fractures.[18] Some investigators recommend a combined approach even in simple vertical talar neck fractures, because in most cases anatomic alignment was supposed to be achieved with a single medial access but an imperfection or lack of reduction was found only after the second incision was made, which otherwise would have been overlooked.[17]

A lateral approach is carried out first because usually this is the tension side of the neck and no comminution is found; thus, the most accurate initial indication of the extent of fracture displacement or rotational malalignment is found laterally. There also is a relatively thickened cortical bone spur, which often provides a key to reduction and temporary pin stabilization in most cases (**Fig. 10**).[29]

Several different lateral accesses are described but 2 are cited more often in the literature.

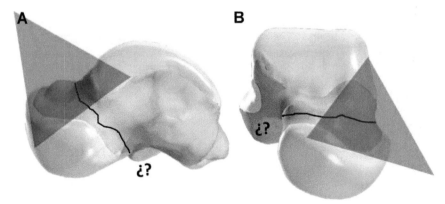

Fig. 7. Direct viewing area by a single approach. (*A*) Dorsal or (*B*) medial side of the neck can be accessed, but full extension of the fracture site cannot be seen.

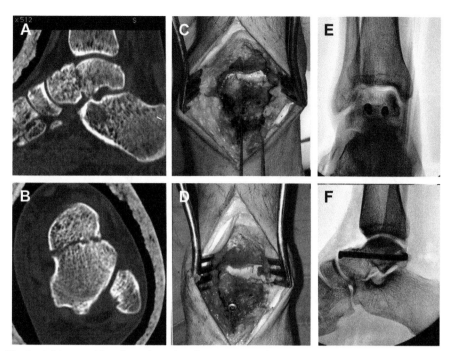

Fig. 8. A 24-year-old male patient. (*A*, *B*) CT scanning shows a simple vertical talar neck fracture with no comminution and minimum initial displacement. (*C*, *D*) Intraoperative views of the reduction and fixation by a single anterior approach. (*E*, *F*) Anatomic reduction confirmed fluoroscopically.

The Ollier approach is more effective for some investigators.[17,30] An incision is performed from the tip of the lateral malleolus to the neck of the talus. Inferior extensor retinaculum is divided, and peroneus tertius and extensor digitorum longus are identified and retracted medially in the superior (distal) part and peroneal tendons posteriorly in the inferior (proximal) part. After partially resecting fat pad over sinus tarsi and detaching and reflecting distally the origin of extensor digitorum brevis, the lateral talar neck can be accessed.

The classic sagittal anterolateral approach (Böhler approach) appears to be more anatomic.[5,6,17–19,22–28] Incision is performed slightly curved from the anterolateral corner of the ankle joint in line with the extensor digitorum longus and peroneus tertius tendons, running toward the sinus tarsi and the base of the fourth metatarsal. Superficial dissection continues to the extensor retinaculum and tendon sheath of the extensor digitorum longus and peroneus tertius tendons. Care is taken to avoid violation of the superficial peroneal nerve proximally. The tendon sheath is incised at the lateral margin of the tendons, and deep dissection is continued to the joint capsules of the ankle and subtalar joints proximally and the extensor digitorum brevis muscle distally. The extensor brevis muscle then is reflected plantarly, thereby exposing the distal portion of the lateral talar neck. The capsules of the ankle and subtalar joints are released dorsally and plantarly, thereby completing a full-thickness flap (**Fig. 11**). If necessary, this approach can be extended proximally with a lateral malleolus osteotomy.

Both lateral approaches provide a clear view of the posterior subtalar facet to ensure that it can be adequately reduced.[5,6,17–19,22–28]

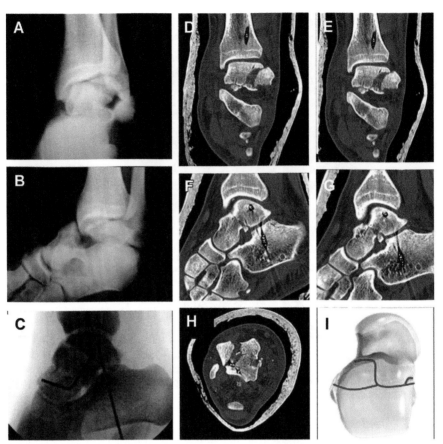

Fig. 9. A 22-year-old male patient. (*A, B*) Initial radiographs. (*C*) Emergency reduction confirmed fluoroscopically. (*D–H*) Post-reduction CT scan shows a complex talar neck fracture with medial comminution and body extension. (*I*) Schematic representation of the fracture pattern.

The anteromedial approach then is initiated, and superficial dissection continues to the extensor retinaculum and joint capsule of the ankle proximally and the talonavicular joint capsule and dorsal margin of the posterior tibial tendon sheath distally (**Fig. 12**).

Fracture reduction must be achieved going from side to side until it is visualized anatomically. The posterior subtalar joint always should be checked by the lateral approach and the medial aspect through the anteromedial access. Definitive fixation is made after perfect reduction of the fracture is obtained (**Fig. 13**). It is recommended to insert the first screw from lateral, because usually there is no comminution in this side of the neck and purchase is better into the thicker cortical bone of this area.[17]

The major concern with a combined medial and lateral approach is the potential threat to talus vascularity, deteriorating the already damaged soft tissue and bloody supply of the talar body.[27,31] Theoretically, the additional surgical insult could increase the potential for the development of osteonecrosis, although this never has been demonstrated.[19,26] Limited soft tissue stripping is mandatory to preserve periosteal

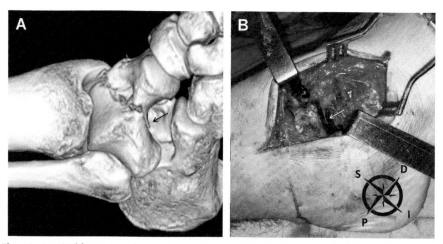

Fig. 10. Cortical bone spur (*arrows*) usually present in the lateral neck. (*A*) A 3-dimensional scan view. (*B*) Intraoperative view.

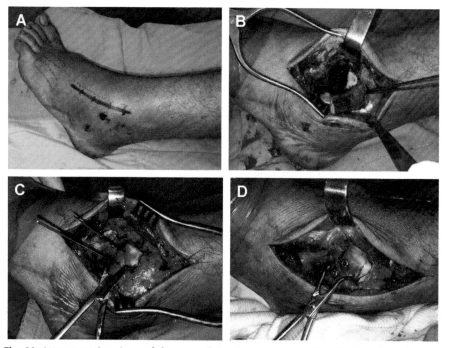

Fig. 11. Intraoperative views of the anterolateral approach used for **Fig. 9** patient. (*A*) Skin incision. Displaced lateral body fragment was (*B*) reduced and (*C*) fixed with pins and two 3.5-mm cannulated screws. (*D*) Then, anatomic reduction of the talar neck fracture on the lateral side was attempted with a Weber clamp.

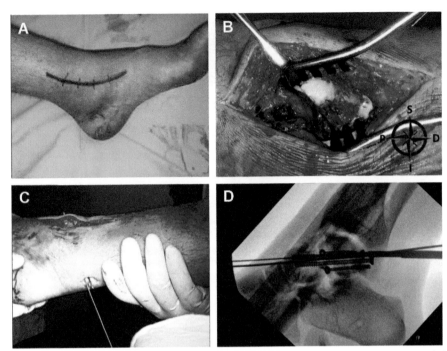

Fig. 12. Same patient as in **Figs. 9** and **11**. Intraoperative views of the anteromedial approach. (*A*) Skin incision. (*B*) Anatomic reduction is check from the medial side. (*C, D*) Definitive fixation was done with 2 posteroanterior 3.5-mm cannulated screws.

blood supply to the involved fragments. It is recommended to limit the extent of subperiosteal dissection into the sinus tarsi laterally and under the talar neck medially, exposing only what is necessary to obtain an anatomic reduction.

Suggested Algorithm

An algorithm for approach selection in talar neck fractures is shown in **Fig. 14**.

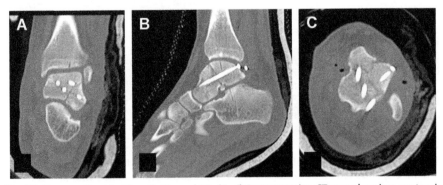

Fig. 13. Same patient in **Figs. 9, 11**, and **12**. (*A–C*) Postoperative CT scan showing anatomic subtalar and neck reduction.

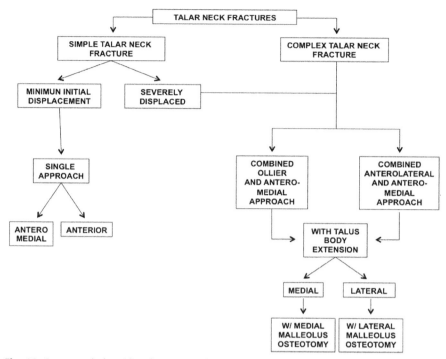

Fig. 14. Suggested algorithm for approach selection in talar neck fractures.

SUMMARY

Adequate approach selection at the time of definitive surgical management of talar neck fractures is crucial for success, because inadequate visualization is a common cause of residual intraarticular malreduction or extraarticular deformity.

Current concepts include an increasing recommendation to use combined lateral and medial approaches, because anatomic reduction not only of the fracture site but also of all the involved joints and axis is necessary due to the strategic position of the talus in the foot and ankle mortise. A single anterior or anteromedial approach, however, could be recommended in selected simple vertical talar neck fractures with no comminution and minimum initial displacement.

A detailed knowledge of the extraosseous and intraosseous vascularity of the talus to understand which arteries must be preserved during surgery and a careful surgical technique are necessary to preserve periosteal blood supply to the involved fracture fragments.

CLINICS CARE POINTS

- A single approach technique does not provide adequate visualization of the fully extension of the fracture site in complex talar neck injuries.
- Combined lateral and medial approaches are strongly recommended for accurate anatomic reduction and axial alignment.
- The potential threat to talus vascularity with a double approach, increasing the risk of osteonecrosis, never has been demonstrated.

DISCLOSURE

The authors do not have any relationship with a commercial company that has a direct financial interest in subject matter or materials discussed in this article or with a company making a competing product.

REFERENCES

1. Baumhauer JF, Alvarez RG. Controversies in treating talus fractures. Orthop Clin North Am 1995;26:335–51.
2. Rammelt S, Zwipp H. Talar neck and body fractures. Injury 2009;40(2):120–35.
3. Lindvall E, Haidukewych G, DiPasquale T, et al. Open reduction and stable fixation of isolated, displaced talar neck and body fractures. J Bone Joint Surg Am 2004;86-A:2229–34.
4. Zwipp H. Severe foot trauma in combination with talar injuries. In: Tscherne H, Schatzker J, editors. Major fractures of the pilon the talus and the calcaneus. New York: Springer-Verlag; 1993. p. 123–35.
5. Rammelt S, Winkler J, Grass R, et al. Reconstruction after talar fractures. Foot Ankle Clin 2006;11(1):61–84, viii.
6. Daniels TR, Smith JW, Ross TI. Varus malalignment of the talar neck. Its effect on the position of the foot and on subtalar motion. J Bone Joint Surg Am 1996; 78(10):1559–67.
7. Sanders DW, Busam M, Hattwick E, et al. Functional outcomes following displaced talar neck fractures. J Orthop Trauma 2004;18:265–70.
8. Vallier HA, Reichard SG, Boyd AJ, et al. A new look at the Hawkins classification for talar neck fractures: which features of injury and treatment are predictive of osteonecrosis? J Bone Joint Surg Am 2014;96:192–7.
9. Miller AN, Prasarn ML, Dyke JP, et al. Quantitative assessment of the vascularity of the talus with gadolinium-enhanced magnetic resonance imaging. J Bone Joint Surg Am 2011;93:1116–21.
10. Lexer E, Kuliga P, Turk W. Untersuchungen uber knochenartevien millelst Rontgenaufnahmen injuzierter knochen und ihre bedeutung fur einzelne pathologische vor- gange am knochensysteme. Berlin: August Hirschwald; 1904. p. 16.
11. Mulfinger GL, Trueta J. The blood supply of the talus. J Bone Joint Surg Br 1970; 52(1):160–7.
12. Wildenauer E. Proceedings: discussion on the blood supply of the talus. Z Orthop Ihre Grenzgeb 1975;113(4):730.
13. Gelberman RH, Mortensen WW. The arterial anatomy of the talus. Foot Ankle 1983;4:64–72.
14. Oppermann J, Franzen J, Spies C, et al. The microvascular anatomy of the talus: a plastination study on the influence of total ankle replacement. Surg Radiol Anat 2014;36(5):487–94.
15. Vani PC, Arthi G, Jessy JP, et al. Vascular foramina of talus: an anatomical study with reference to surgical dissection. Surg Radiol Anat 2019. https://doi.org/10.1007/s00276-019-02394-6.
16. Ohl X, Harisboure A, Hemery X, et al. Long-term follow-up after surgical treatment of talar fractures. Twenty cases with an average follow-up of 7.5 years. Int Orthop 2011;35:93–9.
17. Cronier P, Talha A, Massin P. Central talar fractures—therapeutic considerations. Injury 2004;35. S-B10–S-B22.
18. Fortin PT, Balazsy JE. Talus fractures: evaluation and treatment. J Am Acad Orthop Surg 2001;9(2):114–27.

19. Vallier HA, Nork SE, Barei DP, et al. Talar Neck Fractures: Results and Outcomes. J Bone Joint Surg Am 2004;86A:1616–24.
20. Ziran BH, Abidi NA, Scheel MJ. Medial malleolar osteotomy for exposure of complex talar body fractures. J Orthop Trauma 2001;15:513–8.
21. Ahmad J, Raikin SM. Current Concepts Review: Talar Fractures. Foot Ankle Int 2006;27(6):475–82.
22. Smith PN, Ziran BH. Fractures of the talus. Oper Tech Orthop 1999;9:229–38.
23. Archdeacon M, Wilber R. Fractures of the talar neck. Orthop Clin North Am 2002; 33:247–62.
24. Berlet GC, Lee TH, Massa EG. Talar neck fractures. Orthop Clin North Am 2001; 32:53–64.
25. Daniels TR, Smith JW. Talar neck fractures. Foot Ankle 1993;14:225–34.
26. Fleuriau Chateau P, Brokaw D, Jelen BA, et al. Plate fixation of talar neck fractures: preliminary review of a new technique in twenty-three patients. J Orthop Trauma 2002;16:213–9.
27. Vallier HA. Fractures of the talus: state of the art. J Orthop Trauma 2015;29: 385–92.
28. Rammelt S, Pitakveerakul A. Hindfoot Injuries: How to Avoid Posttraumatic Varus Deformity? Foot Ankle Clin N Am 2019;24:325–45.
29. Sangeorzan BJ, Wagner UA, Harrington RM, et al. Contact characteristics of the subtalar joint: The effect of talar neck misalignement. J Orthop Res 1992;10: 544–51.
30. Maceroli MA, Wong C, Sanders RW, et al. Treatment of Comminuted Talar Neck Fractures With Use of Minifragment Plating. J Orthop Trauma 2016;30:572–8.
31. Clare MP, Maloney PJ. Prevention of Avascular Necrosis with Fractures of the Talar Neck. Foot Ankle Clin N Am 2019;24(1):47–56.

Sinus Tarsi Approach for Calcaneal Fractures
The New Gold Standard?

Gabriel Khazen, MD*, Cesar Khazen Rassi, MD

KEYWORDS

• Calcaneus • Fractures • Sinus tarsi • Approach • Surgical

KEY POINTS

- The sinus tarsi approach allows direct assessment of subtalar joint restoration, with low risk of soft tissue, sural nerve, and lateral calcaneal artery damage.
- Tuberosity fracture fixation using cannulated screws only or sinus tarsi plate provides similar radiographic outcomes and risk of complications to the sinus tarsi approach.
- Recent evidence favoring sinus tarsi rather than the extensile lateral approach has shifted opinion toward this less invasive approach. Now, the sinus tarsi approach might be considered the gold standard for displaced intra-articular calcaneus fracture treatment.

INTRODUCTION

Displaced intra-articular calcaneal fractures (DIACFs) are among the most difficult articular fractures to treat, with a high rate of potential complications. DIACF is not only a subtalar joint problem; calcaneus height loss affects talus pitch and also distorts talonavicular and ankle joint biomechanics.[1] It is crucial to restoring the calcaneus's posterior facet anatomy and calcaneus width, length, and height to reestablish hindfoot biomechanics.

EXTENSILE LATERAL APPROACH

Calcaneus fracture reduction can be performed through an extensile lateral or a minimally invasive approach. Traditionally the extensile lateral approach (ELA) has been recognized as the gold standard method to treat DIACF. It provides excellent fracture visualization and allows surgeons to reduce and fix the displaced fracture fragments. However, a high complication rate has been described with this approach,[2–5] including wound healing complications, deep infection, sural nerve injuries, and

Hospital de Clinicas Caracas, Av Panteón, San Bernardino, Caracas 01050, Venezuela
* Corresponding author.
E-mail address: gabrielkhazen@hotmail.com

Foot Ankle Clin N Am 25 (2020) 667–681
https://doi.org/10.1016/j.fcl.2020.08.003
1083-7515/20/© 2020 Elsevier Inc. All rights reserved.

compromising blood supply from the lateral calcaneal artery at the L-shaped flap corner.

LESS INVASIVE APPROACHES

Different minimally invasive techniques have been described, aiming to avoid soft tissue complications, such as percutaneous reduction and fixation, arthroscopically assisted fracture reduction and fixation, external fixation, and the sinus tarsi approach (STA).[6–8] Weng and colleagues[9] compared percutaneous reduction and screw fixation with plate fixation via STA for calcaneal fractures and found that STA was superior in terms of calcaneal width recovery.

SINUS TARSI APPROACH

The STA allows direct assessment of the subtalar joint restoration, and, by extending the incision distally, the calcaneocuboid joint if needed. It has low risk of damage to the sural nerve and lateral calcaneal artery. However, STA is a more technically demanding procedure, with less calcaneus fracture visualization than ELA. Many studies have described surgical maneuvers[10,11] to achieve better and easier fracture reduction through this approach. Zhao and colleagues[12] described using a lateral Steinmann pin distractor to gain calcaneus length and height. The authors prefer to place a Hintermann distractor from the medial side, which helps to restore the medial calcaneal wall and hindfoot alignment, and a laminar spreader from the talus lateral process to calcaneus anterior process to correct the Gissane angle and reduce the process if needed.

SINUS TARSI APPROACH VERSUS EXTENSILE LATERAL APPROACH

Many studies[13–20] have compared the advantages and disadvantages of ELA and STA to treat DIACF, most of them favoring STA. Yao and colleagues[21] compared the outcome for reduction and internal fixation between these 2 approaches for Sanders type II and type III fractures, finding no differences clinically and radiologically between the two groups. However, wound complication rate (13.3%) in the extensile lateral group was significantly higher compared with the sinus tarsi group.

A meta-analysis by Seat and Seat[22] reported, in only randomized control trials, that there was no statistically significant difference between ELA and STA in postoperative Bohler or Gissane angles. There was a statistically significant difference in wound complications, superficial infection, sural nerve injury, visual analog scale, American Orthopaedic Foot & Ankle Society (AOFAS) scores, operative time, time to operating room, calcaneal height, and postoperative Bohler angle (when all studies were considered), all in favor of the minimal incision approach.

Brandt and colleagues[23] analyzed gait characteristics and functional outcomes during early follow-up between ELA and STA in patients with unilateral intra-articular calcaneal fractures. Results were comparable, with no significant difference regarding biomechanical and functional outcomes. Functional outcomes only revealed significant changes in the physical component of Short Form 36 (SF-36), and STA provides adequate restoration of dynamic foot function.

The authors consider that, for STA, there is no need to wait for the so-called "wrinkle sign to perform surgery, as is suggested for ELA.[3–5] Nevertheless, Li[24] considers it reasonable to wait 6 days from injury for STA to improve soft tissue envelope conditions that may be traumatized and edematous to avoid sural nerve injury.

Park and colleagues[25] showed that a standard STA incision measuring 4 to 5 cm in length made from the tip of distal fibula to the base of the fourth metatarsal was no longer safe to prevent sural nerve damage. Therefore, they suggest that it is safer to make a straight incision distally from just distal to the tip of the fibula to the level of the calcaneocuboid joint and almost horizontal to the sole, which provides adequate exposure to accomplish successful reduction and fixation of calcaneal fractures. Femino and colleagues[26] reported that by avoiding dissection through the deep portion of the superior peroneal retinaculum, the lateral calcaneal artery can be protected, thus preserving the blood supply to the lateral calcaneal skin flap.

STABILIZATION ALTERNATIVES

Many options have been described for stabilizing calcaneus fracture through STA, and even digital precision has been experimentally tested.[27] Zhao and colleagues[12] suggested fixing the fracture with a circular plate to provide maximum lateral wall coverage to restore calcaneus width and solid triangle support by the front, top, and rear to maintain the height and length. However, Zhuang and colleagues[28] reported the same wound complications between the ELA and STA for displaced intra-articular calcaneal fractures when using the same locking compression plate fixation in 384 patients.

Zeman and colleagues[29] compared the use of the locking compression plate through ELA and intramedullary nail fixation through STA with similar fixation results but fewer wound complications with the nail in Sanders II and III fractures. Abdelazeem and colleagues[30] suggest that screw fixation only is sufficient and avoids major wound complication problems. Schepers[31] recommends that less comminuted fractures with adequate bone stock are amenable to screw-only fixation, but, if the construct is not stable enough to allow early motion, then a plate should be added.

Weinraub and David[32] suggested stabilizing the fracture with a sinus tarsi plate. Kir and colleagues,[33] in a prospective randomized study, concluded that plate fixation via STA was associated with a lower rate of implant failure and reoperations, better reconstruction of lateral calcaneal widening, and better functional outcomes in Sanders types 2 and 3 calcaneal fractures compared with screw fixation.

Pitts and colleagues[34] reported radiographic and postoperative outcomes of plate versus screw constructs in reduction and internal fixation of calcaneus fractures via STA, showing no difference in the restoration of the Bohler and Gissane angles. Furthermore, the amount of angular correction achieved by initial reduction showed no statistically significant difference between both groups, and the amount of reduction lost between initial and final postoperative radiographs showed no statistically significant difference between groups. Their data suggest that fixation using cannulated screws alone versus sinus tarsi plate provides similar radiographic outcomes and risk of complications.

All this recent evidence favoring sinus tarsi rather than the ELA to treat DIACF has shifted opinion toward this less invasive approach. STA can now be considered the new gold standard for many surgeons, but it is essential to highlight that, even for expert surgeons, STA can be a challenging procedure. Mainly after a high-energy trauma, hindfoot alignment may be difficult to achieve, and poor reduction and fixation can lead to short hindfoot and varus malunion. Therefore, the authors suggest that, when switching to this less invasive approach, it is important to have some experience in calcaneus fracture treatment through an ELA first, for better understanding of the calcaneus body fracture pattern and its anatomy and to be able to fix it without the need of direct visualization.

SINUS TARSI APPROACH FOR INTRA-ARTICULAR CALCANEUS FRACTURE
Surgical Technique

- Under general or epidural anesthesia, and after ankle nerve block with lidocaine and bupivacaine for postoperative pain control, the patient is positioned in lateral decubitus, and a thigh tourniquet is used. The skin incision is between 4 and 5 cm long and runs 1 cm distal to the tip of the fibula toward the calcaneocuboid joint superior margin. Soft tissues are dissected until the calcaneus lateral rim is visualized, and articular fracture is inspected (**Fig. 1**).
- A Steinmann pin is inserted in the calcaneus tuberosity to distract it and pull it out of varus, recovering length and height. Special care is taken to reduce the calcaneus medial wall, which is performed indirectly by distracting with a Hintermann retractor from the medial talus neck to the medial calcaneus tuberosity, and directly with mini-Hohmann retractors pivoting the medial wall fragments from the STA. A laminar spreader is placed from the talus lateral process to the calcaneus anterior process to correct the Gissane angle and reduce the anterior process if needed (**Figs. 2** and **3**).
- The lateral wall may be retracted slightly to identify and reduce the depressed posterior facet, aligning it under direct visualization with the intact medial part of the posterior facet attached to the sustentaculum tali and is fixed provisionally with Kirschner wires and then with two 3.5-mm cortical screws from the lateral wall underneath the posterior facet to the sustentaculum tali. Direct fluoroscopy is performed during surgery from the same side of the table to assess fracture reduction and fixation (**Figs. 4** and **5**).
- In tongue-type articular fractures, a 3.0-mm Shantz pin is placed posteriorly in the tuberosity to lift the depressed posterior facet correcting Bohler angle, assisted from the STA with a periosteal elevator to reduce under direct visualization the posterior facet, fixing it as explained earlier with two 3.5-mm screws to the sustentaculum tali, or sometimes it can be stabilized directly with a plate (**Fig. 6**).
- The anterior process fracture reconstruction is performed as explained earlier, with a lamina spreader from the talus lateral process to the fractured fragment, reducing the fracture and restoring the Gissane angle; fracture fixation is performed with 3.5-mm screws from the anterior process to the calcaneus medial

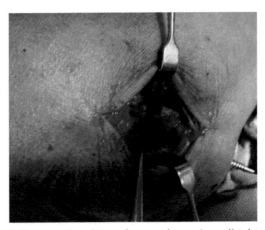

Fig. 1. STA incision is between 4 and 5 cm long and runs 1 cm distal to the tip the fibula toward the calcaneocuboid joint superior margin.

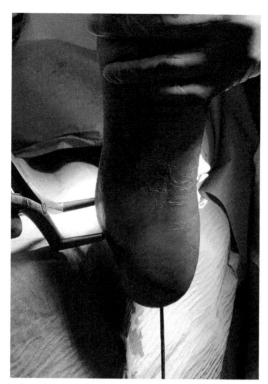

Fig. 2. A Steinmann pin is inserted in the calcaneus tuberosity to distract and pull it out of varus. Special care is taken to reduce the calcaneus medial wall; this is performed indirectly using distraction with a Hintermann retractor from the medial talus neck to the medial calcaneus tuberosity.

or plantar wall. The STA incision can be extended if there is a calcaneocuboid joint fracture to visualize it directly and assess anatomic fracture reduction and fixation with 3.5-mm or 2.7-mm lag screws or 2.7-mm plates and screws (**Figs. 7** and **8**).

- Then, the reduced calcaneus tuberosity fracture is stabilized with either a lateral plate or cannulated screws. Although this may be a source of debate, the authors prefer fixation with axial screws from the tuberosity to the anterior process and sustentaculum tali to maintain fracture reduction. However, in a severely comminuted fracture, we prefer the use of a locking plate in the lateral wall subperiosteally delivered with percutaneous fixation to protect soft tissue envelope biology, the first choice being a distal radius T-angled locking plate, although many other plate options can provide excellent fixation. The Broden view is mandatory to assess posterior facet reduction (**Figs. 9–12**).

- In high-energy Sanders III fractures with severe cartilage damage, and Sanders IV fractures, the authors' preference is performing primary arthrodesis after reconstructing the calcaneus through STA. As Nosewicz and colleagues[35] assumed, even complex fractures can be reduced through this approach) with one or two 6.5-mm or 7.0-mm cannulated screws, avoiding too much compression through the subtalar joint. Most of the time, bone grafting the calcaneus bone defects is not needed (**Fig. 13**).

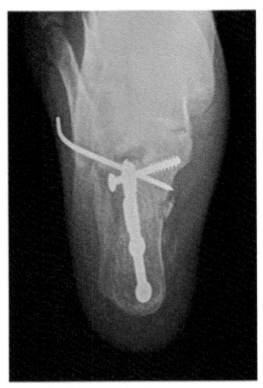

Fig. 3. Medial calcaneal wall correctly reduced.

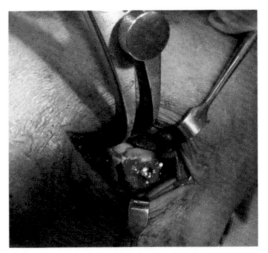

Fig. 4. Depressed posterior facet is reduced, aligning it under direct visualization with the intact medial part of the posterior facet attached to the sustentaculum tali and is fixed with two 3.5-mm cortical screws from the lateral wall underneath the posterior facet to the sustentaculum tali.

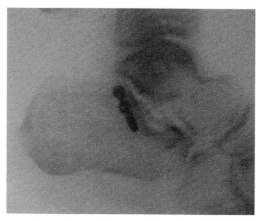

Fig. 5. Direct fluoroscopy is performed during surgery from the same side of the table to assess fracture reduction and fixation.

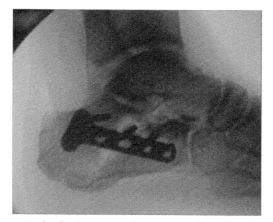

Fig. 6. Tongue-type articular fractures sometimes can be fixed directly with a plate.

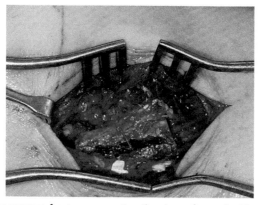

Fig. 7. The anterior process fracture reconstruction is performed with a laminar spreader from the talus lateral process to the fractured fragment, reducing the fracture and restoring the Gissane angle.

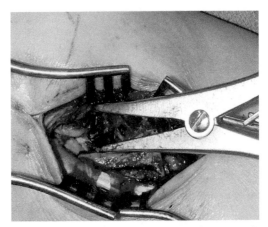

Fig. 8. The anterior process fracture reconstruction is performed with a laminar spreader from the talus lateral process to the fractured fragment, reducing the fracture and restoring the Gissane angle.

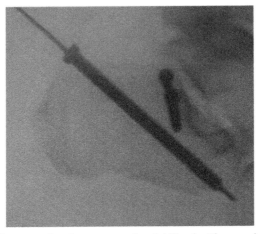

Fig. 9. Reduced calcaneus tuber fracture may be stabilized with cannulated screws.

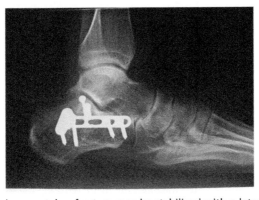

Fig. 10. Reduced calcaneus tuber fracture may be stabilized with a lateral plate.

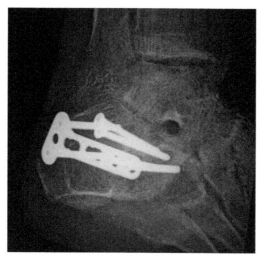

Fig. 11. Broden view is mandatory to assess posterior facet reduction.

- In severely comminuted fractures and osteopenic patients, the authors keep a posterior splint in place for 2 weeks and then start joint motion, keeping all patients non–weight bearing for 6 to 8 weeks. One of the outstanding advantages of the STA approach is that skin over calcaneus lateral wall looks normal after surgery, and rarely has any adhesions the way ELA patients do (**Figs. 14–16**).

COMPLICATIONS

Complications described for STA are related mainly to fracture reduction, fixation, and rarely soft tissue issues.[6–8,35] It was discussed earlier that fracture reduction through STA might be a challenging procedure. Depending on trauma energy and fracture

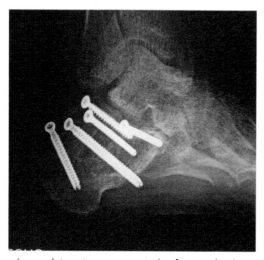

Fig. 12. Broden view is mandatory to assess posterior facet reduction.

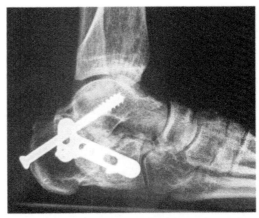

Fig. 13. In high-energy Sanders III fractures with severe cartilage contusion and Sanders IV fractures, the authors prefer primary arthrodesis after reconstructing the calcaneus through STA.

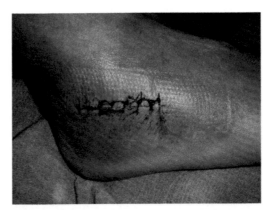

Fig. 14. Skin incision next day after surgery.

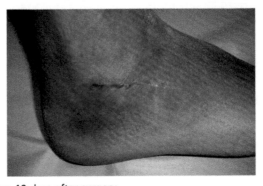

Fig. 15. Skin incision 10 days after surgery.

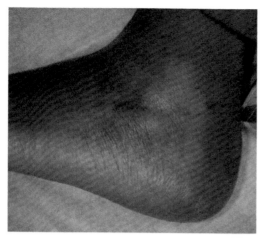

Fig. 16. Skin incision 6 months after surgery.

pattern, hindfoot alignment can be difficult to achieve, and inadequate reduction and/ or fixation can lead to short hindfoot and varus malunion. Choosing an incorrect fixation construct can also lead to poor fixation or fracture reduction loosening between initial and final postoperative radiographs (**Figs. 17** and **18**).

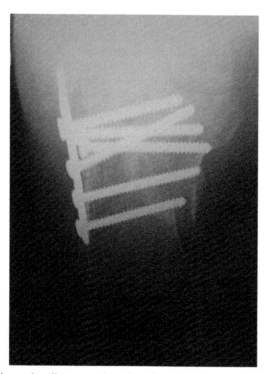

Fig. 17. Medial calcaneal wall incorrectly reduced and hindfoot residual varus.

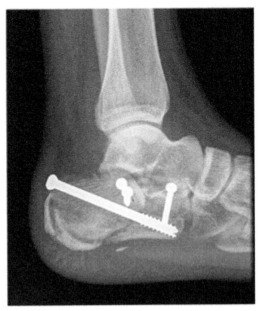

Fig. 18. Poor fixation construct led to poor fixation and fracture reduction loosening between initial and final postoperative radiographs.

Posthuma and colleagues[36] reported a case of traumatic epidermal inclusion cyst after minimally invasive surgery of a displaced intra-articular calcaneal fracture. As discussed earlier in this article, the same wound complications incidence has been described for ELA and STA for displaced intra-articular calcaneal fractures when using the same locking compression plate fixation.[28] Also, wound complications can develop if too much traction is placed on wound edges (**Fig. 19**).

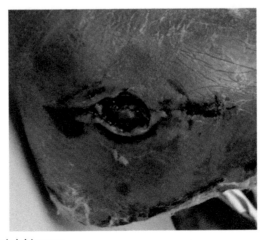

Fig. 19. STA wound dehiscence.

SUMMARY

DIACFs are among the most difficult articular fractures to treat, with a high rate of potential complications.[1] It is crucial to restoring calcaneus posterior facet anatomy as well as calcaneus width, length, and height to restore hindfoot biomechanics. This procedure can be performed through a lateral extensile or an STA.

The ELA provides excellent fracture visualization and allows surgeons to reduce the displaced fracture fragments. However, a high complication rate has been described with this approach,[2–5] including wound healing complications, deep infections, and sural nerve injuries, and for these reasons many studies favor the STA.[13–22] Although STA can be a technically demanding procedure with less calcaneus body and tuberosity fracture visualization, it allows direct assessment of the subtalar joint restoration as well as the calcaneocuboid joint if needed. The use of a Hintermann distractor from the medial side and a lamina spreader through STA can assist in fracture reduction.

Calcaneus tuber fracture can be stabilized with screws only, a lateral plate, or a combination of both.[27–35] The authors prefer fracture fixation with axial screws from the tuberosity to the anterior process and sustentaculum tali. However, in osteopenic patients or severely comminuted fractures, we instead augment with a distal radius T-angled locking plate, subperiosteally delivered with percutaneous fixation to protect soft tissue envelope biology.

All this recent evidence favoring sinus tarsi rather than the ELA to treat DIACF has shifted opinion toward this less invasive approach. Therefore, STA can be considered the new gold standard for the treatment of DIACF.

CLINICS CARE POINTS

- The ELA provides excellent fracture visualization and allows surgeons to reduce and fix the displaced fracture fragments, but a high complication rate has been described with this approach.
- Many studies[13–20] have compared the advantages and disadvantages of the extended lateral approach with STA to treat DIACF, most of them favoring STA.
- Studies have found no difference clinically and radiologically between the 2 groups, but the wound complication rate (13.3%) in the extensile lateral group was significantly higher compared with the sinus tarsi group.

DISCLOSURE

The authors have nothing to disclose.

REFERENCES

1. Sharr PJ, Mangupli MM, Winson IG, et al. Current management options for displaced intra-articular calcaneal fractures: non-operative, ORIF, minimally invasive reduction and fixation or primary ORIF and subtalar arthrodesis. A contemporary review. Foot Ankle Surg 2016;22(1):1–8.

2. Backes M, Schepers T, Beerekamp S, et al. Wound infections following open reduction and internal fixation of calcaneal fractures with an extended lateral approach. Int Orthop 2014;38:767–73.

3. Benirschke SK, Kramer PA. Wound healing complications in closed and open calcaneal fractures. J Orthop Trauma 2004;18:1–6.

4. Kwon JY, Guss D, Lin DE, et al. Effect of delay to definitive surgical fixation on wound complications in the treatment of closed, intra-articular calcaneus fractures. Foot Ankle Int 2015;36(5):508–17.

5. Schepers T. Calcaneal fractures: looking beyond the meta-analyses. J Foot Ankle Surg 2016;55(4):897–8.

6. Giannini S, Cadossi M, Mosca M, et al. Minimally-invasive treatment of calcaneal fractures: a review of the literature and our experience. Injury 2016;47:S138–46.

7. Bremer AK, Kraler L, Frauchinger L, et al. Limited open reduction and internal fixation of calcaneal fractures. Foot Ankle Int 2020;41(1):57–62.

8. Schepers T. The sinus tarsi approach in displaced intra-articular calcaneal fractures: a systematic review. Int Orthop 2011;35(5):697–703.

9. Weng QH, Dai GL, Tu QM, et al. Comparison between percutaneous screw fixation and plate fixation via sinus tarsi approach for calcaneal fractures: an 8-10 year follow-up study. Orthop Surg 2020;12(1):124–32.

10. Arastu M, Sheehan B, Buckley R. Minimally invasive reduction and fixation of displaced calcaneal fractures: surgical technique and radiographic analysis. Int Orthop 2014;38:539–45.

11. Cottom J, Douthett S, McConnell K. Intraoperative reduction techniques for surgical management of displaced intra-articular Calcaneal fractures. Clin Podiatr Med Surg 2019;36(2):269–77.

12. Zhao B, Zhao W, Assan I. Steinmann pin retractor-assisted reduction with circle plate fixation via sinus tarsi approach for intra-articular calcaneal fractures: a retrospective cohort study. J Orthop Surg Res 2019;14:363.

13. Lin J, Xie C, Chen K, et al. Comparison of sinus tarsi approach versus extensile lateral approach for displaced intra-articular calcaneal fractures Sanders type IV. Int Orthop 2019;43(19):2141–9.

14. Schepers T, Backes M, Dingemans SA, et al. Similar anatomical reduction and lower complication rates with the sinus tarsi approach compared with the extended lateral approach in displaced intra-articular calcaneal fractures. J Orthop Trauma 2017;31(6):293–8.

15. Sampath Kumar V, Marimuthu K, Subramani S, et al. Prospective randomized trial comparing open reduction and internal fixation with minimally invasive reduction and percutaneous fixation in managing displaced intra-articular calcaneal fractures. Int Orthop 2014;38(12):2505–12.

16. Zhou HC, Yu T, Ren HY, et al. Clinical comparison of extensile lateral approach and Sinus Tarsi approach combined with medial distraction technique for intra-articular calcaneal fractures. Orthop Surg 2017;9(1):77–85.

17. Jin C, Weng D, Yang W, et al. Minimally invasive percutaneous osteosynthesis versus ORIF for Sanders type II and III calcaneal fractures: a prospective, randomized intervention trial. J Orthop Surg Res 2017;12(1):10.

18. Kline AJ, Anderson RB, Davis WH, et al. Minimally invasive technique versus an extensile lateral approach for intra-articular calcaneal fractures. Foot Ankle Int 2013;34(6):773–80.

19. Khuran A, Dhillon M, Prabhakar S, et al. Outcome evaluation of minimally invasive surgery versus extensile lateral approach in management of displaced intra-articular calcaneal fractures: a randomised control trial. Foot (Edinb) 2017;31: 23–30.

20. Kiewiet NJ, Sangeorzan BJ. Calcaneal fracture management: extensile lateral approach versus small incision technique. Foot Ankle Clin 2017;22(1):77–91.

21. Yao H, Liang T, Xu Y, et al. Sinus tarsi approach versus extensile lateral approach for displaced intra-articular calcaneal fracture: a meta-analysis of current evidence base. J Orthop Surg Res 2017;12:43.

22. Seat A, Seat C. Lateral extensile approach versus minimal incision approach for open reduction and internal fixation of displaced intra-articular calcaneal fractures: a meta-analysis. J Foot Ankle Surg 2020;59(2):356–66.

23. Brand A, Klopfer-Kramer I, Bottger M, et al. Gait characteristics and functional outcomes during early follow-up are comparable in patients with calcaneal fractures treated by either the Sinus Tarsi or the Extended Lateral Approach. Gait Posture 2019;70:190–5.

24. Li S. Wound and Sural nerve complications of the sinus tarsi approach for Calcaneus fracture. Foot Ankle Int 2018;39(9):1106–12.

25. Park J, Chun D, Park K, et al. Can sural nerve injury be avoided in the sinus tarsi approach for calcaneal fracture ? Medicine (Baltimore) 2019;98(42):e17611.

26. Femino J, Vaasenon T, Levin D, et al. Modification of the sinus tarsi approach for open reduction and plate fixation of intra-articular Calcaneus fractures: the limits of proximal extension based upon the vascular anatomy of the lateral Calcaneal artery. Iowa Orthop J 2010;30:161–7.

27. Xu J, He Z, Zhang G, et al. An experimental study on the digital precision of internal fixation via the Sinus Tarsi approach for Calcaneal fractures. J Orthop Surg (Hong Kong) 2019;27(1). 2309499019834072.

28. Zhuang L, Wang L, XU D, et al. Same wound complications between extensile lateral approach and sinus tarsi approach for displaced intra-articular calcaneal fractures with the same locking compression plates fixation: a 9-year follow-up of 384 patients. Eur J Trauma Emerg Surg 2019. https://doi.org/10.1007/s00068-019-01221-2.

29. Zeman J, Zeman P, Matejka T, et al. Comparison of LCP and intramedullary nail osteosynthesis in Calcaneal fractures. Acta Ortop Bras 2019;27(6):288–93.

30. Abdelazeem A, Khedr A, Abousayed M, et al. Management of displaced intra-articular calcaneal fractures using the limited open sinus tarsi approach and fixation by screws only technique. Int Orthop 2014;38:601–6.

31. Schepers T. Sinus tarsi approach with screws-only fixation for displaced intra-articular calcaneal fractures. Clin Podiatr Med Surg 2019;36(2):211–24.

32. Weinraub GM, David MS. Sinus tarsi approach with subcutaneously delivered plate fixation for displaced intra-articular calcaneal fractures. Clin Podiatr Med Surg 2019;36(2):225–31.

33. Kir M, Ayanoglu S, Cabuk L, et al. Mini-plate fixation via sinus tarsi approach is superior to cannulated screw in intra-articular calcaneal fractures: A prospective randomized study. Orthop Surg 2018;26(3):1–7.

34. Pitts C, Almaguer A, Wilson J, et al. Radiographic and postoperative outcomes of plate versus screw constructs in open reduction and internal fixation of calcaneus fractures via the Sinus Tarsi. Foot Ankle Int 2019;40(8):929–35.

35. Nosewicz T, Knupp M, Barg A, et al. Mini-open sinus tarsi approach with percutaneous screw fixation of displaced calcaneal fractures: a prospective computed tomography-based study. Foot Ankle Int 2012;33(11):925–33.

36. Posthuma JJ, de Ruiter KJ, de Jong VM, et al. Traumatic epidermal inclusion cyst after minimal invasive surgery of a displaced intra-articular calcaneal fracture: a case report. J Foot Ankle Surg 2018;57(6):1253–5.

Fixation by Open Reduction and Internal Fixation or Primary Arthrodesis of Calcaneus Fractures: Indications and Technique

Tim Schepers, MD, PhD

KEYWORDS

- Extended lateral approach • Sinus tarsi approach • Primary arthrodesis • Outcome
- Complications

KEY POINTS

- The management of displaced intraarticular calcaneal fractures should be centralized in experienced and high-volume centers.
- Surgeons treating calcaneal fractures should be able to implement more than 1 technique.
- Anatomic reduction is associated with improved outcome in displaced intraarticular calcaneal fractures, and the sinus tarsi approach is becoming the new gold standard.
- If anatomic reduction cannot be obtained, in selected cases, a primary arthrodesis is a valid option.
- Primary arthrodesis should be performed only in combination with restoration of overall anatomy of the calcaneus.

INTRODUCTION

Since one of the earliest descriptions of calcaneal fractures by Hippocrates (about 400 BC) and their treatment with cerate (wax plus lard) and compressive bandages, the discussion on treatment has not been settled yet. Even though we have several randomized trials, even more metaanalyses, and countless case series at our disposal, there is no universal treatment protocol to date.

Since the 1990s, the gold standard in treating displaced intraarticular calcaneal fractures (DIACFs) has become the extended lateral approach (ELA).[1] This technique is, however, shaded by a rather high complication rate. Several large series reported percentages greater than 15% wound complication. Large variations in reported wound complications exist throughout the literature and throughout geographic regions.[2]

Trauma Unit, Amsterdam UMC Location AMC, Room G5-250, Meibergdreef 9, 1105 AZ Amsterdam, The Netherlands
E-mail address: t.schepers@amsterdamumc.nl

Foot Ankle Clin N Am 25 (2020) 683–695
https://doi.org/10.1016/j.fcl.2020.08.008
1083-7515/20/© 2020 The Author(s). Published by Elsevier Inc. This is an open access article under the CC BY license (http://creativecommons.org/licenses/by/4.0/).

foot.theclinics.com

Especially in the last decade, the sinus tarsi approach (STA) has regained interest in the treatment of DIACFs. A review published in 2011 on the STA contained data from 8 series published between 2000 and 2010.[3] This number more than doubled in a follow-up review from 2014.[4] One of the earliest reports of a subfibular approach was by Palmer[5] in 1948, who credited Lenormant and Wilmoth. The incision described by Palmer was a curved incision, 6 cm in length, beneath the fibula (limited Kocher approach).[6] The peroneal tendon sheet was incised, and the tendons were displaced anteriorly. Lutz and colleagues[7] showed that the direct lateral approaches as propagated by Palmer and Stephenson puts the thin anastomotic arch between the peroneal and lateral tarsal artery on the outside of the heel at risk. Currently, a 3- to 5-cm straight incision is made from the tip of the fibula toward the base of the fourth metatarsal. The sural nerve and the peroneal tendons are held distally from the incision.[8]

Even though numerous percutaneous techniques were among the first operative strategies and are still in practice, the author believes they should be reserved for less complex fractures, in the case of arthroscopically assisted surgery or for patients who are at increased risk for significant wound complications in open approaches. Therefore, the percutaneous procedures are left out of the current review.

Besides the open reduction and internal fixation (ORIF) via the ELA or STA following reconstruction of the calcaneus, a different treatment approach can be offered, the primary arthrodesis following ORIF.[9] The current review deals with the surgical treatment of DIACFs. Both ORIF and primary arthrodesis via ELA and STA are addressed.

Treatment Goals

The main goals of treatment of displaced calcaneal fractures are as follows:

- A tailor-made plan: choose the correct treatment strategy for the right patient and fracture type.
- Allow for an early return to previous levels of activity, including sports, or as close as possible.
- In the case of surgical management, obtain a (near) anatomic reduction of the overall anatomy (height, width, axis) and to restore the congruency of the joint surfaces (subtalar and calcaneocuboid).
- Reach the previous goals at the lowest rate of complications (early and late).

The only way to assure achieving all the above-named goals is an adequate surgeon caseload. Sanders and colleagues[1] showed that the learning curve for calcaneal fractures is 35 to 50 cases. In addition, some have shown that with prolonged surgery, the infection rates were higher,[10,11] which is very likely linked to the experience of the surgeon, with an increase in wound complications in less experienced surgeons, as was shown in other studies as well.[12,13] A cutoff value of at least 1 calcaneal fracture treated surgically per month to lower the rate of complications was found in a meta-analysis by Poeze and colleagues.[14] In addition, no universal treatment or surgical approach exists that can be applied to treat all fractures of the calcaneus.[15] Therefore, surgeons responsible for the treatment of DIACFs should be able to perform various different techniques to suit all patients fit for surgery and all fractures that are expected to fare better with operative treatment.

Indications for surgery

Whether a DIACF should be treated operatively depends on several factors. First, patient characteristics regarding significant comorbidities (eg, uncontrolled diabetes, peripheral vascular disease, systemic immune suppressive agents, heavy smoking, substance abuse), low physical demands, or personality issues compromising compliance may warrant nonoperative management.[16] In addition, the geographic setting (patients living in rural areas or unsuited level of expertise of the hospital) may be insufficient to guarantee adequate surgical treatment and after-treatment.

If the patient is fit for surgery, the soft tissues are adequately recovered from the initial trauma, and the expertise of the team is adequate, one could opt for surgical treatment in DIACFs. Loss of height with a Böhler angle less than 15°, posterior subtalar joint incongruence of 2 mm or more, widening of 5 mm or more, varus of more than 5°, or valgus of more than 10° are accepted indications for surgical intervention.[17] In a systematic review by Rammelt and colleagues,[18] the current evidence regarding the when and how in surgery for DIACFs was collected. Numerous clinical studies showed a relation between a failure to restore Böhler angle, joint step-offs of more than 2 mm, and gaps of more than 3 mm and biomechanical disturbances or clinical worse results. This need for anatomic reduction is backed up by several biomechanical studies.[19–23]

Historical overview of primary arthrodesis

To understand how the primary arthrodesis came to be, it is worthwhile to take a short trip through the long history of this procedure. A technique adopted because many were unhappy with the results of the (surgical) management of their time, primary arthrodesis has been around for more than a century. The dogma of that time was that an anatomic reduction of the calcaneal fracture was impossible, and without anatomic reduction, the outcome would always be poor.[24,25] Many have credited the Dutchman Willem Jacob Van Stockum for reporting the first primary arthrodesis in DIACFs in 1911. In his speech at the Dutch Surgical Society, he told his peers to have performed the fusion a few times, mainly due to the fact that he was convinced that the cause for persistent pain following crush injuries of the calcaneus was situated in the subtalar joint.[26] He then presented a case of a bilateral talar fracture in a female patient. Because of persistent complaints following closed reduction and casting, similar to the complaints of a calcaneal fracture, and varus deformity, a "primary" subtalar arthrodesis was performed after approximately 7 months (October 1908). Two years later, the patient requested a similar procedure on the contralateral side.[26,27]

In this time period, surgical treatment strategies like those by Cotton (reduction with a mallet), Conn (traction), Böhler (closed reduction and traction device), and Westhues (percutaneous reduction) dominated the realm of calcaneal fracture treatment. However, Conn[28] reported in 1926 that he too used the primary fusion on occasion, and that for both recent and old cases the subtalar fusion deserved a much more general acceptance than accorded at that time. One year later, in 1927, Wilson reported on 26 cases treated by primary arthrodesis, ranging from 4 days to 5 years (!) after the initial trauma.[29] To paraphrase Wilson: "when treating fracture one should anticipate future difficulties before they arise, with regards to recent calcaneal fractures there is sufficient certainty of future trouble to warrant arthrodesis with reconstruction to avoid prolonged disability."[29] Nutter[30] reviewed the available literature a few years later and stated that it would seem that this most baffling surgical problem is in the process of solution, referring to the primary arthrodesis. In addition, others have noticed an earlier return to work with a primary subtalar fusion (PSF).[31] Becker[32] showed that the motion in the subtalar joint is limited following a calcaneal fracture in most patients, thereby justifying arthrodesis.

Different techniques have been described to perform the subtalar fusion, but the one used most frequently in the 1940s and 1950s was the one described by Gallie[33] via a posterolateral approach and creating a slot, or mortise, in the talus and calcaneus at the subtalar joint. This slot is then filled with a bone graft from the anteromedial tibia.[33] This technique has been used with various modifications (graft from the posterior tibia,[34] or from the iliac crest[35]). In most papers, regarding primary or early fusions, an isolated subtalar fusion is performed by the surgeon[29,32,33,35]; however, others propagate a triple fusion with or without excision of the navicular bone.[28,34,36]

A paper that received much attention was that by Lindsay and Dewar.[37] They pointed out that surgically treated patients (including primary arthrodesis) had a more prolonged time to return to work. However, upon closer look, many of the primary arthrodesis were in fact delayed primary (postprimary) fusions with a significant delay in treatment itself.[37,38] The timing of the primary arthrodesis has been a point of discussion. Some stated that it can only be a primary fusion when it is the first and only initial treatment. In contrast to several others who attempted a (percutaneous/traction) reduction, judged the accuracy on follow-up images, and if deemed insufficient, an arthrodesis was scheduled. Performing an arthrodesis soon after attempting a reduction first can be seen as an early arthrodesis (contrary to a secondary fusion after fracture healing).[24,39] Harris[34] used a 2-stage procedure, reduction first, and based on the postoperative radiographs, a decision whether a primary fusion should be performed. He subsequently reports that the most impressive results were obtained in those cases in whom the subtalar joint had been fused.[34]

None of the studies use a clear definition of primary or early, and there is currently still no unambiguous terminology. A suggested definition could be that

- A primary arthrodesis is a fusion without previous treatment within 4 weeks before the healing of fracture fragments.
- An early arthrodesis (<3 months) is a staged procedure with a subtalar fusion following previous attempts at reduction but still well before one develops complaints of the initial treatment.
- A delayed primary fusion (>3–6 months), for example, because of poor soft tissues, delay referral/diagnosis.
- A secondary subtalar fusion is used for the treatment of complaints of malunion and/or arthritis after a significantly longer period of follow-up (>1 year) with or without primary surgical treatment.

Most of the PSFs were accompanied by remodeling of the calcaneus (either during the same time or in a separate procedure before the fusion). However, some reported that no reduction was attempted at all.[40,41] It is currently accepted as mandatory that before the fusion of the subtalar joint a complete reconstruction of the overall shape of calcaneus has to be pursued.[42,43]

The combined results of the case series on primary arthrodesis published between 1990 and 2010 are reported in a systematic review from 2012.[9] At total of 7 case series and 1 abstract were identified, reporting on 120 patients with 128 severely comminuted calcaneal fractures. With an average follow-up of 28 months, a union rate of 97% was shown. Weighted American Orthopaedic Foot and Ankle Society (AOFAS) hindfoot score was 77.4 (range 72.4–88) on average. The maximum AOFAS following subtalar fusion is 94 points. Three studies reported on return to work, ranging from 75% to 100%. In the case series using the ELA to perform the reduction and fusion, 27% of the patients suffered from a complication.[9]

After 2010, the total number of publications specifically dealing with the primary arthrodesis in calcaneal fractures is limited.[44–50] All publications except for the randomized controlled trial (RCT) by Buckley are level 3 or 4 evidence at best (see "Clinical outcome").

Indications for primary arthrodesis

For most cases, the decision making regarding the primary fusion takes place before the surgery. Depending on the severity of the injury and certain patient characteristics, the patient is counseled on the different treatment options. **Table 1** shows the various criteria used to opt for a primary fusion, which is considered and discussed preoperatively with the patient if 2 or more of the following fracture or patient characteristics are present.

Anatomically reducing the subtalar joint in highly comminuted fractures is less likely. Sanders and colleagues[1] reported that 23% of type III fractures (7 out of 30) and 70% of type IV fractures (8 out of 11) required secondary subtalar arthrodesis. However, with longer follow-up, even less comminuted fractures are at significant risk for secondary arthritis and subsequent fusion (~20% in Sanders type 2 and ~50% in Sanders type 3 fractures).[51]

Buckley and colleagues[52] also showed that the more severely injured calcaneal fractures (Sanders 3 or 4, and Böhler angle <0) were at a higher risk of secondary fusions.[53]

Open fractures and locked fracture dislocations are also linked to less favorable outcomes and more likely to get a fusion at some point.[54,55] Patients with a secondary infection (following open fractures or due to initial treatment) are linked to higher subtalar fusion rates as well.[14,55] One reason to opt for a primary arthrodesis is to prevent the trouble of a painful result from the initial treatment, a delay in secondary subtalar fusion (often not before 1 year after the initial treatment), and the subsequent rehabilitation from this secondary surgery. The patient perspective is very important in the decision making (shared decision making) as to whether to opt for a primary arthrodesis. Eisenstein and colleagues[46] studied the patient perspective. First, they performed a literature search in what outcome to expect from ORIF or ORIF + PSF. They then proceeded to perform an expected value decision analysis in 100 healthy volunteers. In other words, they asked the volunteers what treatment option they would prefer given the pooled probabilities for different outcome in treatment from the literature review. In all different scenarios, the expected value decision analysis favored ORIF + PSF as the optimal treatment for complex DIACF.[46]

Surgical techniques

Regarding the ELA and the STA, many excellent papers exist that explain the surgical techniques in detail:

- Suggested reading for the surgical technique of the ELA: Refs.[1,56–58]
- Suggested reading for the surgical technique of the STA: Refs.[8,59–61]

The surgical technique for primary arthrodesis has been described less often. It follows many of the steps for ORIF via either the ELA (**Fig. 1**) or STA (**Fig. 2**).[9,59] A

Table 1 Indications for primary arthrodesis	
Injury Characteristics	**Patient Characteristics**
Sanders type 3 or 4	Age >65
Locked fracture dislocations	Lower physical demand
Böhler angle < 0	Doubts on compliance
Open fractures (grade 3)	Comorbidities (diabetes, smoking, obesity)
Extensive damage to cartilage	Patients request (shared decision making)
Delay in treatment	Polytrauma

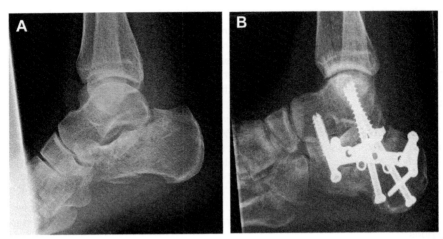

Fig. 1. Primary subtalar arthrodesis following reconstruction via ELA. (*A*) Preoperative, (*B*) postoperative.

complete reconstruction of the overall anatomy should precede the arthrodesis of the posterior subtalar joint (ORIF + PSF).

The following is the preferred technique of the author:

The patient is positioned in a lateral decubitus position on a beanbag on the contralateral side (**Fig. 3**A). A radiolucent table is used. The injured leg is flexed at the knee, and the contralateral leg is in a straight position. The beanbag can be raised at the level of the ankle. As it supports the ankle, the foot is free; this allows for adding varus of the hindfoot during the procedure to look inside the subtalar joint.

A tourniquet is placed 1 hand-width below the knee joint, to assure the common peroneal nerve is not injured, and is only inflated (to 100 mm Hg above the systolic blood pressure with a maximum level of 250 mm Hg) during the reconstruction and fixation of the joint part of the procedure if deemed necessary.

The image intensifier is located at the opposite side of the table. With the foot slightly elevated in the horizontal plane, a lateral image can be obtained; when lifting the

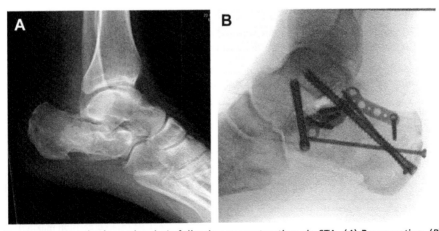

Fig. 2. Primary subtalar arthrodesis following reconstruction via STA. (*A*) Preoperative, (*B*) postoperative.

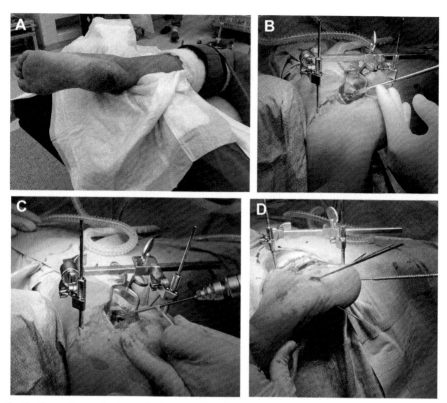

Fig. 3. Operative technique of primary arthrodesis via STA. (*A*) Lateral decubitus position on beanbag. (*B*) Removing cartilage using chisels. (*C*) Creating drill holes on both sides of the subtalar joint. (*D*) Screw placement for subtalar fusion (see text).

forefoot 45° and extending or flexing the ankle, a series of Brodén views can be made. If the leg is extended and externally rotated at the hip while pointing the toes to the ceiling and in addition tilting the C-arm, an axial view is provided.[59]

The STA is made from 5 mm below the tip of the distal fibula toward the base of the fourth metatarsal. It is usually between 3 and 4 cm in length. In the case of calcaneo-cuboid joint involvement, the incision can be lengthened more distally. The peroneal tendons sheet is preserved as much as possible, and tendons are held plantar-ward. The sural nerve is not routinely explored, but if encountered, it is freed up and protected. Following debridement, the subtalar joint and the crucial angle of Gissane are visualized. A subperiosteal flap is created using a broad periosteal elevator and a small blade.

At this stage, a decision is made whether joint reconstruction is feasible, for example, if large fragments of loose cartilage are identified. In severely comminuted fractures, or in cases whereby 2 or more of the criteria listed in **Table 1** are met, the option of a primary arthrodesis has been discussed before the surgery with the patient as part of the shared decision-making process. In case of a primary arthrodesis, the subtalar joint is meticulously debrided. In joint-depression fractures, the lateral portion of the joint can be temporarily taken out to be debrided. The medial portion of the sub-talar joint is debrided first. Using chisels and burrs, the bone is denuded (see **Fig. 3**B). In addition, 2.0-/2.5-mm drill holes are made on both sides of the joint (**Fig. 3**C). In the case of Sanders type 3 or 4, the central fragments are debrided outside the patient, as they are usually too mobile to debride inside. Following the removal of all cartilage from the joint fragments, a small periosteal elevator is inserted via the STA into the fracture line to exit medially. The medial fragment is subsequently lifted and pushed against the talus. A 1.6-mm Kirschner wire is inserted from medial-plantar through the medial sustentaculum part of the fractured calcaneus and driven into the talus to create a constant/fixed part medially (**Fig. 4** A). The pin placement is orthogonal in relation to the tuberosity to adjust for any varus/valgus malalignment. In case a 5-mm Schanz pin is used, it can either be inserted from posterior or from lateral in the most distal/plantar portion of the tuberosity, taking the varus position of the tuber into account. After reducing the tuberosity, one or two 1.6-mm Kirschner wires are inserted on the medial side of the tuber into the sustentaculum, which is subsequently checked on fluoroscopy in the axial plane, to ensure correct neutral alignment of the calcaneal axis (see **Fig. 4**B,C). To gain more access to the subtalar joint, either a small distractor or a 5-mm Schanz pin can be used. In the case of a small distractor, it is mounted with 3.0-mm half-pins from the talar neck to the distal part of the tuberosity of the calcaneus (**Fig. 4**D).

Any removed joint fragments are now reinserted and aligned anatomically. Reduction is checked fluoroscopically, and anatomic reduction of height is met when Böhler angle and Gissane angle are restored. Fragments are held in place using 2 K-wires just

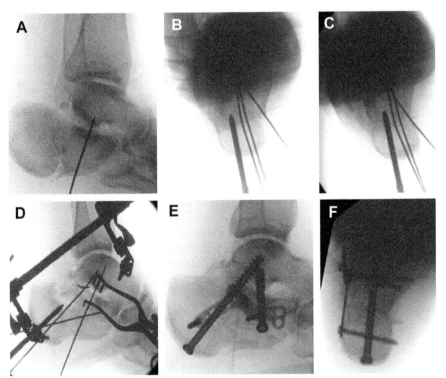

Fig. 4. Peroperative steps. (*A*) Reduction and stabilization of sustentaculum tali (constant fragment). (*B*) Reduction of tuberosity and axial alignment first attempt. (*C*) Final reduction and temporary fixation of tuberosity. (*D*) Use of small distractor to correct height. (*E*) Insertion of K-wires for large cannulated screws and plate fixation. (*F*) Insertion of large cannulated screws to fuse subtalar joint.

underneath the joint toward the sustentaculum. Subsequently, two or three 3.0 K-wires for the cannulated screws (7.3 to 7.5 mm) are added for the subtalar fusion. Inserting the guidewires at this stage ensures that the screws that are inserted here-after from lateral to medial are not interfering with the cannulated screws. Before inserting the cannulated screws for the subtalar joint fusion, screws of a small plate are placed to stabilize the reduction, and to prevent pushing the joint fragments apart while inserting the 7.3- to 7.5-mm cannulated screws (**Fig. 4**E,F). In comminuted frac-ture, caution is warranted that the large-diameter screws do not produce too much compression, because this will cause loss of height. One fully threaded positioning screw is often used because it does not cause compression (see **Fig. 3**D). Bone graft-ing is rarely used. Any remaining bulging of the lateral wall is now compressed inwards using a large periosteal elevator. Any hematoma is washed out, and the subcutis and skin are closed meticulously.

Clinical outcomes

There are currently more systematic reviews and metaanalyses than RCT in calcaneal fracture treatment.[62] All large randomized studies comparing operative with nonoper-ative use the ELA[52,63,64] with wound complication rates between 19% and 23% in the operative group.[52,63,64]

More recently, the STA is becoming more and more popular. Obtaining a similar quality of reduction at a significantly lower complication rate is the main incentive.

Studies comparing ELA versus STA show at least similar outcome and similar reduction at significantly lower complication rates in favor of the STA.[8,60,61,65-67]

Unfortunately, not many studies comparing ORIF versus ORIF + PSF are currently available. The study by Buckley and colleagues[45] is an RCT; however, it is small, and they were unable to include the required number of patients. They concluded that there were no significant differences between ORIF and ORIF + PSF at 2 years. They, however, noticed that patients with PSF healed more quickly and might benefit from fewer secondary procedures and less lost time from work.[45] The other compar-ative study is by Dingemans and colleagues.[44] They also observed no statistical sig-nificant difference in functional outcome between patients with ORIF and patients with primary arthrodesis after a minimal follow-up of 18 months.

These outcome scores were confirmed by Holm and colleagues[47] in a noncompar-ative study on primary fusions. The average AOFAS score in these 3 series ranged from 66 to 78 points.[44,45,47]

DISCUSSION

Calcaneal fracture remains a complex injury. There is not 1 single treatment option to manage all different fractures. The current review focuses on ORIF with or without PSF. Anatomic reduction is associated with improved outcome in DIACFs, and in light of the similar reduction rates and significantly lower rates of wound complications, the STA is likely the new gold standard. If anatomic reduction cannot be obtained following ORIF, a primary arthrodesis is a valid option. In addition, there are several factors associated with poorer outcome, which may be indications for primary arthrodesis as well. However, the primary arthrodesis should be performed only when preceded by restoration of overall anatomy of the calcaneus.

The evidence displayed in the current review is mainly level 3 and level 4. Future di-rections regarding the primary arthrodesis in DIACFs should be aimed at strength-ening the available evidence for primary fusion. Fusion criteria, as shown in **Table 1**, should be validated. In addition, there is a strong need for more comparative (RCT) studies comparing ORIF via STA versus ORIF via STA + PSF.

In conclusion, the ORIF of DIACFs, in the right hands, yields the best results if anatomic reduction is obtained and wound complications are avoided. In cases with severe comminution or when anatomic reduction cannot be obtained, a primary subtalar arthrodesis is a valuable option, if the overall anatomy of the calcaneus is corrected first.

CLINICS CARE POINTS

- Open reduction and internal fixation via the sinus tarsi approach yields similar results at a significant lower complication rate compared with the extended lateral approach.
- The primary arthrodesis following ORIF is a valuable addition in the treatment of comminuted displaced intraarticular calcaneal fractures and in specific cases.

DISCLOSURE

The author has nothing to disclose.

REFERENCES

1. Sanders R, Fortin P, DiPasquale T, et al. Operative treatment in 120 displaced intraarticular calcaneal fractures. Results using a prognostic computed tomography scan classification. Clin Orthop Relat Res 1993;(290):87–95.
2. Backes M, Spierings KE, Dingemans SA, et al. Evaluation and quantification of geographical differences in wound complication rates following the extended lateral approach in displaced intra-articular calcaneal fractures - a systematic review of the literature. Injury 2017;48(10):2329–35.
3. Schepers T. The sinus tarsi approach in displaced intra-articular calcaneal fractures: a systematic review. Int Orthop 2011;35(5):697–703.
4. Schepers T. Towards uniformity in communication and a tailor-made treatment for displaced intra-articular calcaneal fractures. Int Orthop 2014;38(3):663–5.
5. Palmer I. The mechanism and treatment of fractures of the calcaneus; open reduction with the use of cancellous grafts. J Bone Joint Surg Am 1948; 30A(1):2–8.
6. Stephenson JR. Treatment of displaced intra-articular fractures of the calcaneus using medial and lateral approaches, internal fixation, and early motion. J Bone Joint Surg Am 1987;69(1):115–30.
7. Lutz M, Gabl M, Horbst W, et al. [Wound margin necroses after open calcaneal reconstruction. Anatomical considerations of surgical approach]. Unfallchirurg 1997;100(10):792–6.
8. Schepers T, Backes M, Dingemans SA, et al. Similar anatomical reduction and lower complication rates with the sinus tarsi approach compared with the extended lateral approach in displaced intra-articular calcaneal fractures. J Orthop Trauma 2017;31(6):293–8.
9. Schepers T. The primary arthrodesis for severely comminuted intra-articular fractures of the calcaneus: a systematic review. Foot Ankle Surg 2012;18(2):84–8.
10. Ding L, He Z, Xiao H, et al. Risk factors for postoperative wound complications of calcaneal fractures following plate fixation. Foot Ankle Int 2013;34(9):1238–44.
11. Koski A, Kuokkanen H, Tukiainen E. Postoperative wound complications after internal fixation of closed calcaneal fractures: a retrospective analysis of 126 consecutive patients with 148 fractures. Scand J Surg 2005;94(3):243–5.

12. Court-Brown CM, Schmied M, Schutte BG. Factors affecting infection after calcaneal fracture fixation. Injury 2009;40(12):1313–5.
13. Schepers T, Den Hartog D, Vogels LM, et al. Extended lateral approach for intra-articular calcaneal fractures: an inverse relationship between surgeon experience and wound complications. J Foot Ankle Surg 2013;52(2):167–71.
14. Poeze M, Verbruggen JP, Brink PR. The relationship between the outcome of operatively treated calcaneal fractures and institutional fracture load. A systematic review of the literature. J Bone Joint Surg Am 2008;90(5):1013–21.
15. Magnuson PB, Stinchfield F. Fracture of the os calcis. Am J Surg 1938;42:685–92.
16. Rammelt S, Zwipp H. Calcaneus fractures: facts, controversies and recent developments. Injury 2004;35(5):443–61.
17. Zwipp H, Pasa L, Zilka L, et al. Introduction of a new locking nail for treatment of intraarticular calcaneal fractures. J Orthop Trauma 2016;30(3):e88–92.
18. Rammelt S, Sangeorzan BJ, Swords MP. Calcaneal fractures - should we or should we not operate? Indian J Orthop 2018;52(3):220–30.
19. Barrick B, Joyce DA, Werner FW, et al. Effect of calcaneus fracture gap without step-off on stress distribution across the subtalar joint. Foot Ankle Int 2017;38(3):298–303.
20. Mulcahy DM, McCormack DM, Stephens MM. Intra-articular calcaneal fractures: effect of open reduction and internal fixation on the contact characteristics of the subtalar joint. Foot Ankle Int 1998;19(12):842–8.
21. Sangeorzan BJ, Ananthakrishnan D, Tencer AF. Contact characteristics of the subtalar joint after a simulated calcaneus fracture. J Orthop Trauma 1995;9(3):251–8.
22. Wagner UA, Ananthakrishnan D, Sangeorzan BJ, et al. Influence of talar neck and intra-articular calcaneal fractures on subtalar joint mechanics. Foot Ankle Surg 1996;2:19–26.
23. Xu C, Liu H, Li M, et al. A three-dimensional finite element analysis of displaced intra-articular calcaneal fractures. J Foot Ankle Surg 2017;56(2):319–26.
24. Schumpelick W. [Treatment of severe calcaneum fracture by early arthrodesis]. Arch Orthop Unfallchir 1953;46(1):66–77.
25. Whittaker AH. Treatment of fractures of the os calcis by open reduction and internal fixation. Am J Surg 1947;74(5):687–96.
26. Van Stockum WJ. Operatieve behandeling van de breuk van den calcaneus en den talus. Ned Tijdschr Geneeskd 1911;III:1723–4.
27. Van Stockum WJ. Operative behandlung der calcaneus und talusfraktur. Zentralbl Chir 1912;39:1438–9.
28. Conn HR. Fractures of the os calcis: diagnosis and treatment. Radiology 1926;6(3):228–35.
29. Wilson PD. Treatment of fractures of the os calcis by arthrodesis of the subastragalar joint. JAMA 1927;89(20):1676–83.
30. Nutter JA. Treatment of fractures of the os calcis by arthrodesis of the subastragalar joint. Can Med Assoc J 1930;22:247.
31. Spiers HW. Comminuted fractures of the os calcis. JAMA 1938;110(1):28–31.
32. Becker F. Primare arthrodese bei der behandlung von fersenbeinbruchen. Zentralbl Chir 1951;76:834–7.
33. Gallie WE. Subastragalar arthrodesis in fractures of the os calcis. J Bone Joint Surg 1943;25:731–6.
34. Harris RI. Fractures of the os calcis: their treatment by tri-radiate traction and subastragalar fusion. Ann Surg 1946;124(6):1082–99.

35. Hall MC, Pennal GF. Primary subtalar arthrodesis in the treatment of severe fractures of the calcaneum. J Bone Joint Surg Br 1960;42-B:336–43.

36. Bankart ASB. Fractures of the os calcis. Lancet 1942;240(6207):175.

37. Lindsay WR, Dewar FP. Fractures of the os calcis. Am J Surg 1958;95(4):555–76.

38. Tanke GM. Fractures of the calcaneus. A review of the literature together with some observations on methods of treatment. Acta Chir Scand Suppl 1982;505:1–103.

39. Ehalt W. Our current therapy of fresh calcaneus fractures. Arch Orthop Unfallchir 1965;57:133–6 [in German].

40. Holsscher AA. Primaire en secundaire arthrodese bij fracturen van de calcaneus. Amsterdam (the Netherlands): Thesis; 1965.

41. Potenza V, Caterini R, Farsetti P, et al. Primary subtalar arthrodesis for the treatment of comminuted intra-articular calcaneal fractures. Injury 2010;41(7):702–6.

42. Malik AK, Solan M, Sakellariou A, et al. Primary subtalar arthrodesis for the treatment of comminuted intra-articular calcaneal fractures [Injury 41;2010:702-706]. Injury 2011;42(4):431–2 [author reply: 432–3].

43. Myerson MS. Primary subtalar arthrodesis for the treatment of comminuted fractures of the calcaneus. Orthop Clin North Am 1995;26(2):215–27.

44. Dingemans SA, Meijer ST, Backes M, et al. Outcome following osteosynthesis or primary arthrodesis of calcaneal fractures: a cross-sectional cohort study. Injury 2017;48(10):2336–41.

45. Buckley R, Leighton R, Sanders D, et al. Open reduction and internal fixation compared with ORIF and primary subtalar arthrodesis for treatment of Sanders type IV calcaneal fractures: a randomized multicenter trial. J Orthop Trauma 2014;28(10):577–83.

46. Eisenstein ED, Kusnezov NA, Waterman BR, et al. Open reduction and internal fixation (ORIF) versus ORIF and primary subtalar arthrodesis for complex displaced intraarticular calcaneus fractures: an expected value decision analysis. OTA Int 2018;1(2):1–7.

47. Holm JL, Laxson SE, Schuberth JM. Primary subtalar joint arthrodesis for comminuted fractures of the calcaneus. J Foot Ankle Surg 2015;54(1):61–5.

48. Fuentes-Viejo D, Cellarier G, Lauer P, et al. Primary or secondary subtalar arthrodesis and revision of calcaneal nonunion with minimally invasive rigid internal nail fixation for treatment of displaced intra-articular calcaneal fractures. Clin Podiatr Med Surg 2019;36(2):295–306.

49. Facaros Z, Ramanujam CL, Zgonis T. Primary subtalar joint arthrodesis with internal and external fixation for the repair of a diabetic comminuted calcaneal fracture. Clin Podiatr Med Surg 2011;28(1):203–9.

50. Lopez-Oliva F, Sanchez-Lorente T, Fuentes-Sanz A, et al. Primary fusion in worker's compensation intraarticular calcaneus fracture. Prospective study of 169 consecutive cases. Injury 2012;43(Suppl 2):S73–8.

51. Sanders R, Vaupel ZM, Erdogan M, et al. Operative treatment of displaced intra-articular calcaneal fractures: long-term (10-20 years) results in 108 fractures using a prognostic CT classification. J Orthop Trauma 2014;28(10):551–63.

52. Buckley R, Tough S, McCormack R, et al. Operative compared with nonoperative treatment of displaced intra-articular calcaneal fractures: a prospective, randomized, controlled multicenter trial. J Bone Joint Surg Am 2002;84-A(10):1733–44.

53. Csizy M, Buckley R, Tough S, et al. Displaced intra-articular calcaneal fractures: variables predicting late subtalar fusion. J Orthop Trauma 2003;17(2):106–12.

54. Spierings KE, Min M, Nooijen LE, et al. Managing the open calcaneal fracture: a systematic review. Foot Ankle Surg 2019;25(6):707–13.

55. Backes M, Schep NW, Luitse JS, et al. The effect of postoperative wound infections on functional outcome following intra-articular calcaneal fractures. Arch Orthop Trauma Surg 2015;135(8):1045–52.
56. Backes M, Schepers T, Beerekamp MS, et al. Wound infections following open reduction and internal fixation of calcaneal fractures with an extended lateral approach. Int Orthop 2014;38(4):767–73.
57. Zwipp H, Rammelt S, Barthel S. [Fracture of the calcaneus]. Unfallchirurg 2005; 108(9):737–47 [quiz: 748].
58. Eastwood DM, Langkamer VG, Atkins RM. Intra-articular fractures of the calcaneum. Part II: open reduction and internal fixation by the extended lateral transcalcaneal approach. J Bone Joint Surg Br 1993;75(2):189–95.
59. Schepers T. Sinus tarsi approach with screws-only fixation for displaced intra-articular calcaneal fractures. Clin Podiatr Med Surg 2019;36(2):211–24.
60. Xia S, Lu Y, Wang H, et al. Open reduction and internal fixation with conventional plate via L-shaped lateral approach versus internal fixation with percutaneous plate via a sinus tarsi approach for calcaneal fractures - a randomized controlled trial. Int J Surg 2014;12(5):475–80.
61. Yeo JH, Cho HJ, Lee KB. Comparison of two surgical approaches for displaced intra-articular calcaneal fractures: sinus tarsi versus extensile lateral approach. BMC Musculoskelet Disord 2015;16:63.
62. Schepers T. Calcaneal fractures: looking beyond the meta-analyses. J Foot Ankle Surg 2016;55(4):897–8.
63. Agren PH, Wretenberg P, Sayed-Noor AS. Operative versus nonoperative treatment of displaced intra-articular calcaneal fractures: a prospective, randomized, controlled multicenter trial. J Bone Joint Surg Am 2013;95(15):1351–7.
64. Griffin D, Parsons N, Shaw E, et al. Operative versus non-operative treatment for closed, displaced, intra-articular fractures of the calcaneus: randomised controlled trial. BMJ 2014;349:g4483.
65. Li LH, Guo YZ, Wang H, et al. Less wound complications of a sinus tarsi approach compared to an extended lateral approach for the treatment of displaced intraarticular calcaneal fracture: a randomized clinical trial in 64 patients. Medicine (Baltimore) 2016;95(36):e4628.
66. Zhou HC, Yu T, Ren HY, et al. Clinical comparison of extensile lateral approach and sinus tarsi approach combined with medial distraction technique for intra-articular calcaneal fractures. Orthop Surg 2017;9(1):77–85.
67. Nosewicz TL, Dingemans SA, Backes M, et al. A systematic review and meta-analysis of the sinus tarsi and extended lateral approach in the operative treatment of displaced intra-articular calcaneal fractures. Foot Ankle Surg 2019; 25(5):580–8.

How to Identify Unstable Lisfranc Injuries? Review of Diagnostic Strategies and Algorithm Proposal

German Joannas, MD[a,b,c], Jorge Filippi, MD, MBA[d,e,*]

KEYWORDS

- Lisfranc • Tarsometatarsal • Instability • Midfoot arthrodesis • Imaging • Injury
- Diagnosis

KEY POINTS

- Misdiagnosed Lisfranc injuries can be as high as 50%, leading to chronic pain, functional impairment, and posttraumatic arthritis. Subtle or incomplete lesions are the most problematic group for an adequate diagnosis.
- When clinical suspicion for a midfoot injury is present, all efforts must be done to rule out Lisfranc instability. Conventional non–weight-bearing radiographs can overlook up to 30% of unstable cases.
- Abduction stress radiographs and anteroposterior monopodial comparative weight-bearing radiographic views are very useful to identify instability, and they are recommended as the initial study for a potentially unstable Lisfranc injury.
- Computed tomography gives detailed information about fracture patterns and comminution, but its role in detecting occult instability is unclear.
- MRI can predict instability but it is expensive and not readily available in the acute setting.

INTRODUCTION

The incidence of reported injuries to the Lisfranc joint is estimated at 1 per 55,000 people per year.[1] Misdiagnosed Lisfranc injuries can be as high as 50%, leading to chronic

[a] Foot and Ankle Division "CEPP", Instituto Dupuytren, Av. Belgrano 3402, Ciudad Autónoma de Buenos Aires CP 1078, Argentina; [b] Foot and Ankle Division, Orthopaedics Department, Centro Artroscópico Jorge Batista SA, Pueyrredón 2446 1er piso, Ciudad Autónoma de Buenos Aires (CABA) CP 1119, Argentina; [c] Instituto Barrancas, Hipolito Yrigoyen 902, Quilmes, CP 1878, Buenos Aires, Argentina; [d] Department of Orthopedic Surgery, Foot and Ankle Unit, Clinica Las Condes, Estoril 450, Las Condes, Santiago 7591047, Chile; [e] Department of Orthopedic Surgery, Foot and Ankle Unit, Hospital del Trabajador, Ramon Carnicer 185, Providencia, Santiago 7501239, Chile
* Corresponding author. Estoril 450, Las Condes, Santiago 7591047, Chile.
E-mail address: jfilippi@clinicalascondes.cl

Foot Ankle Clin N Am 25 (2020) 697–710
https://doi.org/10.1016/j.fcl.2020.08.011
1083-7515/20/© 2020 Elsevier Inc. All rights reserved.

foot.theclinics.com

pain, functional impairment, and posttraumatic arthritis.[2–6] Subtle or pure ligamentous lesions are the most problematic group for an adequate diagnosis because plain radiographs are not capable of addressing potential instability.

Comparative weight-bearing (WB) radiographs, abduction stress views, and MRI have been used to address tarsometatarsal (TMT) instability.[7–11]

A precise evaluation of instability is also needed during surgery to decide which joints to stabilize. Stress maneuvers under anesthesia or direct view of the joints are very helpful. Deciding on which joints to treat has important repercussions in terms of hardware usage, cartilage disruption (ie, when transarticular screws are used), and time of surgery.

This article reviews the current evidence in diagnostic tools for Lisfranc instability and presents a diagnostic algorithm for these injuries.

RELEVANT ANATOMY AND BIOMECHANICS

The TMT complex includes bony and ligamentous structures. The metatarsals display in the transverse plane as a Roman arch with the second metatarsal as the cornerstone giving inherent bone stability. It is divided into 3 functional and anatomic areas, medial column comprising the first metatarsal (M1) and medial cuneiform (C1) joint, middle column comprising the second (M2) and third metatarsal (M3) joint with intermediate (C2) and lateral cuneiform (C3), and the lateral column comprising fourth (M4) and fifth metatarsal (M5) joint with the cuboid. The lateral column has the highest degree of motion with 13 mm, and the middle column is the more stable with only 0.6 mm of dorsoplantar movement.[12]

The most clinically relevant ligament is the C1-M2 (Lisfranc) ligament. It has 3 components, dorsal, interosseous, and plantar, the interosseous being the strongest.[13,14] Its importance is that it is the only structure that connects the medial and middle column since the absence of an M1-M2 interosseous ligament.[15,16]

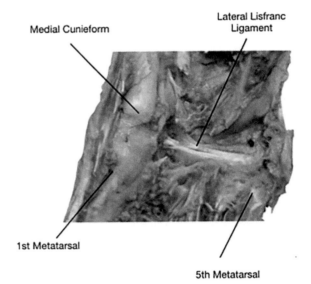

Fig. 1. Anatomic preparation of the lateral Lisfranc ligament (Liverpool ligament). (*From* Mason L, Jayatilaka MLT, Fisher A, et al. Anatomy of the lateral plantar ligaments of the transverse metatarsal arch. Foot Ankle Int. 2020;41(1):109–14; with permission).

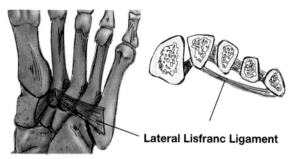

Lateral Lisfranc Ligament

Fig. 2. The lateral Lisfranc ligament (Liverpool ligament). (*From* Mason L, Jayatilaka MLT, Fisher A, et al. Anatomy of the lateral plantar ligaments of the transverse metatarsal arch. Foot Ankle Int. 2020;41(1):109–14; with permission).

Interosseous ligaments are present between each of the metatarsals from the second to the fifth. The presence of intermetatarsal ligaments explains the conjoined behavior of the middle and the lateral columns in certain types of injuries. A study by Mayne and colleagues[17] suggested that when intermetatarsal ligaments are intact, stabilizing the medial cuneiform to the second metatarsal base combined with stabilization of the fourth and fifth TMT joints with K-wires will stabilize the first and third TMT joints.

Recently, Mason and colleagues described the lateral Lisfranc ligament ("The Liverpool ligament"). This newly described structure provides a connection through the long plantar ligament of both the transverse and the longitudinal arches. This ligament connects the plantar aspect of M2 to M5, and the investigators hypothesized that this could be the reason why the lateral column can get stabilized after fixation of the middle column. They suspected that in most of the homolateral and divergent types of TMT injuries, the lateral Lisfranc ligament remains intact and explains the physiopathology for this type of injury[18] (**Figs. 1 and 2**).

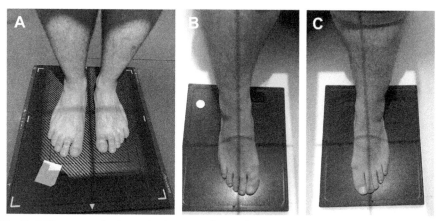

Fig. 3. Different methods to obtain WB radiographs. (*A*) Bipedal WB comparative view in the same cassette. Note that the beam is centered in the area between both feet. (*B, C*) Monopodial WB comparative view on both feet. In this case, the beam is centered in the second metatarsal.

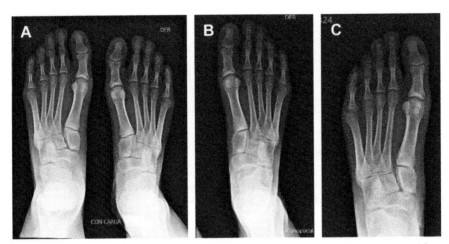

Fig. 4. Patient with pain in the left foot after direct trauma. (*A*) Bipedal WB view with no evident displacement on the left foot. (*B*) Monopodial WB view of the right (noninjured) foot. (*C*) Monopodial WB view of the injured foot that reveals intercuneiform and C1-M2 instability.

The complex anatomy of the midfoot with several ligament interconnections and inherent bone stability makes it difficult to diagnose a subtle Lisfranc instability accurately. This can explain the multiple and different injury patterns of the midfoot and also gives an explanation of the fact that during surgery after stabilizing the middle column, sometimes the others get stability without fixation.

DIAGNOSTIC STUDIES
Conventional Radiographs

Conventional radiographs provide important information about Lisfranc injuries. However, undiagnosed and misdiagnosed lesions can easily occur. Rankine and

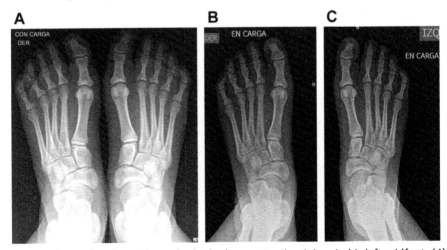

Fig. 5. Radiographs of a patient who had a hyperextension injury in his left midfoot. (*A*) Bipedal WB view with a nonconclusive asymmetry of the C1-M2 distance. (*B*) Monopodial WB view of the right (noninjured) foot. (*C*) Monopodial WB view of the left (injured) foot that shows more evidently the increase in C1-M2 distance.

colleagues[19] reported that non-WB radiographs correctly identified only 68.9% of Lisfranc injuries.

On the anteroposterior (AP) view, the central beam is centered on M2, with 15° of caudal angulation, and in the oblique (OB) view, the foot has an internal rotation of 30°.[4]

Anatomic alignment on the AP and OB views is as follows: the lateral border of M1 aligns with the lateral border of C1, the medial border of the base of the M2 aligns with the medial border of the C2, the medial and lateral border of the M3 should align with the medial and lateral border of C3, and the medial border of the base of the M4 should be in line with the medial side of the cuboid.[5,20]

The presence of the "fleck sign" has been identified as pathognomonic for C1-M2 instability. It represents an avulsion fracture of the Lisfranc ligament from M2. Although it is commonly seen in unstable injuries, its absence does not rule out instability.[2,21]

Malalignment at the second TMT joint, with lateral displacement of the base of M2 with respect to C2, and a diastasis of more than 2 mm between the bases of M1 and M2 are indicators of instability.[5,22]

Rankine and colleagues[23] showed that 29° of craniocaudal angulation in the AP view optimizes the view of the second TMT joint and suggests its routine use when studying midfoot injuries.

A study by Seo and colleagues identified signs of instability in comparative non-WB radiographs. They compared the radiographic findings with intraoperative instability. Avulsion of the base of M2 (fleck sign) and C1-M2 and C1-C2 diastasis were found to have 100% of specificity for intraoperative instability. The sensitivity was 48%, 92%, and 60% respectively. The fleck sign was only present in 47% of this series. For M1-C1 instability, abnormal preoperative findings were present in only 43% of the cases with intraoperative first ray instability.[24]

Weight-bearing Radiographs

WB views are used to improve the diagnostic capabilities of conventional radiographs by adding physiologic stress to the TMT joints.[4] Examination of the contralateral uninjured foot is very helpful to detect asymmetries. Classically, more than 2 mm of difference in C1-M2 or M1-M2 distance with the contralateral foot may be an indicator of instability. Thomas and colleagues determined the value of the Lisfranc joint width in a standardized adult population in 100 healthy volunteers with WB views. The mean C1-M2 distance was 5.6 mm (95% confidence interval [CI] 5.39–5.81), and the mean difference between both feet was 0.7 mm (95% CI 0.63–0.77).[20]

Even though its extended use has been referenced in many studies, a detailed description of how to take WB views is hard to find. There are several options to take WB AP views: bipedal WB in the same cassette, bipedal WB in a different cassette, or monopodial WB. Each of them will provide a different view angle, and the degree of stress to the TMT joint could change.

To our knowledge, no study has compared these methods.

Our preferred method to obtain standing feet radiographs is with monopodial WB. This technique allows the standardizing of WB, and the central beam is oriented to the foot instead of the area between both feet (**Fig. 3**). **Figs. 4 and 5** show 2 cases in which the Lisfranc instability is more evident on the monopodial WB view than the bipedal comparative view.

When a patient with high clinical suspicion of a Lisfranc injury is not able to put weight on the injured foot, and the conventional non-WB radiographs do not show findings, WB images can be ordered 7 to 10 days after the injury during follow-up.

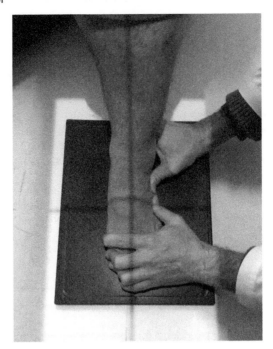

Fig. 6. Abduction stress views (*left*).

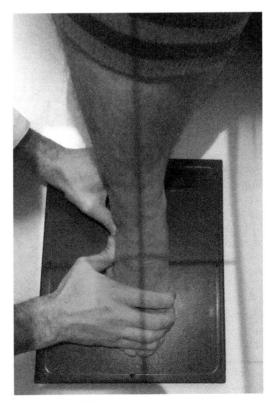

Fig. 7. Abduction stress views (*right*).

Abduction Stress Views

As noted previously, non-WB radiographs can overlook up to 40% of Lisfranc instability. Regarding this problem, stress views have been described to improve these mediocre results. Abduction maneuvers were suggested by some investigators in the early 90s.[25,26] In 1998, Coss and colleagues described the parameters of

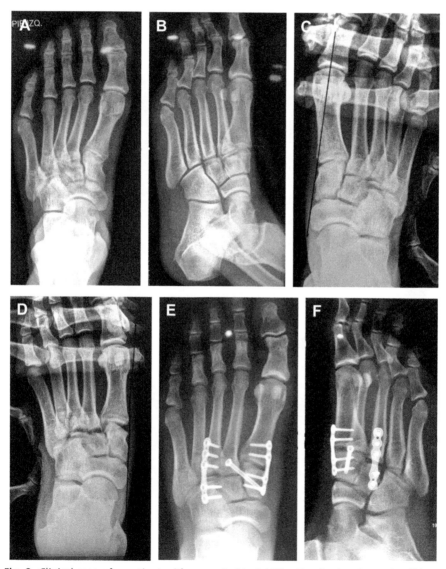

Fig. 8. Clinical case of a patient with suspected instability. Standard radiographs did not show any abnormalities. Abduction stress views revealed instability of M1-C1, M2-C1, and M3-C3. (*A*) Preoperative AP view. (*B*) Preoperative OB view. (*C*) Negative Abduction stress view. (*D*) Positive abduction stress view (instability of M1-C1, M2-C1, and M3-C3). (*E*) Postoperative surgery AP view: position screw M2C1 and plating for M1C1 and M3C3. (*F*) Postoperative surgery OB view.

abnormal abduction stress views. They compared findings in 9 cadaveric feet who had sequential sectioning of midfoot ligaments with 20 healthy volunteers. In 39 of 40 healthy feet, a line tangential to the medial aspect of the navicular and C1 (medial column line [MCL]) intersected the base of M1 on abduction stress radiographs. Three of 4 cadavers with isolated sectioning of the Lisfranc ligament had disruption of MCL. In all 9 cadavers, sectioning of the Lisfranc ligament in combination with the dorsal TMT ligaments produced a disruption of the MCL on abduction stress, whether or not, the plantar ligaments had yet been sectioned. On simulated AP WB views, M1-M2 distances did not widen more than 1.5 mm, even with completely sectioned ligaments.[9]

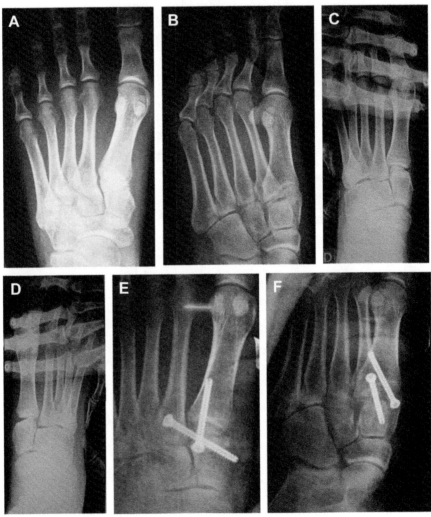

Fig. 9. Clinical case of a patient with hidden injury. Standard radiographs did not show any abnormalities. Abduction stress views revealed instability of M1-C1 and M2-C1. (*A*) Preoperative AP view. (*B*) Preoperative OB view. (*C*) Negative abduction stress view. (*D*) Positive abduction stress view (instability of M1-C1 and M2-C1). (*E*) Postoperative surgery AP view: position screw M2C1 and M1C1. (*F*). Postoperative surgery OB view.

Another cadaveric study compared WB radiographs with manual abduction stress views in feet with sequential ligament sectioning. They concluded that stress views showed qualitatively greater displacement when used to evaluate instability compared with WB views.[27]

The use of the abduction stress view is not widespread, possibly for the pain elicited during the examination and the need for trained personnel. In the authors' experience, this can be done without anesthesia and is very reliable to demonstrate instability. The inconvenience of needing a qualified operator is real, and this method can be done only when an orthopedic physician is available to perform and evaluate the stress

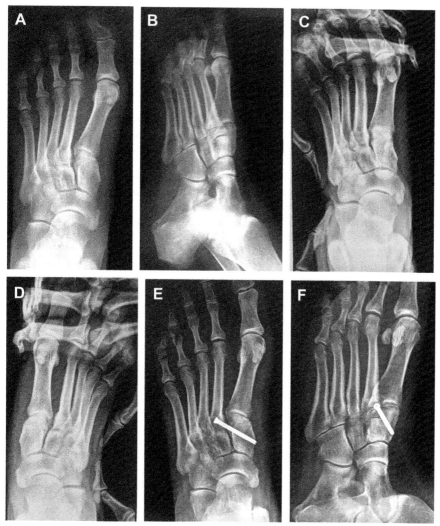

Fig 10. Clinical case of a patient with suspected instability. Standard radiographs did not show any abnormalities. Abduction stress views revealed instability of M2-C1 and "fleck sign." (*A*) Preoperative AP view. (*B*) Preoperative OB view. (*C*) Negative abduction stress view. (*D*) Positive abduction stress view (instability of M2-C1 and fleck sign). (*E*) Postoperative surgery AP view: *ONLY one* position screw M2C1. (*F*) Postoperative surgery OB view.

maneuvers. **Figs. 6 and 7** show our preferred method for acquiring the abduction stress view.

Taking into consideration all these aspects, it is still believed that this is a powerful tool to diagnose an occult instability preoperatively, it helps in the decision for surgery and surgical planning, and that it should be used when possible. **Figs. 8–10** show 3 cases with apparently normal conventional radiographs and the instability of medial and middle column after stress views.

Computed Tomography

CT provides excellent visualization of bone details and helps to detect occult fractures or subtle articular subluxation and determine the degree of comminution and articular extension of the fracture. In a study, CT detected twice tarsal fractures and TMT joint malalignment and 60% more metatarsal fractures than conventional radiographs.[28]

However, conventional CT is not a dynamic study; therefore, it has the same limitations as non-WB radiographs in terms of identifying occult instability. Also, no consensus exists in the literature as to how the distance of the C1 and M2 articulation should be defined and measured[5] nor what the normal range of this value should be when evaluated by CT.[10]

An interesting study showed, in 117 patients with clinical signs compatible with midfoot injury, that in patients with positive findings in WB radiographs 54% had a negative or equivocal CT report. On the other hand, 12% of equivocal or negative WB radiographs had a positive CT. They concluded that relying on the CT report alone, a significant proportion of subtle injuries would have been misdiagnosed, and CT did not provide any additional information for patients with a positive WB film and detected only a small percentage of additional injuries.[29]

WB-CT has had great attention lately, especially in foot and ankle surgery.[30] To our knowledge, no clinical studies have been published regarding WB-CT and Lisfranc injuries. The authors only found one article that analyzed CT findings of simulated WB in 16 cadavers. After sequential ligament sectioning, they found an increase of MC-M2 and M1-M2 distance, and this value was higher when more ligaments were sectioned.[7]

CT gives excellent information about fracture details and is very helpful to determine the degree of comminution, especially in high-energy or complex midfoot injuries.[10] The authors recommend to take a CT as a complement for WB or stress views and not as the first line of study. In the future, the use of WB-CT in this type of injury is promising because it could combine high detail imaging with stress to the TMT joint.

MRI

MRI offers a detailed view of the ligaments and bony anatomy in the midfoot. Several investigators have demonstrated that injuries to Lisfranc ligaments are highly correlated with MRI findings.[5,10,11,16,28] Although it is not a dynamic study, a high degree of predictability for instability has been described. Raikin and colleagues,[31] in a clinical study with 20 patients, showed that when the plantar C1-M2-M3 ligament is torn or has a grade 2 sprain it highly suggests an unstable midfoot, also when this ligament is intact on MRI it suggests a stable TMT joint (**Fig. 11**). Only one case report has been published on WB MRI in Lisfranc injuries[8]; therefore, more studies are needed to have a better understanding of this alternative.

Unfortunately, MRI has some drawbacks. It is costly and not always available in the acute setting, interpretation errors could over- or underestimate the level of injury, and it is not a dynamic study.[10] Because most of the unstable Lisfranc lesions can be ruled out with WB or stress radiographs, the authors consider that MRI must be

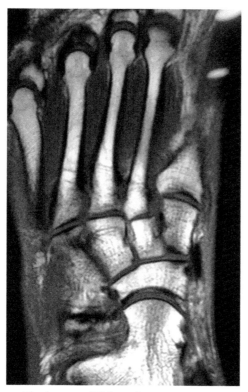

Fig. 11. MR axial view with absence of Lisfranc ligament.

recommended when WB or stress radiographs are normal in patients with a high clinical index of suspicion.

THE AUTHORS' RECOMMENDATION AND ALGORITHM

Based on the available evidence and the authors' hospitals' experience, they suggest the following diagnostic algorithm (**Fig. 12**).

Conventional radiographs are the first line for the study in any patient with clinical suspicion of Lisfranc instability such as plantar ecchymosis, swollen midfoot, WB pain, and history with a compatible mechanism of injury. According to the radiographic findings and the classification described by Arrondo and colleagues,[32] the injuries can be divided into hidden or evident. When evident or high-energy injury is present, CT evaluation is indicated for surgery planning to decide whether osteosynthesis or arthrodesis will be the final treatment.

When the information of the radiographs is not clear or negative (hidden injuries), it is recommended to use comparative abduction stress radiographs. It is believed that it is the most effective method to evaluate the potential instability in the 3 columns of the midfoot. This maneuver provides essential information about C1-M2 (Lisfranc ligament), C1-M1, and M3-C3 stability. When the abduction stress view is positive for instability, it is not necessary to do any other study, and surgery is indicated. If the stress view is negative and a high clinical suspicion is present, the authors consider

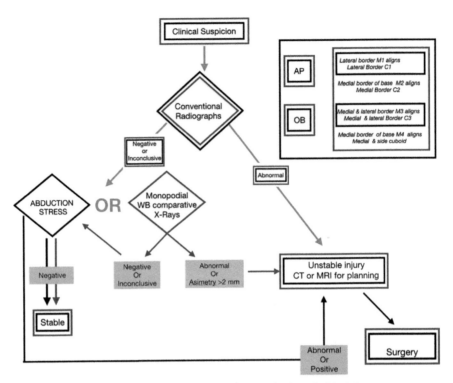

Fig. 12. Diagnostic algorithm: the authors' preference is given in black boxes.

the use of MRI. If MRI shows an intact Lisfranc ligament, conservative treatment is indicated, and when the plantar C1-M2-M3 is torn, surgery is indicated.

If the abduction stress view cannot be performed, the authors suggest the use of comparative monopodial WB radiographs instead. Even though it does not produce as much stress as the abduction test, it is very helpful and can reveal occult instability as well.

SUMMARY

Undetected or misdiagnosed Lisfranc injuries are frequent and lead to bad results, chronic pain, functional impairment, and arthritis. The complex anatomy of the midfoot explains the multiple and different injury patterns. Subtle injuries are the most challenging in terms of diagnosis. When clinical suspicion is present, all efforts must be done to rule out Lisfranc instability. CT gives detailed information about fracture patterns and comminution, but its role in detecting occult instability is unclear. Because conventional radiographs can overlook up to one-third of occult injuries, the use of dynamic or stress methods is mandatory. The authors recommend to start with the abduction stress radiographs because they provide a thorough understanding of the midfoot instability and they believe is the best method to differentiate a stable injury from an unstable one. If the abduction stress radiographs cannot be performed, the authors recommend the use of monopodial WB comparative radiographs. If the aforementioned studies are negative and there is a high clinical suspicion, MRI findings could help to decide if surgical treatment is necessary.

CLINICS CARE POINTS

- Up to 30% of unstable Lisfranc injuries look normal in non-weightbearing x-rays.
- Abduction stress radiographs by trained personnel are very useful to address instability. In the authors' experience, there is no need for anesthesia.
- Comparative monopodial weightbearing x-rays is an excellent alternative to get stress views.
- CT and MRI are useful for preoperative planning, but the surgical decision must be based on dynamic studies.

DISCLOSURE

The authors have nothing to disclose.

REFERENCES

1. Lee CA, Birkedal JP, Dickerson EA, et al. Stabilization of Lisfranc joint injuries: a biomechanical study. Foot Ankle Int 2004;25(5):365–70.
2. Desmond EA, Chou LB. Current concepts review: Lisfranc injuries. Foot Ankle Int 2006;27(8):653–60.
3. Aronow MS. Treatment of the missed Lisfranc injury. Foot Ankle Clin 2006;11(1): 127–142, ix.
4. Weatherford BM, Anderson JG, Bohay DR. Management of tarsometatarsal joint injuries. J Am Acad Orthop Surg 2017;25(7):469–79.
5. Siddiqui NA, Galizia MS, Almusa E, et al. Evaluation of the tarsometatarsal joint using conventional radiography, CT, and MR imaging. Radiographics 2014; 34(2):514–31.
6. Kuo RS, Tejwani NC, Digiovanni CW, et al. Outcome after open reduction and internal fixation of Lisfranc joint injuries. J Bone Joint Surg Am 2000;82(11): 1609–18.
7. Penev P, Qawasmi F, Mosheiff R, et al. Ligamentous Lisfranc injuries: analysis of CT findings under weightbearing. Eur J Trauma Emerg Surg 2020. https://doi.org/10.1007/s00068-020-01302-7.
8. Gunio DA, Vulcano E, Benitez CL. Dynamic stress MRI of midfoot injuries: measurable morphology and laxity of the sprained lisfranc ligament during mechanical loading: a case report. JBJS Case Connect 2019;9(3):e0228.
9. Coss HS, Manos RE, Buoncristiani A, et al. Abduction stress and AP weightbearing radiography of purely ligamentous injury in the tarsometatarsal joint. Foot Ankle Int 1998;19(8):537–41.
10. Sripanich Y, Weinberg MW, Krähenbühl N, et al. Imaging in Lisfranc injury: a systematic literature review. Skeletal Radiol 2020;49(1):31–53.
11. Ablimit A, Ding H-Y, Liu L-G. Magnetic resonance imaging of the Lisfranc ligament. J Orthop Surg Res 2018;13(1):282.
12. Ouzounian TJ, Shereff MJ. In vitro determination of midfoot motion. Foot Ankle 1989;10(3):140–6.
13. Johnson A, Hill K, Ward J, et al. Anatomy of the lisfranc ligament. Foot Ankle Spec 2008;1(1):19–23.
14. Panchbhavi VK, Molina D 4th, Villarreal J, et al. Three-dimensional, digital, and gross anatomy of the Lisfranc ligament. Foot Ankle Int 2013;34(6):876–80.
15. de Palma L, Santucci A, Sabetta SP, et al. Anatomy of the Lisfranc joint complex. Foot Ankle Int 1997;18(6):356–64.

16. Castro M, Melão L, Canella C, et al. Lisfranc joint ligamentous complex: MRI with anatomic correlation in cadavers. AJR Am J Roentgenol 2010;195(6):W447–55.

17. Mayne AIW, Lawton R, Dalgleish S, et al. Stability of Lisfranc injury fixation in Thiel cadavers: Is routine fixation of the 1st and 3rd tarsometatarsal joint necessary? Injury 2017;48(8):1764–7.

18. Mason L, Jayatilaka MLT, Fisher A, et al. Anatomy of the lateral plantar ligaments of the transverse metatarsal Arch. Foot Ankle Int 2020;41(1):109–14.

19. Rankine JJ. The diagnostic accuracy of plain radiographs in Lisfranc injury and the potential value of a cranial caudal projection. Clin Radiol 2011;S3. https://doi.org/10.1016/j.crad.2011.07.006.

20. Thomas JL, Kopiec A, Mark K, et al. Radiographic value of the Lisfranc diastasis in a standardized population. Foot Ankle Spec 2019. https://doi.org/10.1177/1938640019890738. 193864001989073.

21. Myerson MS, Fisher RT, Burgess AR, et al. Fracture dislocations of the tarsometatarsal joints: end results correlated with pathology and treatment. Foot Ankle 1986;6(5):225–42.

22. Foster SC, Foster RR. Lisfranc's tarsometatarsal fracture—dislocation. Radiology 1976;120(1):79–83.

23. Rankine JJ, Nicholas CM, Wells G, et al. The diagnostic accuracy of radiographs in Lisfranc injury and the potential value of a craniocaudal projection. AJR Am J Roentgenol 2012;198(4):W365–9.

24. Seo D-K, Lee H-S, Lee KW, et al. Nonweightbearing radiographs in patients with a subtle Lisfranc injury. Foot Ankle Int 2017;38(10):1120–5.

25. Hansen ST. Foot injuries. In: Browner BD, Jupiter JB, Levine AM, et al, editors. Skeletal trauma, vol. 2, 1st edition 1992;. p. 1977–80.

26. Myerson M. The diagnosis and treatment of injuries to the Lisfranc joint complex. Orthop Clin North Am 1989;20(4):655–64.

27. Kaar S, Femino J, Morag Y. Lisfranc joint displacement following sequential ligament sectioning. J Bone Joint Surg Am 2007;89(10):2225–32.

28. Preidler KW, Peicha G, Lajtai G, et al. Conventional radiography, CT, and MR imaging in patients with hyperflexion injuries of the foot: diagnostic accuracy in the detection of bony and ligamentous changes. AJR Am J Roentgenol 1999;173(6):1673–7.

29. Kennelly H, Klaassen K, Heitman D, et al. Utility of weight-bearing radiographs compared to computed tomography scan for the diagnosis of subtle Lisfranc injuries in the emergency setting. Emerg Med Australas 2019;31(5):741–4.

30. Conti MS, Ellis SJ. Weight-bearing CT scans in foot and ankle surgery. J Am Acad Orthop Surg 2020. https://doi.org/10.5435/JAAOS-D-19-00700.

31. Raikin SM, Elias I, Dheer S, et al. Prediction of midfoot instability in the subtle Lisfranc injury. Comparison of magnetic resonance imaging with intraoperative findings. J Bone Joint Surg Am 2009;91(4):892–9.

32. Schepers T, Rammelt S. Classifying the Lisfranc injury: literature overview and a new classification. Fuß & Sprunggelenk 2018;16(3):151–9. https://doi.org/10.1016/j.fuspru.2018.07.003.

Subtle Lisfranc Injuries: Fix It, Fuse It, or Bridge It?

Jorge Briceno, MD[a], Anna-Kathrin Leucht, MD[b],
Alastair Younger, MB, ChB, MSc, ChM, FRCSC[c,d,e],
Andrea Veljkovic, MD, BComm, MPH, FRCSC[c,d,e,*]

KEYWORDS

- Tarsometatarsal joint injuries • Subtle Lisfranc injuries • Low-energy Lisfranc

KEY POINTS

- Subtle Lisfranc injuries are difficult to diagnose and frequently missed; therefore, high clinical suspicion and close follow-up are required to ensure the expected evolution.
- Conservative treatment is recommended for injuries with demonstrated stability only.
- Surgical treatment is mandatory for all the unstable injuries; however, the best surgical technique remains controversial.
- In athletes, surgical stabilization may confer a more reproducible result and potential faster return to play.
- Many surgical techniques are available for subtle Lisfranc injuries. Surgeons must select the most appropriate treatment of each patient based on the instability pattern, the physical demand of the patient, and their own surgical experience.

INTRODUCTION

Lisfranc injuries include a broad spectrum of traumatic injuries affecting the tarsometatarsal (TMT) joint complex. The highly variable presentation of these injuries, in terms of energy and severity, makes it difficult to compare the effectiveness of alternate treatments. At present, there is no consensus on the best management of subtle TMT injuries.

Despite the lack of definitions, subtle Lisfranc injuries (SLIs) refer to low-energy injuries that affect TMT joint, including potentially purely ligamentous injuries or periarticular avulsion fractures. The most frequent scenario in SLI is the involvement and subsequent compromise of the plantar interosseous ligament, or Lisfranc ligament,

[a] Department of Orthopedic Surgery, Pontificia Universidad Catolica de Chile. Diagonal Paraguay 362, Postal code: 8330077, Santiago, Región Metropolitana, Chile; [b] Department of Orthopaedics and Traumatology, Cantonal Hospital of Winterthur, Buchnerstrasse 1, 8006 Zurich, Switzerland; [c] Department of Orthopaedics, Division of Distal Extremities, University of British Columbia, Vancouver, British Columbia, Canada; [d] Department of Orthopedics, St. Paul's Hospital, UBC, Vancouver, Canada; [e] Footbridge Centre for Integrated Orthopaedic Care Inc., Footbridge Clinic, 221-181 Keefer Place, Vancouver, British Columbia V6B 6C1, Canada
* Corresponding author. 221–181 Keefer Place, Vancouver, British Columbia V6B 6C1, Canada.
E-mail address: docveljkovic@yahoo.com

Foot Ankle Clin N Am 25 (2020) 711–726
https://doi.org/10.1016/j.fcl.2020.08.014
1083-7515/20/© 2020 Elsevier Inc. All rights reserved.
foot.theclinics.com

which traverses the articulation between the second metatarsal base and the medial cuneiform. Compromise of the Lisfranc ligament can result in widening of the first intermetatarsal space, but it is common to observe mild intercuneiform instability or avulsive fractures at the base of other metatarsals without gross loss of TMT and intercuneiform joint congruence. Lisfranc ligament injury results in loss of stability of the transverse arch, diastasis between the medial and middle columns of the foot, and ultimately midfoot collapse, pain, and arthrosis.[1]

The diagnosis of SLI can be challenging. Imaging findings can be minimal and subject to interpretation considering the limitations of the different techniques. These injuries are frequently missed because initial radiographs can be normal in up to 50% of cases,[2] so a high clinical suspicion is required to indicate additional study. In contrast, because of the difficulties of determining the stability of the injury, surgery for SLI can be easily overindicated based on rotational asymmetries or questionable gaping on the weight-bearing radiographs. Standing computed tomography (CT) may better elucidate the issue as it relates to minor but relevant alterations in intimate bony congruency based on applied weight-bearing forces.

Multiple studies have shown that the most predictive factor for a successful outcome is the maintenance of anatomic alignment.[3–10] However, the best treatment to achieve this objective and assess the subsequent result remains controversial. The selection of the appropriate surgical technique can be difficult because, even with good diagnosis and proper treatment, these injuries can lead to chronic pain and result in a permanent disability.

This article discusses the management of SLIs focused on the treatment alternatives. It does not address the diagnosis strategies because they are discussed extensively in another article in this issue.

CONSERVATIVE TREATMENT

There is no controversy in the literature over the treatment of stable tarsometatarsal injuries. Most publications suggest that midfoot sprains with no evident displacement or widening on weight-bearing radiographs can be treated nonsurgically with excellent results and a high rate of return to sports.[2,7,11]

The treatment usually consists of a period of 6 to 8 weeks of protected weight bearing either in a short-leg cast or walker boot. Considering the diagnostic difficulties in determining the stability of the injury, most investigators suggest a close follow-up and repeated standing radiographs in 7 to 14 days after the initial diagnosis when the pain permits full weight bearing.[6,12,13]

Several case series studies have reported the results of conservative treatment. Faciszewski and colleagues (1990) reviewed the cases of 15 patients with a subtle tarsometatarsal injury, with evident diastasis between the first and second metatarsal bases (2–5 mm). Eleven patients were treated conservatively, 3 of them requiring subsequent TMT fusion. The investigators found no correlation between the severity of the diastases and the patients' functional results.

Curtis and colleagues[7] (1993), in a retrospective series of 19 low-energy injuries sustained during athletic activity, reported the results of 14 patients with injuries considered stable and consequently treated conservatively. The worst results in this series were observed in the group with conservative treatment, 4 cases with fair/regular functional results, and 1 extra patient with poor results requiring TMT fusion after the conservative treatment. Three patients with conservative treatment could not return to sports. Interestingly, inferior outcomes were found in patients with a delayed diagnosis.

Shapiro and colleagues[11] (1994), in another small retrospective series in athletic injuries with documented diastasis between the first and second metatarsal, reported excellent results and return to sports in 7 out of 8 patients treated conservatively. After a minimal follow-up of 1 year (average follow-up of 34 months), all the patients were practicing their sports with no sequelae. Although this study supported nonoperative treatment even for SLI with minor displacement, most of the current literature does not support this treatment.

Nunley and Vertullo[2] (2002) reviewed the cases of 15 patients with athletic injuries. The cases were classified based on weight-bearing radiographs; if the injury was nondisplaced, the diagnosis was confirmed using bone scans. All the displaced injuries underwent operative treatment with early percutaneous fixation or late open reduction and internal fixation (ORIF). Patients with nondisplaced injuries (n = 7) were treated nonoperatively with excellent results and full return to sports at 11 to 16 weeks after the injury.

Despite these studies showing good results, in a more recent study, Crates and colleagues[13] (2015) reported a high rate of failure in patients with SLI treated nonsurgically. In this retrospective case series, 20 patients (55%) required surgery after failed conservative treatment. However, the failure of conservative treatment and surgical fixation was decided by the senior author based on the persistence of pain. The lack of a clear definition of treatment failure makes this high rate of failure difficult to extrapolate to other settings. Interestingly, they report excellent outcomes after surgical treatment with screws or suture-button devices with no patients requiring fusion despite delayed fixation.

Although these studies report successful nonoperative treatment of SLI even in the case of minor displacement, it has been shown in multiples studies that the most important factor predictive of favorable outcome is stable anatomic reduction. In the authors' opinion, conservative treatment should be preserved for patients with demonstrated stability on imaging studies and physical examination. Close follow-up is recommended with serial weight-bearing radiographs and further physical examination assessment. In general, for higher-demand patients, such as elite athletes whose sports require midfoot torque, surgical fixation provides a more reliable/reproducible result and allows sooner return to play. The type of fixation used by the authors depends on the physical and radiographic examination and the timing of the injury and the presentation.

SURGICAL TREATMENT

Despite advances in surgical techniques, surgical treatment of Lisfranc injuries is still challenging considering the high incidence of posttraumatic arthrosis and chronic pain, even in successfully treated patients.[14]

Multiple studies have shown that the most important goal of treatment is restoring anatomic and stable joint alignment. Therefore, surgical treatment is indicated for all the Lisfranc injuries with proven instability. Although several techniques have shown successful outcomes, surgeons must choose the best treatment option to restore the alignment and stability of the foot according to the severity of the injury and functional demands of the patient. To date, the best surgical technique for low-energy Lisfranc injuries remains controversial.

ORIF has historically been considered the gold standard treatment of SLI. However, in the last decade, several studies have reported equivalent or better results in patients treated with primary arthrodesis (PA).[15–17] Nonetheless, the outcome measure in some of these studies was subsequent hardware removal, which is not a relevant outcome measure to prognosticate which surgical technique is superior. In recent years, the use of reconstructive techniques with sutures or autograft tendon reconstruction has become more popular in the treatment of subtle instability to preserve the normal motion of the TMT joints and reduce the risk of hardware removal.

Percutaneous Surgery

Many investigators consider that closed reduction under fluoroscopy cannot guarantee an optimal reduction. There are some anecdotal reports of failed closed reduction by an entrapped tendon or ligament, but, usually, they were described in high-energy injuries.[18,19] More often, the interposition of a fracture fragment from the base of the second metatarsal can prevent anatomic closed reduction. Any mechanical block impeding the reduction requires conversion to an open procedure. Probably the most challenging problem in the setting of an SLI is the missed inaccurate reduction at the moment of fixation that cannot be seen under fluoroscopy.

Despite the difficulties in guaranteeing an anatomic reduction, the few case series reporting surgical outcomes after closed reduction and percutaneous fixation show good clinical results (**Fig. 1**).

Perugia and colleagues[20] (2002) reviewed the results of 42 patients treated with percutaneous fixation. This series mixed cases of different energy and severity, and several configurations of screws were used. The average American Orthopaedic Foot and Ankle Society (AOFAS) midfoot score was 81, with an average follow-up of 58 months. In 17 cases, the reduction was considered nearly anatomic, but there were no differences in outcome scores comparing anatomic with nearly anatomic reduction.

Wagner and colleagues[9] (2013) published the results of 22 patients with low-energy injuries treated with percutaneous screw fixation. In this series, 50% of the cases (11) required fixation of the first TMT joint and 5 cases had percutaneous fixation of the third TMT joint. Although the primary objective was to evaluate the results of early weight bearing after percutaneous fixation, they reported excellent outcomes (AOFAS

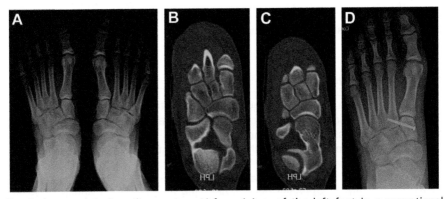

Fig. 1. Acute subtle bony/ligamentous Lisfranc injury of the left foot in a recreational athlete presented within the first 3 weeks after injury. (*A*) Weight-bearing comparative radiograph with a clear widening between the medial cuneiform and the second metatarsal base (1–3 mm; see **Figs. 5–8**). (*B–C*) Preoperative CT performed to rule out nonvisible fractures on the radiographs, showing excellent joint alignment without weight bearing. (*D*) Postoperative radiograph after percutaneous reduction and fixation with a cannulated screw. In order to accept a percutaneous fixation technique, the surgeon must ensure that the Lisfranc interval is completely reduced or open reduction is warranted.

average was 94 points) with an anatomic or near-anatomic reduction in all patients and no soft tissue complications.

More recently, Vosbikian and colleagues[21] (2017), in another retrospective study, showed the results after percutaneous fixation with a minimal follow-up of 3 years. This series reported the results of 31 out of 38 patients treated, 7 lost in follow-up, with an average Foot and Ankle Ability Measure (FAAM) score of 94.2 (range 40–100). No patient required additional operative procedures and no wound complication was reported.

In order to reduce the risk of inadequate reduction in percutaneous techniques, our group has used arthroscopic assistance either for fixation or fusion.[22] The surgical technique was described by Escudero and colleagues[22] (2018), where a 2.4-mm to 2.9-mm arthroscope is inserted into the first web space and the reduction is assessed by a combination of arthroscopy and fluoroscopy. Fixation can be performed with screws or suture-button devices (**Figs. 2** and **3**). Fusion is preferred for select patients, such as older or obese patients, or potentially when the bases of metatarsals are comminuted. This technique can be performed in the same way with arthroscopic assistance by adding a small burr to prepare the articular surfaces.

Because of the risk of a missed subtle malreduction, many surgeons advocate open reduction for all unstable injuries. Despite this, most of the information about surgical outcomes after Lisfranc fixation comes from case series mixing injuries of different severities. Furthermore, the importance of residual minimal gaping in the setting of SLI is unknown.

Flexible Fixation

Rigid fixation can prevent the normal motion in the Lisfranc joint complex. The senior author feels that rigid fixation is paramount in the ligamentous Lisfranc and can be augmented by flexible fixation as required. Rigid fixation is also a more stable construct in the bony variant. This loss of motion or accommodation capacity is particularly important for the first TMT joint and can be a relevant concern when treating active patients or athletes (see **Fig. 3**). Instability in the TMT can be addressed well with anchor-suture-anchor suspensory constructs and can be augmented with a bridge plate if required (**Figs. 4–8**). Mulier and colleagues[23] (2002) showed in their retrospective investigation comparing ORIF versus arthrodesis for severe Lisfranc injuries that the PA group complained of more stiffness. Reinhardt and colleagues[24] (2012), in another retrospective case series study of 25 selective fusions, found that 3 patients (12%) had degenerative changes in the adjacent joints at 42-month follow-up.

In recent years, multiple techniques and small case series have reported good results using flexible fixation. All these techniques try to preserve a more normal motion in the midfoot and to reduce screw breakage and need for hardware removal.

In 2009, Panchbhavi and colleagues[25] showed that suture-button fixation (TightRope) can provide similar stability to that provided by screw fixation in cadaver specimens after isolated transection of the Lisfranc ligament. Subsequently, similar findings have been shown by Pelt and colleagues[26] and Ahmed and colleagues[27] comparing the Mini TightRope system.

Brin and colleagues[28] (2010) reported the results of a small case series of 5 athletes (including Olympic and professional athletes) with low-energy Lisfranc injuries treated with TightRope. In this series, the TightRope was used from the medial cuneiform to the base of the second metatarsal. In addition, 3 of the patients required first TMT fixation with a transarticular screw. There were no complications or loss of reduction at a

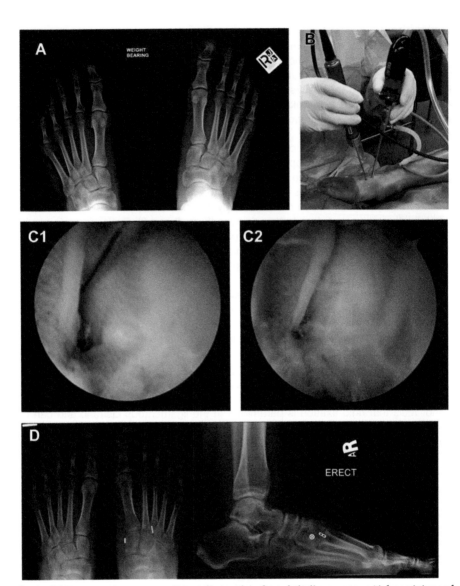

Fig. 2. (*A*) Preoperative comparative radiographs of a subtle ligamentous Lisfranc injury of the right foot in an elite athlete. (*B*) Arthroscopic assistance in the reduction for percutaneous fixation. (*C1* and *C2*) Arthroscopic visualization of the second TMT joint before and after reduction. (*D*) Postoperative radiographs after arthroscopically assisted reduction and percutaneous fixation with TightRope.

follow-up of 1 year. They had excellent clinical results, with full return to sports at 6 months in all the patients and high satisfaction in 4 out of the 5 patients. One patient had moderate results despite no technical issues in that case.

It is the senior authors opinion that the TMT joint can be addressed and stabilized well with anchor-suture-anchor constructs or bridge plate constructs, avoiding the need to violate the joint with transarticular screw fixation (see **Figs. 2** and **3**). In patients presenting after 2 weeks, the senior author advocates reflecting the capsule back off

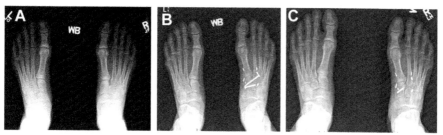

Fig. 3. (*A*) Elite athlete presenting 6 weeks after the injury (see **Fig. 5** for subacute injuries, >2 weeks and <3 months). (*B*) Treatment with ORIF: screw fixation Lisfranc and intercuneiform. Flexible fixation was used to augment screw fixation because of the severe injury pattern and delayed presentation of the patient. Metal hardware removal (*C*) was planned for 3 months postoperative.

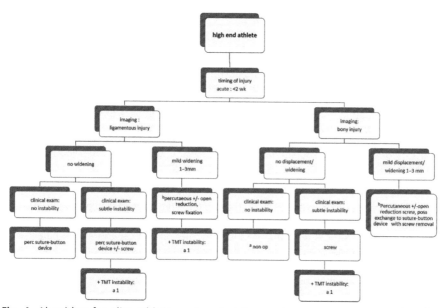

Fig. 4. Algorithm for elite athletes and acute injury. a 1, suspensory suture and anchor technique ± bridge plate. Clinical first TMT/Lisfranc instability: comparison of mobility with the contralateral side with more than 25% of dorsal translation/general motion being considered unstable. [a]Non-operative treatment: stiff-soled, rocker-bottom shoes, night splint, heel lift, graphite plate. Physiotherapy: work on gastrocnemius stretching, dynamic arch control, tibialis posterior strength, no midfoot torque. [b]In order to accept a percutaneous fixation technique, the surgeon must ensure that the Lisfranc interval is completely reduced or open reduction is warranted. The sooner the surgeon can complete the case, the more successful the percutaneous procedure will be. [c]Exchange to suture-button device with removal of screw at minimum of 3 months with ligamentous and 6 weeks for bony injury. Minor bony avulsion might need to be treated as a ligamentous injury. Exchange from screw to flexible devices is done in concerning injury patterns, ligamentous injuries, and significant planovalgus deformity.

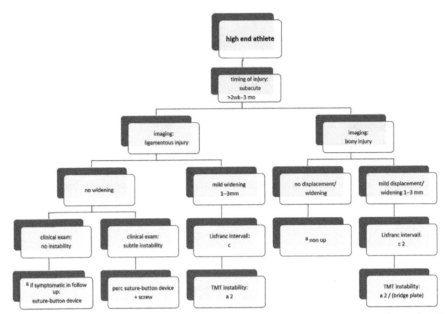

Fig. 5. Algorithm for elite athletes and subacute injury. a 2, open reduction, peal capsule off the first TMT dorsal/medial preparation of bone, advancement of capsule anchor–suture anchor technique ± bridge plate; c, open reduction, amputation of Lisfranc ligament (1 mm) of medial cuneiform, preparation medial cuneiform, fixation with screws and suspensory suture-button devices; c 2, open reduction, resection bony block to reduction ± amputation of Lisfranc ligament (1 mm) at the base of second, preparation medial cuneiform, fixation with screws and suspensory suture-button devices. Clinical first TMT/Lisfranc instability: comparison of mobility with the contralateral side with more than 25% of dorsal translation/general motion being considered unstable. Footnotes as in **Fig. 4.**

the first TMT from distal to proximal off the proximal first metatarsal, preparing the underlying bone with a burr, and then advancing the capsule distally and securing it with suture bridge constructs (**Fig. 9**). The Lisfranc interval can be addressed nicely with flexible fixation, sometimes augmented with more rigid screws. In more chronic cases, greater than 2 weeks, amputation of 1 mm of the Lisfranc ligament with preparation of the underlying bone may be required in order to allow closure of the Lisfranc interval (see **Fig. 9**). In some cases, first and second TMT instability persists with continued gaping, an in these cases we include flexible fixation between the first and second metatarsals to control the deforming force and augment our fixation. See **Figs. 3 and 9**.

Charlton and colleagues[29] in 2015 used suture-button fixation in 7 high-level athletes with SLIs after 6 months of failed conservative treatment. At 6 months postoperatively, no patients reported residual deficits. The AOFAS midfoot scores improved from 65 to 97 points. Despite the small number of cases, suture-button fixation showed excellent results for delayed fixation in athletes with SLIs and avoided the need for subsequent implant removal. The senior author advocates reconstruction versus fusion in high-end athletes even after 3 months (see **Figs. 6** and **8**). Jain and colleagues[30] (2017), in another small clinic series treating 5 professional soccer and rugby players with SLIs with a suture-button device, showed excellent results with

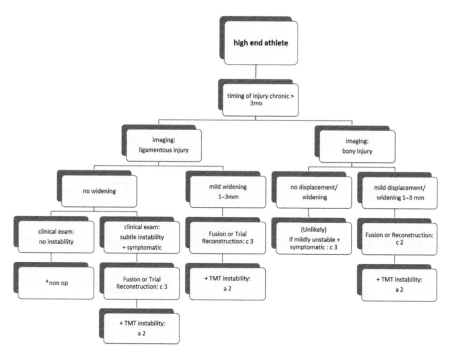

Fig. 6. Algorithm for elite athletes and chronic injury. b, suspensory suture-button device and/or screw/anchor-suture-anchor construct; c 3, open peel ligament directly of medial cuneiform with no ligament amputation, preparation medial cuneiform, fixation with screws and suspensory suture-button devices. Clinical first TMT/Lisfranc instability: comparison of mobility with the contralateral side with more than 25% of dorsal translation/general motion being considered unstable. Footnotes as in **Fig. 4**.

no loss of reduction at the final follow-up. All the patients returned to full elite-level competition. The mean time to return to training was 16.1 weeks (range, 14–17 weeks) and to full competition was 20.4 weeks (range, 18–24 weeks).

Recently, Kwon and colleagues[31] published a novel and inexpensive flexible technique creating a tension band with sutures and using 2 screws as posts. This technique avoids the damage of transarticular fixation and is particularly useful for subtle instability of the first TMT.

Rigid Fixation

Transarticular screw fixation has been the traditional surgical technique used in the management of unstable low-energy Lisfranc injuries. However, the associated cartilage damage and the possible loosening and breakage of the screws have promoted the use of stronger constructs such as bridging dorsal plates or a combination of both methods. With the development of new implants, such as low-profile, segment-specific locked plates, more rigid stabilization can be achieved, even in cases with comminution, and avoid damage to the articular cartilage[5] (**Fig. 10**).

Surprisingly, despite extensive literature reporting results from clinical series, few studies have attempted to compare the results of plates versus screws. Again, the retrospective nature of the available studies, with the evident selection bias and the inclusion of cases of different severities; make it difficult to draw valid conclusions about the superiority of one treatment over another.

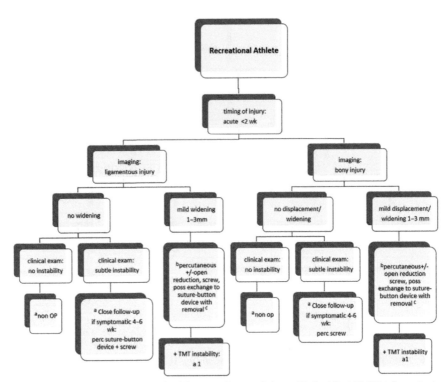

Fig. 7. Algorithm for recreational athletes and acute injury. Clinical first TMT/Lisfranc instability: comparison of mobility with the contralateral side with more than 25% of dorsal translation/general motion being considered unstable. Footnotes as in **Fig. 4**.

Hu and colleagues[32] (2014) published a prospective study evaluating dorsal bridge plating versus screw fixation in 60 patients. They concluded that fixation with dorsal plates has better outcomes compared with transarticular screws when using the AOFAS midfoot score. Nonetheless, most of the patients in this cohort had severe Lisfranc injuries, with just 8 patients (13%) with low-energy injuries. Anatomic reduction was achieved in 90% of patients in the plate fixation group compared with 80% in the screw fixation group. More patients in the screw fixation group developed arthritic degeneration seen at the time of device removal. Furthermore, a slightly higher percentage of patients underwent secondary arthrodesis in the screw fixation group.

In a recent retrospective study, Lau and colleagues[5] compared the results of 50 patients treated with transarticular screws (28%), dorsal bridge plating (38%), or a combination of both fixations (34%). They did not report how many cases were high-energy or low-energy Lisfranc injuries. Similar functional outcomes were reported despite the treatment used and concluded that functional outcomes are most dependent on the quality of reduction and not the choice of fixation implant used.

The limited literature available on the best fixation option precludes making an evidence-based recommendation. In this situation, surgeons must choose the fixation method according to surgical experience and the functional demands of the patient.

Fixation Versus Fusion

The high rate of posttraumatic degenerative changes in TMT joints, even in successfully treated patients, has led multiple investigators to suggest that arthrodesis

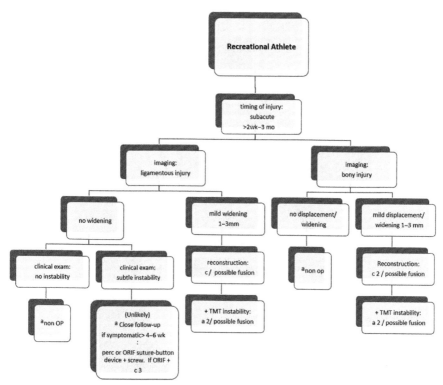

Fig. 8. Algorithm for recreational athletes and subacute injury. Clinical first TMT/Lisfranc instability: comparison of mobility with the contralateral side with more than 25% of dorsal translation/general motion being considered unstable. Footnotes as in **Fig. 4**.

should be considered the preferred treatment of these injuries. In particular, purely ligament injuries have been shown to evolve more rapidly to posttraumatic osteoarthritis.[14,8]

Ly and Coetzee[33] published in 2006 a randomized prospective study of 41 patients with isolated primarily ligamentous Lisfranc joint injuries and compared ORIF (n = 20) with primary fusion. They noted a more rapid recovery, better foot outcome scores, and improved return to function in patients who underwent PA as opposed to ORIF. In addition, the ORIF group had 16 patients who required hardware removal at 6 months postoperatively, and 5 patients with high-energy Lisfranc later underwent midfoot arthrodesis. The fusion group rated their postoperative activity levels at 92% of their preinjury levels, compared with the ORIF group rating of 65%. The conclusions were that fusion provides a quicker recovery, superior function recovery, and fewer secondary procedures compared with ORIF. It is the senior author's opinion that, in the acute and semichronic (3 weeks to 3 months) intervals, similar outcomes can be obtained with joint preservation reconstruction in both high-end and recreational athletes for ligamentous injuries, avoiding the need for fusion (see **Figs. 5** and **9**).

Subsequently, Henning and colleagues,[17] in another prospective randomized study, compared PA with ORIF, including patients with either combined osseous-ligamentous or purely ligamentous Lisfranc injuries. Their series of 32 patients

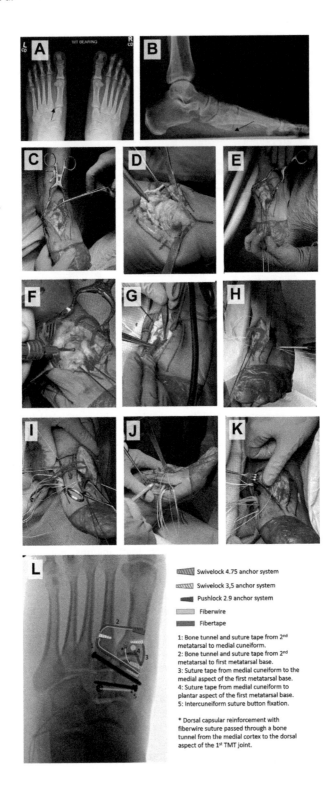

Swivelock 4.75 anchor system
Swivelock 3,5 anchor system
Pushlock 2.9 anchor system
Fiberwire
Fibertape

1: Bone tunnel and suture tape from 2nd metatarsal to medial cuneiform.
2: Bone tunnel and suture tape from 2nd metatarsal to first metatarsal base.
3: Suture tape from medial cuneiform to the medial aspect of the first metatarsal base.
4: Suture tape from medial cuneiform to plantar aspect of the first metatarsal base.
5: Intercuneiform suture button fixation.

* Dorsal capsular reinforcement with fiberwire suture passed through a bone tunnel from the medial cortex to the dorsal aspect of the 1st TMT joint.

comparing ORIF (n = 14) with PA (n = 18) showed no difference between groups at any time point. At a mean follow-up of 53 months, telephone surveys revealed patient satisfaction rates of 90% in the ORIF group and 92% in the PA group. As part of the ORIF protocol, the hardware was removed routinely. Seventy-nine percent of the ORIF patients and 17% of the primary partial arthrodesis patients underwent hardware removal, and, therefore, this variable could not be assessed in this study.

Smith and colleagues[15] performed a systematic review and a meta-analysis in 2016, comparing ORIF with primary fusion for acute Lisfranc injuries. They concluded that the ORIF group had a statistically significant higher rate of hardware removal compared with the fusion group. There was no significant difference in patient-reported outcomes, revision surgery, and risk of nonanatomic alignment between the 2 groups. The investigators reported design errors in all the studies included, and mention a possible bias in the results of the meta-analysis.

More recently, Cochran and colleagues[34] (2017) retrospectively compared primary fusion versus ORIF for low-energy Lisfranc injuries in a cohort of 32 young athletic patients on active military duty (average age of 28 years). Fusion was performed in 14 patients and ORIF in 18. The implant removal rates, fitness test scores, return to military duty rates, and FAAM scores were compared. The investigators concluded that low-energy Lisfranc injuries treated with PA had a lower implant removal rate, an earlier return to full military activity, and better fitness test scores after 1 year, but there was no difference in FAAM scores after 3 years. Seybold and Coetzee[14] recommend the use of arthrodesis for injuries with significant intra-articular comminution or purely ligamentous injuries that involve the entire medial and middle columns. They recommend ORIF and subsequent hardware removal as the preferred treatment of patients with flexible midfoot at baseline, and they suggest a lower threshold to fuse the first and second TMT joints in patients with cavus foot because these patients have a very stiff midfoot at baseline and the functional loss is minimal.

Despite these studies showing comparable or even better outcomes with primary fusion, TMT arthrodesis may result in serious complications such as ray shortening, malreduction, and associated metatarsalgia. These complications can be avoided with joint preservation techniques, as advocated by the senior author. In addition, stiffness of the foot following arthrodesis procedures, especially involving multiple TMT joints, may not be desirable for young athletic patients.

Fig. 9. Elite athlete presented more than 3 months after the injury who was treated with ORIF with Lisfranc screw fixation and intercuneiform screw, but a flexible ligament augmentation was also performed with suture tape (see **Fig. 6**C3 trial reconstruction). (*A, B*) Preoperative radiographs showing mild intermetatarsal widening and plantar gaping of TMT joint. (*C*) Identification and preservation of the dorsal capsule of the first TMT joint. (*D*) Medial approach showing disruption of the medial TMT capsule. (*E*) Reduction and transient fixation under direct visualization. (*F*) Periosteal removal from the first metatarsal base with a burr for subsequent capsule reattachment and augmentation with suture. (*G*) Amputation of residual dorsal Lisfranc ligament. (*H*) Use of a suture tape and fixation in the second metatarsal with a PushLock anchor system (Arthrex). (*I*) Use of an intercuneiform suture-button device. (*J*) Use of a SwiveLock anchor system (Arthrex) for fixation of the suture tape passing through a tunnel from the second metatarsal to the medial cuneiform. (*K*) Augmentation with fiber wire of the dorsal capsule repair. (*L*) Intraoperative fluoroscopy summarizing the tunnels and suture tape used for trial reconstruction.

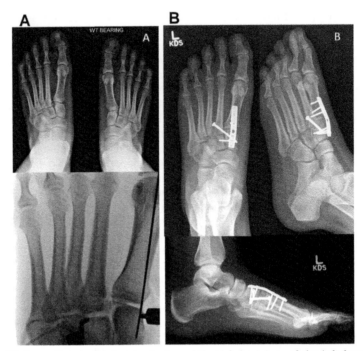

Fig. 10. (*A*) Recreational athlete who had a subtle Lisfranc injury of the left foot with an avulsion fracture of the second metatarsal base and intraoperative fluoroscopy showing the TMT instability. (*B*) Postoperative radiographs after ORIF with a small fragment plate and screws.

SUMMARY

Lisfranc injuries are challenging even in their most subtle form. Difficulties in diagnosis and the broad spectrum of injuries involved require surgeons to make decisions based on their own experience and to choose well-performed surgical techniques that adequately recover joint alignment and stability. At present, available information does not show superiority of one treatment over another. Hence, the selection of treatment should be individualized to the requirements and experience of each center. Comparative studies with clear definitions are needed to provide higher-quality evidence-based recommendations.

CLINICS CARE POINTS

- Conservative treatment requires a close follow up with serial weight-bearing radiographs and further physical examination.
- Percutaneous fixation of subtle Lisfranc injuries may fail due to limited visualization of an inaccurate reduction. Consider an open procedure when not achieving a proper reduction easily.
- The Lisfranc interval can be addressed nicely with flexible fixation devices, preserving motion and avoiding hardware removal in selected patients. Flexible fixation can be used in isolation, associated with a more rigid construct, or as a ligament augmentation after hardware removal.
- When performing primary Lisfranc fusions, preserving the length and the alignment of the metatarsal bones is of paramount importance.

DISCLOSURE

A. Veljkovic is a paid speaker for Arthrex, Inc. and has participation in stocks or stock options of Therapia and Arthritis Innovation Corporation. J. Briceno has nothing to disclose. A.-K. Leucht has nothing to disclose. A. Younger reports grants and personal fees from Wright medical, grants and personal fees from Acumed PLC, grants from Synthes, personal fees from Axolotyl, grants and personal fees from Zimmer, and grants from Arthrex.

REFERENCES

1. Aronow MS. Treatment of the missed Lisfranc injury. Foot Ankle Clin 2006;11(1): 127–42, ix.
2. Nunley JA, Vertullo CJ. Classification, investigation, and management of midfoot sprains: Lisfranc injuries in the athlete. Am J Sports Med 2002;30(6):871–8.
3. Hardcastle PH, Reschauer R, Kutscha-Lissberg E, et al. Injuries to the tarsometatarsal joint. Incidence, classification and treatment. J Bone Joint Surg Br 1982; 64(3):349–56.
4. Kirzner N, Zotov P, Goldbloom D, et al. Dorsal bridge plating or transarticular screws for Lisfranc fracture dislocations: A retrospective study comparing functional and radiological outcomes. Bone Joint J 2018;100B(4):468–74.
5. Lau S, Guest C, Hall M, et al. Functional outcomes post lisfranc injury - transarticular screws, dorsal bridge plating or combination treatment? J Orthop Trauma 2017;31:447–52.
6. Myerson MS, Cerrato R. Current management of tarsometatarsal injuries in the athlete. Instr Course Lect 2009;58:583–94. Available at: http://www.ncbi.nlm. nih.gov/pubmed/19385569. Accessed July 1, 2018.
7. Curtis MJ, Myerson M, Szura B. Tarsometatarsal joint injuries in the athlete. Am J Sports Med 1993;21(4):497–502.
8. Kuo RS, Tejwani NC, Digiovanni CW, et al. Outcome after open reduction and internal fixation of Lisfranc joint injuries. J Bone Joint Surg Am 2000;82(11): 1609–18.
9. Wagner E, Ortiz C, Villalón IE, et al. Early weight-bearing after percutaneous reduction and screw fixation for low-energy lisfranc injury. Foot Ankle Int 2013; 34(7):978–83.
10. Teng AL, Pinzur MS, Lomasney L, et al. Functional outcome following anatomic restoration of tarsal-metatarsal fracture dislocation. Foot Ankle Int 2002;23(10): 922–6.
11. Shapiro MS, Wascher DC, Finerman GAM. Rupture of Lisfranc's ligament in athletes. Am J Sports Med 1994;22(5):687–91.
12. Krause F, Schmid T, Weber M. Current swiss techniques in management of lisfranc injuries of the foot. Foot Ankle Clin 2016;21(2):335–50.
13. Crates JM, Barber FA, Sanders EJ. Subtle lisfranc subluxation: results of operative and nonoperative treatment. J Foot Ankle Surg 2015;54(3):350–5.
14. Seybold JD, Coetzee JC. Lisfranc injuries: when to observe, fix, or fuse. Clin Sports Med 2015;34(4):705–23.
15. Smith N, Stone C, Furey A. Does open reduction and internal fixation versus primary arthrodesis improve patient outcomes for lisfranc trauma? a systematic review and meta-analysis. Clin Orthop Relat Res 2016;474(6):1445–52.
16. Coetzee JC, Ly TV. Treatment of primarily ligamentous Lisfranc joint injuries: primary arthrodesis compared with open reduction and internal fixation. Surgical technique. J Bone Joint Surg Am 2007;89:122–7. Pt 1 Su(3).

17. Henning JA, Jones CB, Sietsema DL, et al. Open reduction internal fixation versus primary arthrodesis for lisfranc injuries: a prospective randomized study. Foot Ankle Int 2009;30(10):913–22.
18. DeBenedetti MJ, Evanski PM, Waugh TR. The unreducible Lisfranc fracture. Case report and literature review. Clin Orthop Relat Res 1978;136:238–40. Available at: http://www.ncbi.nlm.nih.gov/pubmed/729290. Accessed March 25, 2020.
19. Karaindros K, Arealis G, Papanikolaou A, et al. Irreducible Lisfranc dislocation due to the interposition of the tibialis anterior tendon: Case report and literature review. Foot Ankle Surg 2010;16(3):e68–71.
20. Perugia D, Basile A, Battaglia A, et al. Fracture dislocations of Lisfranc's joint treated with closed reduction and percutaneous fixation. Int Orthop 2003;27(1):30–5.
21. Vosbikian M, O'Neil JT, Piper C, et al. Outcomes after percutaneous reduction and fixation of low-energy lisfranc injuries. Foot Ankle Int 2017;38(7):710–5.
22. Escudero MI, Symes M, Veljkovic A, et al. Low-energy lisfranc injuries in an athletic population: a comprehensive review of the literature and the role of minimally invasive techniques in their management. Foot Ankle Clin 2018;23(4):679–92.
23. Mulier T, Reynders P, Dereymaeker G, et al. Severe Lisfrancs injuries: primary arthrodesis or ORIF? Foot Ankle Int 2002;23(10):902–5.
24. Reinhardt KR, Oh LS, Schottel P, et al. Treatment of Lisfranc fracture-dislocations with primary partial arthrodesis. Foot Ankle Int 2012;33(1):50–6.
25. Panchbhavi VK, Vallurupalli S, Yang J, et al. Screw fixation compared with suture-button fixation of isolated Lisfranc ligament injuries. J Bone Joint Surg Am 2009;91(5):1143–8.
26. Pelt CE, Bachus KN, Vance RE, et al. A biomechanical analysis of a tensioned suture device in the fixation of the ligamentous lisfranc injury. Foot Ankle Int 2011;32(4):422–31.
27. Ahmed S, Bolt B, Mcbryde A, et al. Comparison of standard screw fixation versus suture button fixation in lisfranc ligament injuries. Foot Ankle Int 2010. https://doi.org/10.3113/FAI.2010.0892.
28. Brin YS, Nyska M, Kish B. Lisfranc injury repair with the TightRope™ device: A short-term case series. Foot Ankle Int 2010;31(7):624–7.
29. Charlton T, Boe C, Thordarson DB. Suture Button Fixation Treatment of Chronic Lisfranc Injury in Professional Dancers and High-Level Athletes. J Dance Med Sci 2015;19(4):135–9.
30. Jain K, Drampalos E, Clough TM. Results of suture button fixation with targeting device aid for displaced ligamentous Lisfranc injuries in the elite athlete. Foot 2017;30:43–6.
31. Briceno J, Stupay KL, Moura B, et al. Flexible fixation for ligamentous lisfranc injuries. Injury 2019;50(11):2123–7.
32. Hu SJ, Chang SM, Li XH, et al. Outcome comparison of Lisfranc injuries treated through dorsal plate fixation versus screw fixation. Acta Ortop Bras 2014;22(6):315–20.
33. Ly TV, Coetzee JC. Treatment of primarily ligamentous lisfranc joint injuries: primary arthrodesis compared with open reduction and internal fixation: a prospective, randomized study. J Bone Joint Surg Am 2006;88(3):514.
34. Cochran G, Renninger C, Tompane T, et al. Primary arthrodesis versus open reduction and internal fixation for low-energy lisfranc injuries in a young athletic population. Foot Ankle Int 2017;38(9):957–63.

Primary Arthrodesis for High-Energy Lisfranc Injuries

Alexandre Leme Godoy-Santos, MD, PhD[a,b,*],
Cesar de Cesar Netto, MD, PhD[c]

KEYWORDS

- Lisfranc • Trauma • Injury • Fixation • Arthrodesis • Treatment

KEY POINTS

- The treatment of patients presenting with complex foot injuries and associated high-energy Lisfranc injuries could be categorized in 2 phases: early damage control and definitive treatment.
- The goals of treatment are to obtain a painless, plantigrade, and stable foot, with return to preinjury function.
- No statistically significant difference comparing primary arthrodesis versus open reduction and internal fixation in terms of work/sports return, complications and patient satisfaction rates.
- However, primary arthrodesis patients showed better functional scores.
- Anatomic reduction is a key factor for improved outcomes.

INTRODUCTION

Lisfranc injuries are named after Jacques Lisfranc de Saint-Martin, who described a partial amputation of the foot at the level of the tarsometatarsal joints (TMTJ).[1] They are composed of a broad spectrum of injuries ranging from minor sprains and isolated ligamentous injuries, to grossly unstable and multiligamentous lesions, possibly accompanied by fractures and/or fracture-dislocations.[2]

The definitions and classifications of these injuries has changed over time, with the most commonly used classifications systems being proposed by classification systems developed by Quenu and Kuss, Nunley and Vertullo, Chiodo and Myerson, and Lau and Guest.[3–6] Almost 100 years after the first classification system was described, there is still no clear consensus on how these injuries should be defined.[7]

[a] Department of Orthopedic Surgery, Faculdade de Medicina, Universidade de São Paulo, Rua Dr Ovídio Pires de Campos 333, Cerqueira Cesar, Sao Paulo, São Paulo 05403-010, Brazil; [b] Hospital Israelita Albert Einstein, São Paulo, São Paulo, Brazil; [c] Department of Orthopedics and Rehabilitation, University of Iowa, 200 Hawkins drive, Iowa City, IA 52242, USA
* Corresponding author.
E-mail address: alexandrelemegodoy@gmail.com

Foot Ankle Clin N Am 25 (2020) 727–736
https://doi.org/10.1016/j.fcl.2020.08.010
1083-7515/20/© 2020 Elsevier Inc. All rights reserved.

The reported incidence of Lisfranc injuries is around 9.2/100.000 person-years, and two-thirds of the injuries are nondisplaced (<2 mm displacement in fracture or joint) and usually caused by low-energy mechanisms. Most common injury patterns are tumbling or slipping, direct trauma to the dorsal aspect of the midfoot, motor vehicle accidents, a fall from heights, and sports activities.[8]

Some authors classify these injuries as "high energy" and "low energy" based on the trauma mechanism.[7,9,10] Myerson and colleagues[11] defined low-energy injures as midfoot sprains with partial incongruity of the TMTJ (type B), whereas high-energy injures present as homolateral (type A) or divergent (type C) displacements in the setting of dislocations or fracture-dislocations. The high-energy injuries are usually linked with mechanical energy dissipation through the soft tissues, and possible concomitant edema, blistering, and foot compartment syndrome.[12]

Subtle Lisfranc injuries are challenging and may present with instability without frank displacement, and undiagnosed patients can develop post-traumatic arthritis[13] Whenever diagnosed, unstable and/or displaced injuries should be considered for surgical treatment, aiming avoid progressive deformity, dysfunction and secondary arthritis.[14–17] Operative treatment options include open reduction and internal fixation (ORIF), open reduction with hybrid internal and external fixation, closed reduction with percutaneous internal or external fixation, and primary arthrodesis (PA).[18] There is some debate regarding the ideal surgical treatment technique and fixation constructs: rigid or flexible, provisional or definitive, and permanent or removable.[19] The goals of treatment are to obtain a painless, plantigrade, and stable foot, with return to preinjury function.[20] Anatomic reduction is a key factor for improved outcomes and decreased rates of post-traumatic arthritis.[21]

WHEN SHOULD I CHOOSE A PRIMARY ARTHRODESIS PROCEDURE FOR HIGH-ENERGY LISFRANC INJURIES?

In the current literature there are 12 relevant studies assessing the subject: 2 randomized clinical trials, 7 nonrandomized clinical trials, and 2 systematic reviews and meta-analysis on acute Lisfranc injuries comparing outcomes of ORIF versus PA, totalizing 547 patients studied.[16,17,22–31]

There was no statistically significant difference in most of the outcomes when comparing PA versus ORIF in terms of return to work, return to sports, and patient satisfaction rates. Likewise, no differences in the rate of complications were noted, especially in regard rates to postoperative infection.[16,17,22–31] However, patients who underwent PA showed better functional scores than patients underwent ORIF.[28] The high level of study heterogeneity should be considered for adequate interpretation of the results.

Patients treated with ORIF were at increased risk of additional procedures, mainly considering hardware removals and secondary fusions. The combined findings from these studies suggest that PA may be associated with lower rates of pain, better functional results and less need for revision surgery when compared with ORIF.[16,17,22–31]

Cochran and colleagues[24] focused their study on the outcomes in a specific population, namely, athletic young adults. The authors reported the best outcomes after PA rather than ORIF. In light of those results, we would recommend PA as the preferred option for high-energy Lisfranc injuries, such as Myerson types A and C2, especially in young adults.[13,17,24] Relative contraindications for PA would include pediatric injuries, incomplete ligamentous disruptions (stable Lisfranc Injuries), unidirectional instability, and extra-articular fractures of the cuneiforms and/or proximal metatarsals, with questioned ligamentous disruption.[13,22,29]

COST EFFECTIVENESS OF PRIMARY ARTHRODESIS AND OPEN REDUCTION INTERNAL FIXATION

Albright and colleagues[32] observed the total lifetime cost for treatment with ORIF was U$127,294 on average and the costs on patients undergoing PA was lower, with a mean value of U$99,445. The authors reported a total effectiveness for treatment with PA of 18.68 quality-adjusted life-years versus 17.66 quality-adjusted life-years for patients treated with ORIF.

In another retrospective study by Barnds and colleagues,[33] the authors evaluated the cost comparison and complication rate of Lisfranc injuries treated with open with either ORIF or PA. The authors observed an increased average cost of care associated with PA when compared with ORIF, as well as an increased overall complication rate with PA (30.2% vs 23.1% for ORIF); however, the rates of hardware removal independent of complications was greater (43.6%) for ORIF than for PA (18.4%). The average cost of patients in the ORIF group not requiring hardware removal was $3,688 versus $4,311 in the patients requiring hardware removal.

HIGH-ENERGY LISFRANC INJURIES

The term complex foot injuries is reserved for fractures with severe soft tissue damage, vascular and nerve injuries, usually associated with articular involvement and fracture comminution (**Fig. 1**A–C), and higher risk for complications.[34] High-energy Lisfranc injuries are common in these settings. The literature shows a high rates of association between polytrauma and complex foot injuries, with numbers around 32% to 52%, a situation considered as a predictor of unfavorable functional prognosis in

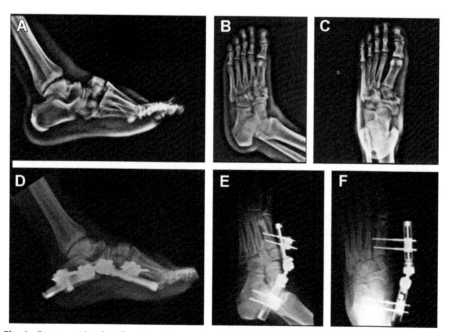

Fig. 1. Preoperative (*A–C*) and postoperative (*D–F*) lateral, oblique, and anteroposterior conventional radiographic images of high-energy Lisfranc fracture-dislocation. Initial damage control surgical treatment with closed reduction and external fixation to preserve medial column length and alignment.

polytraumatized patients, deserving special attention in the acute and follow-up settings, and aggressive recommended treatment guidelines similar to diaphyseal fractures of long bones.[34,35]

The treatment of patients presenting with complex foot injuries and associated high-energy Lisfranc injuries could be categorized in 2 phases: initial/early damage control treatment and definitive treatment. The initial or immediate treatment has several goals and can be divided into 3 overlapping substages: prevention of progression of ischemia and soft tissue necrosis, prevention of infection, and consideration for salvage procedure or amputation.[36] The presence of compartment syndrome should be assessed and, if confirmed, emergently treated with fasciotomy. Early fasciotomy is associated with lower rates of morbidity and with better outcomes.[34] Early total care should be adopted in selected cases with simpler fracture patterns, clean wounds and in the presence of an experienced team, trained and comfortable with the definitive procedures, and when both the patient's systemic condition and the local soft tissue conditions are adequate.[34,36]

Staged treatment should be preferred in all other situations, with initial treatment based on aggressive irrigation and debridement of wounds, early soft tissue coverage and rigid (temporary) fracture fixation using external fixation or Kirschner wires (**Fig. 1D–F**). [37,38]

When planning for definitive treatment, the following principles should be considered: anatomic reduction of axial, sagittal, and coronal alignment of the medial, middle, and lateral columns of the foot; starting the reduction and from proximal to distal and from medial to lateral; primary fusions for severe cartilage injury or gross instability; and stable internal fixation.[34,35,39]

SURGICAL APPROACHES FOR PRIMARY ARTHRODESIS

Patient is placed in a supine position, with a bump under the ipsilateral thigh to neutralize the external rotation of the lower limb. A tourniquet is applied in the proximal thigh. Similar surgical approaches are described for PA and ORIF.[40] The pattern of the injury, instability, and fragmentation determines the exact location and the need for 2 or 3 longitudinal incisions.

Classically, the first longitudinal incision is made between the first and second metatarsals (between the extensor hallucis longus tendon and extensor hallucis brevis tendon) (**Fig. 2A–C**), the structures at risk are the dorsalis pedis artery and the deep fibular nerve.[40] This approach allows adequate access to the first and second TMTJ. The second dorsolateral incision is centered over the fourth TMTJ (**Fig. 2D, G; Fig. 3D, 3E**), roughly in line with the fourth metatarsal. It is positioned laterally to EDL and EDB tendons, and the structures at risk are the superficial peroneal nerve branches and medial branches of the sural nerve. The surgeon can adequately reduce the third, fourth, and fifth TMTJ and visualize cuboid fractures.[2,40] Alternatively, a third medial incision (along the medial column) can be used for additional reduction landmarks and fixation. When a medial longitudinal incision is used, the 2 dorsal incisions should be made slightly lateral, one between second and third metatarsal and the other between the fourth and fifth metatarsal (**Fig. 2E; see Fig. 3D, E**), to preserve a wider skin bridge in between each incision. Alternatively, a singled dorsal transverse approach can also be used (**Fig. 2F**).[41–44]

Efforts should always be made to preserve an adequate skin bridge, as wide as possible. However, as long as careful dissection with no undermining of the skin bridge is performed, blood supply and skin bridge viability are usually not compromised.

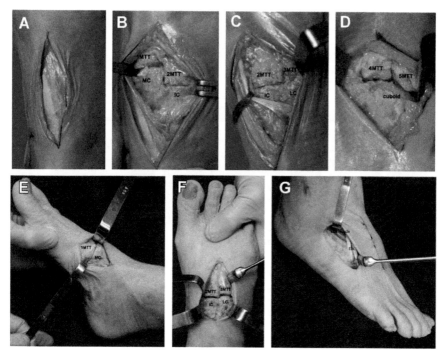

Fig. 2. Anatomic dissection of the TMTJs through classic (*A–D*) and alternative approaches (*E–G*). 1MTT, first metatarsal; 2MTT, second metatarsal; 3MTT, third metatarsal; EDB, extensor digitorum brevis; EDL, extensor digitorum longus; IC, intermediate cuneiform; LC, lateral cuneiform; MC, medial cuneiform.

Reduction Strategies

When performing PA, before proceeding with anatomic reduction of the foot columns, it is important to prepare articular surfaces properly. The goal is only to remove the cartilage and to expose subchondral bone. After removal of all chondral tissue, a 2.0-mm drill or small osteotome can then be used to fenestrate the subchondral bone plate and stimulate bone marrow bleeding to promote healing on the entire joint surface.[40]

The reduction strategy must take into account the best reference or landmark with preserved anatomy, with integrity of the bone architecture, length, and articular alignment. As mentioned elsewhere in this article, it is usually recommended to start the reduction medially (first or second rays) and proximally and then work laterally and distally.[18] If there is any question regarding the preinjury alignment, the contralateral foot can be used for comparison.[45]

The first ray and first TMTJ reduction could be performed using a pointed reduction clamp (Weber) followed by provisional K-wire stabilization, confirmed under direct visualization and under fluoroscopy guidance. The next step would be to reduce the space between the first and second metatarsals. The enlarged toothed reduction forceps can be used with that intention. A good intraoperative landmark is the adequate reduction of the space between the second metatarsal base and the medial cuneiform. Provisional K-wires are used to stabilize the reduction. The second TMTJ is then reduced and stabilized by provisional K-wire fixation.

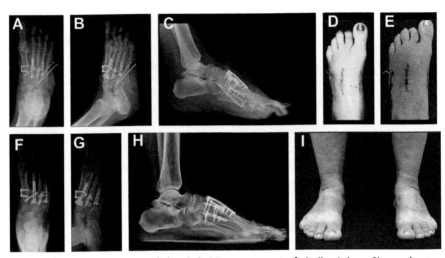

Fig. 3. Postoperative images of the definitive treatment of similar injury. Six weeks non-weightbearing anteroposterior, oblique, and lateral conventional radiographs demonstrating PA of the first, second and third TMTJ using plate and screws, as well as K-wire fixation of the fourth and fifth TMTJ (*A–C*). Alternate triple approach used (*D, E*). Twelve weeks weightbearing anteroposterior, oblique, and lateral conventional radiographs after hardware removal of the lateral column, with adequate healing of the first, second and third TMTJ (*F–H*). Adequate functional comparative alignment of the feet, with complete healing of the surgical approaches (*I*).

After stabilization of the medial 2 rays, the stability of the third, fourth, and fifth rays should be reassessed. Intercuneiform should also be evaluated. It is not uncommon for the third ray to be unstable. If so, it should be reduced and stabilized similarly. If the fourth and fifth rays are unstable, they are reduced under direct visualization and/or under fluoroscopy and stabilized with K-wires. These 2 rays are usually spared and not included in the PA.[18,40]

Definitive Fixation Methods

There are several definitive fixation methods for Lisfranc arthrodesis, once anatomic reduction and provisional fixation are achieved.[18,40,45]

The first TMTJ is classically fixed by compression screw placed from the dorsal proximal first metatarsal basis into the plantar medial cuneiform. It could be done with 3.5-mm noncannulated, or a 4.0/4.5-mm cannulated screw. A second screw (from the dorsal medial cuneiform through the plantar base of the first metatarsal) or a dorsal locking or nonlocking plate could be used to neutralize forces.[18,45]

After the second metatarsal is properly reduced into the keystone formed between the base of the first metatarsal and the medial cuneiform, the articular surface of the intermediate cuneiform, and the lateral surface of the lateral cuneiform and the third metatarsal, its fixation is performed with a compression screw placed from the medial area of the medial cuneiform (**Fig. 3**A–C), through the base of the second metatarsal. A solid fully threaded 4.0-mm screw with a lag technique is our preferred fixation. A smaller diameter screw can be used, but there is risk regarding the option for weaker constructs.[18,45] The second TMTJ can be fixed with a compression screw placed from the dorsal proximal second metatarsal into the plantar intermediate cuneiform. It could be done with 3.5-mm solid screw, or a 4.0/4.5-mm cannulated screw. A second screw (from the dorsal intermediate cuneiform through the plantar base of the second metatarsal) or a dorsal locking or nonlocking plate could also be used to neutralize forces.[45,46]

Similarly, the third TMTJ is usually fixed with a compression screw 3.0- or 3.5-mm solid or cannulated, from dorsal to plantar, with the entry point either distally at the proximal third metatarsal, or proximally at the lateral cuneiform. A dorsal neutralization plate can also be used after screw fixation.[45,46]

The fourth and fifth TMTJ are usually spared during Lisfranc arthrodesis. When the more medial TMT joints are reduced and stabilized, the lateral TMT joints often fall back into place in a reduced position. As stated elsewhere in this article, having some motion at these joints is extremely helpful for normal foot function and fine-tuning the positioning of the forefoot, mainly on uneven ground.[13] If the lateral column is still unstable and stabilization is required, the classic choice would be fixing the fourth and the fifth metatarsals to the cuboid using provisional K-wire fixation, which are usually percutaneously placed and removed after 6 to 8 weeks (**Fig. 3**F–H).[40,45–47] Alternatively, screws can be used in very unstable conditions, with placement usually from the base of the fourth or fifth metatarsal into the cuboid. However, because these joints are best left mobile, the screws are removed after 6 to 8 weeks.[46,47]

Regarding choice between cannulated and solid screws, clinical data comparing fixation methods have demonstrated increased incidence of hardware failure and screw breakage when using cannulated screws.[47] However, biomechanical cadaveric studies showed similar compression force and resistance to deformation under load when comparing cortical and cannulated screws. Therefore, the use of cannulated screws is acceptable and can simplify the surgical procedure without sacrificing the strength of the fixation.[48] Our preference is still for solid compression screws.

It is important to emphasize that adequate compression and alternative fixation can be achieved using external compression devices, such as Hintermann's spreaders, and fixation with dorsal plates and positional fully threaded screws, or with specialized midfoot compression plates.[40,45–47]

Postoperative Management

Patients are usually placed in a short leg splint for 4 to 6 weeks, remaining nonweight-bearing during this time. Patients then slowly progress from partial to full weightbearing over the next 4 to 6 weeks wearing a walker boot. Full weightbearing usually is permitted after 12 weeks.[28]

Patients are seen at 2, 4, and 12 weeks, and after 12 months postoperatively, monitoring for wound complications, maintenance of achieved reduction, fusion rate, hardware loosening/failure, ability to progress weightbearing and return to prior level of activities. Radiographic incidences that are frequently assessed include anteroposterior, lateral, and oblique radiographic views (see **Fig. 3**F–H).

Once there is clinical and radiographic confirmation of timed interval healing of the fusions of the medial and intermediate columns, with a stable midfoot, the fourth and fifth TMT percutaneous fixation could be removed, usually after 8 to 12 weeks.[18,49] If needed, screws and plates could be removed after clinical and radiographic confirmation that fractures and fusion sites have completely healed. Recommended time is around 10 to 14 months postoperatively following the index procedure, and computed tomography scan confirmation is advisable.[22,28,47–50]

Physical therapy can be started after 6 to 10 weeks from the surgical treatment, with a focus on swelling control and range of motion exercises for the ankle, hindfoot, and toes, as well muscle strengthening of intrinsic and extrinsic foot muscles, ankle, and

CORE, as well as gait training (**Fig. 3l**). Custom-made orthotics can be prescribed on an as-needed basis, depending on residual symptoms.

SUMMARY

Lisfranc injuries continue to be an important source of pain and disability for patients worldwide. Over the past several years, published literature has debated regarding preferential use ORIF versus PA. Controversy persists as to whether high-energy Lisfranc injuries are best treated with PA. Our opinion is that PA should not be considered an inferior option and is strongly recommended for high-energy injuries.

Regardless of the technique chosen, high-energy injuries should be treated respecting important principles of initial soft tissue damage control and timed definitive treatment ensuring anatomic reduction and stable fixation for the medial and intermediate columns and preservation of motion in the lateral column.

CLINICS CARE POINTS

- Do not miss the diagnosis.
- Surgical planning based on clinical findings and images.
- Take care with surgical approaches.
- Properly reduced tarsometatarsals joints.
- Follow staged postoperative protocol.

DISCLOSURE

The authors have nothing to disclose.

REFERENCES

1. Fischer LP. Jacques Lisfranc de saint-martin (1787-1847). Hist Sci Med 2005;39: 17–34 [in French].
2. Welck MJ, Zinchenko R, Rudge B. Lisfranc injuries. Injury 2015;46:536–41.
3. Chiodo CP, Myerson MS. Developments and advances in the diagnosis and treatment of injuries to the tarsometatarsal joint. Orthop Clin North Am 2001;32:11–20.
4. Lau SC, Guest C, Hall M, et al. Do columns or sagittal displacement matter in the assessment and management of Lisfranc fracture dislocation? an alternate approach to classification of the Lisfranc injury. Injury 2017;48:1689–95.
5. Nunley JA, Vertullo CJ. Classification, investigation, and management of midfoot sprains: Lisfranc injuries in the athlete. Am J Sports Med 2002;30:871–8.
6. Sobrado MF, Saito GH, Sakaki MH, et al. Epidemiological study on Lisfranc injuries. Acta Ortop Bras 2017;25:44–7.
7. Rosenbaum A, Dellenbaugh S, Dipreta J, et al. Subtle injuries to the Lisfranc joint. Orthopedics 2011;34:882–7.
8. Ponkilainen VT, Laine HJ, Maenpaa HM, et al. Incidence and characteristics of midfoot injuries. Foot Ankle Int 2019;40:105–12.
9. Rajapakse B, Edwards A, Hong T. A single surgeon's experience of treatment of Lisfranc joint injuries. Injury 2006;37:914–21.
10. Renninger CH, Cochran G, Tompane T, et al. Injury characteristics of low-energy Lisfranc injuries compared with high-energy injuries. Foot Ankle Int 2017;38: 964–9.
11. Myerson MS, Fisher RT, Burgess AR, et al. Fracture dislocations of the tarsometatarsal joints: end results correlated with pathology and treatment. Foot Ankle 1986;6:225–42.

12. Rammelt S, Zwipp H. Focus on midfoot injuries. Eur J Trauma Emerg Surg 2010; 36:189–90.

13. Coetzee JC. Making sense of Lisfranc injuries. Foot Ankle Clin 2008;13: 695–704, ix.

14. Smith N, Stone C, Furey A. Does open reduction and internal fixation versus primary arthrodesis improve patient outcomes for Lisfranc trauma? a systematic review and meta-analysis. Clin Orthop Relat Res 2016;474:1445–52.

15. Lau S, Howells N, Millar M, et al. Plates, screws, or combination? radiologic outcomes after Lisfranc fracture dislocation. J Foot Ankle Surg 2016;55:799–802.

16. Kuo RS, Tejwani NC, Digiovanni CW, et al. Outcome after open reduction and internal fixation of Lisfranc joint injuries. J Bone Joint Surg Am 2000;82:1609–18.

17. Kirzner N, Teoh W, Toemoe S, et al. Primary arthrodesis versus open reduction internal fixation for complete Lisfranc fracture dislocations: a retrospective study comparing functional and radiological outcomes. ANZ J Surg 2019;90(4):585–90.

18. Moracia-Ochagavia I, Rodriguez-Merchan EC. Lisfranc fracture-dislocations: current management. EFORT Open Rev 2019;4:430–44.

19. Mulcahy H. Lisfranc injury: current concepts. Radiol Clin North Am 2018;56: 859–76.

20. Watson TS, Shurnas PS, Denker J. Treatment of Lisfranc joint injury: current concepts. J Am Acad Orthop Surg 2010;18:718–28.

21. Rammelt S, Schneiders W, Schikore H, et al. Primary open reduction and fixation compared with delayed corrective arthrodesis in the treatment of tarsometatarsal (Lisfranc) fracture dislocation. J Bone Joint Surg Br 2008;90:1499–506.

22. Alcelik I, Fenton C, Hannant G, et al. A systematic review and meta-analysis of the treatment of acute Lisfranc injuries: open reduction and internal fixation versus primary arthrodesis. Foot Ankle Surg 2019;26(3):299–307.

23. Buda M, Hagemeijer NC, Kink S, et al. Effect of fixation type and bone graft on tarsometatarsal fusion. Foot Ankle Int 2018;39:1394–402.

24. Cochran G, Renninger C, Tompane T, et al. Primary arthrodesis versus open reduction and internal fixation for low-energy Lisfranc injuries in a young athletic population. Foot Ankle Int 2017;38:957–63.

25. Dubois-Ferriere V, Lubbeke A, Chowdhary A, et al. Clinical outcomes and development of symptomatic osteoarthritis 2 to 24 years after surgical treatment of tarsometatarsal joint complex injuries. J Bone Joint Surg Am 2016;98:713–20.

26. Hawkinson MP, Tennent DJ, Belisle J, et al. Outcomes of Lisfranc injuries in an active duty military population. Foot Ankle Int 2017;38:1115–9.

27. Henning JA, Jones CB, Sietsema DL, et al. Open reduction internal fixation versus primary arthrodesis for Lisfranc injuries: a prospective randomized study. Foot Ankle Int 2009;30:913–22.

28. Ly TV, Coetzee JC. Treatment of primarily ligamentous Lisfranc joint injuries: primary arthrodesis compared with open reduction and internal fixation. A prospective, randomized study. J Bone Joint Surg Am 2006;88:514–20.

29. Magill HHP, Hajibandeh S, Bennett J, et al. Open reduction and internal fixation versus primary arthrodesis for the treatment of acute Lisfranc injuries: a systematic review and meta-analysis. J Foot Ankle Surg 2019;58:328–32.

30. Mulier T, Reynders P, Dereymaeker G, et al. Severe Lisfrancs injuries: primary arthrodesis or ORIF? Foot Ankle Int 2002;23:902–5.

31. Qiao YS, Li JK, Shen H, et al. Comparison of arthrodesis and non-fusion to treat Lisfranc injuries. Orthop Surg 2017;9:62–8.

32. Albright RH, Haller S, Klein E, et al. Cost-effectiveness analysis of primary arthrodesis versus open reduction internal fixation for primarily ligamentous Lisfranc injuries. J Foot Ankle Surg 2018;57:325–31.

33. Barnds B, Tucker W, Morris B, et al. Cost comparison and complication rate of Lisfranc injuries treated with open reduction internal fixation versus primary arthrodesis. Injury 2018;49:2318–21.

34. Schepers T, Rammelt S. Complex foot injury: early and definite management. Foot Ankle Clin 2017;22:193–213.

35. Zelle BA, Brown SR, Panzica M, et al. The impact of injuries below the knee joint on the long-term functional outcome following polytrauma. Injury 2005;36:169–77.

36. Probst C, Richter M, Lefering R, et al. Incidence and significance of injuries to the foot and ankle in polytrauma patients–an analysis of the trauma registry of DGU. Injury 2010;41:210–5.

37. Chandran P, Puttaswamaiah R, Dhillon MS, et al. Management of complex open fracture injuries of the midfoot with external fixation. J Foot Ankle Surg 2006;45:308–15.

38. Klaue K. The role of external fixation in acute foot trauma. Foot Ankle Clin 2004;9:583–594, x.

39. Tran T, Thordarson D. Functional outcome of multiply injured patients with associated foot injury. Foot Ankle Int 2002;23:340–3.

40. Coetzee JC, Ly TV. Treatment of primarily ligamentous Lisfranc joint injuries: primary arthrodesis compared with open reduction and internal fixation. Surgical technique. J Bone Joint Surg Am 2007;89(Suppl 2 Pt.1):122–7.

41. Herscovici D Jr, Scaduto JM. Acute management of high-energy Lisfranc injuries: a simple approach. Injury 2018;49:420–4.

42. Philpott A, Lawford C, Lau SC, et al. Modified dorsal approach in the management of Lisfranc injuries. Foot Ankle Int 2018;39:573–84.

43. Schepers T, Oprel PP, Van Lieshout EM. Influence of approach and implant on reduction accuracy and stability in Lisfranc fracture-dislocation at the tarsometatarsal joint. Foot Ankle Int 2013;34:705–10.

44. Vertullo CJ, Easley ME, Nunley JA. The transverse dorsal approach to the Lisfranc joint. Foot Ankle Int 2002;23:420–6.

45. Boffeli TJ, Collier RC, Schnell KR. Combined medial column arthrodesis with open reduction internal fixation of central column for treatment of Lisfranc fracture-dislocation: a review of consecutive cases. J Foot Ankle Surg 2018;57:1059–66.

46. Desmond EA, Chou LB. Current concepts review: Lisfranc injuries. Foot Ankle Int 2006;27:653–60.

47. Stavlas P, Roberts CS, Xypnitos FN, et al. The role of reduction and internal fixation of Lisfranc fracture-dislocations: a systematic review of the literature. Int Orthop 2010;34:1083–91.

48. Rozell JC, Chin M, Donegan DJ, et al. Biomechanical comparison of fully threaded solid cortical versus partially threaded cannulated cancellous screw fixation for Lisfranc injuries. Orthopedics 2018;41:e222–7.

49. Fan MQ, Li XS, Jiang XJ, et al. The surgical outcome of Lisfranc injuries accompanied by multiple metatarsal fractures: a multicenter retrospective study. Injury 2019;50:571–8.

50. Weatherford BM, Bohay DR, Anderson JG. Open reduction and internal fixation versus primary arthrodesis for Lisfranc injuries. Foot Ankle Clin 2017;22:1–14.

Jones Fracture in the Nonathletic Population

Michelle M. Coleman, MD, PhD, Gregory P. Guyton, MD*

KEYWORDS

- Proximal fifth metatarsal • Jones fracture • Tuberosity fracture • History
- Nomenclature • Treatment • Screw fixation • Bone grafting

KEY POINTS

- Zone 1 fractures have excellent healing potential and may be treated nonoperatively with a weightbearing as tolerated protocol.
- "Jones fractures" may refer to proximal fifth metatarsal fractures in zones 2 and 3.
- Zone 2 fractures are truly acute injuries, whereas zone 3 fractures commonly occur in the presence of a chronic stress reaction. Zone 2 fractures may heal well with nonoperative or operative treatment. Zone 3 fractures typically require operative treatment.
- Axial screw fixation is an effective operative treatment of Jones fractures, but the optimal screw design remains unclear.
- Bone grafting and bone marrow aspirate concentrate injection are emerging adjuvant treatments for patients with zone 2 or zone 3 injuries at high risk for nonunion or refracture.

INTRODUCTION

Fractures of the proximal fifth metatarsal are common injuries with a unique history. Controversies abound because of confusing nomenclature and recent advances in the understanding of the fracture subtypes.

ANATOMY

The bony anatomy of the proximal fifth metatarsal includes the metatarsal shaft (diaphysis), the base, and the tuberosity (styloid) (**Fig. 1**). The fifth metatarsal base articulates with the cuboid and with the fourth metatarsal base. Stability of these joints is provided by capsular ligaments, dorsal and plantar cubometatarsal ligaments, and the lateral band of the plantar aponeurosis. Because of flat articulations and ligamentous tensioning, a larger amount of sagittal motion is possible through fourth and fifth

Department of Orthopaedic Surgery, MedStar Union Memorial Hospital, 3333 North Calvert Street, Suite 400, Baltimore, MD 21218, USA
* Corresponding author.
E-mail address: lyn.camire@medstar.net

Foot Ankle Clin N Am 25 (2020) 737–751
https://doi.org/10.1016/j.fcl.2020.08.012

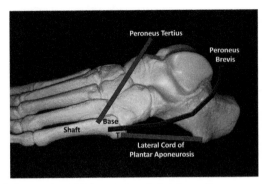

Fig. 1. Anatomy of the proximal fifth metatarsal. T, tuberosity.

cubometatarsal joints compared with the other tarsometatarsal joints. The tuberosity flares laterally and plantarly, although its size and shape vary.

The peroneus tertius inserts along the dorsal surface of the metatarsal shaft distal to the tuberosity. The peroneus brevis tendon inserts broadly along the dorsolateral aspect of the tuberosity. The lateral band of the plantar aponeurosis inserts along the plantar-lateral aspect of the tuberosity. The mechanism of tuberosity fractures was initially believed to be an avulsion because of the pull of the peroneus brevis tendon. A more recent cadaver study demonstrated that avulsion is rather caused by the strong attachment of the lateral band of the plantar aponeurosis.[1]

The blood supply of the proximal fifth metatarsal is supplied to the base and tuberosity via metaphyseal arteries.[2,3] The proximal diaphysis is perfused via a nutrient artery that sends branches proximally. The metaphyseal-diaphyseal junction represents a watershed region between these two vascular supplies. As discussed in additional detail later, proximal fifth metatarsal fractures are currently classified by three anatomic zones as described by Lawrence and Botte.[4]

EPIDEMIOLOGY AND RISK FACTORS

The incidence of proximal fifth metatarsal fractures is incompletely understood. In one population study of 534,715 persons over 1 year, 218 patients were treated for proximal fifth metatarsal fractures. This suggests an annual incidence of approximately 1 per 2500 persons.[5] Approximately 82% of these injuries were zone 1 proximal tuberosity avulsion fractures, and 18% were either zone 2 or zone 3 fractures. In another study of 898 proximal fifth metatarsal fractures treated over 5 years at a single institution, 73% were tuberosity fractures, 19% were zone 2 fractures, and 8% were zone 3 proximal diaphyseal stress fractures.[6]

Early retrospective studies and many case reports have reported proximal fifth metatarsal fractures to be most common in young male athletes.[7–9] However, more recent larger population studies suggest that all three types of proximal fifth metatarsal fractures may be more common in women than men.[6,10] Kane and colleagues[6] reported that 72% of their 898 fractures occurred in women. Pugliese and colleagues[10] reported that 73% of their 149 fractures occurred in women. Women accounted for approximately 73% of zone 1 fractures, 68% to 73% of zone 2 fractures, and 68% to 75% of zone 3 fractures in these studies.

Studies have found conflicting results in terms of anatomic risk factors for fracture. In one study of zone 2 fractures among 51 National Football League (NFL) players (96 feet), a higher risk for fracture was found for individuals with long, narrow, and straight fifth metatarsals with metatarsus adductus.[11] Other studies have found metatarsus adductus to be a risk factor for slower healing of zone 2 fractures[12] and a risk factor for refracture of zone 2 fractures.[13] Whereas some studies report a high coincidence of hindfoot varus alignment and Jones fractures,[14] studies with a comparison group have not shown an association with hindfoot alignment and fracture risk.[15] Having a higher medial longitudinal arch (pes cavus) was associated with Jones fractures in a case-control study of 60 soccer players.[16]

WHAT IS A JONES FRACTURE?

Fractures of the proximal fifth metatarsal were first described by Robert Jones in 1902.[17] This article presented six fractures caused by "indirect violence," but the quality of x-rays was poor and no concise definition or anatomic description was given (**Fig. 2**). At least one fracture was a proximal diaphyseal stress fracture, with radiographs demonstrating cortical hypertrophy and widening of the fracture line.[17]

In 1960, Stewart[18] reviewed the existing literature regarding Jones fractures and presented his case series of 51 fractures. He proposed a classification system for proximal fifth metatarsal fractures that included two types: fractures of the styloid process and fractures at the "junction of the shaft and base" (**Fig. 3**).

In 1975, Dameron[19] reported a case series of 120 fractures of the proximal fifth metatarsal. Dameron defined a Jones fracture as a fracture through the tuberosity, which he equated to the flare of the fifth metatarsal. This imprecision contributed to some confusion in later published reports. Importantly, Dameron reported uniform healing of 100 tuberosity fractures with nonoperative treatment. He reported that proximal diaphyseal fractures have variable and prolonged healing, often requiring bone grafting.

In 1978, Kavanaugh and coworkers[7] presented a case series of 23 injuries which they called Jones fractures. They performed anatomic dissections of five amputation

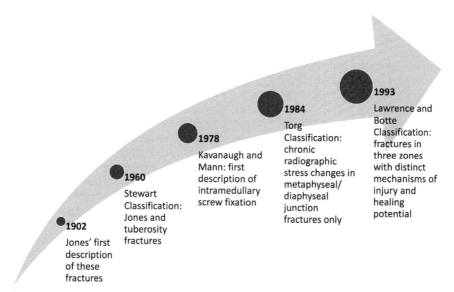

Fig. 2. Historical milestones of fifth proximal metatarsal fractures.

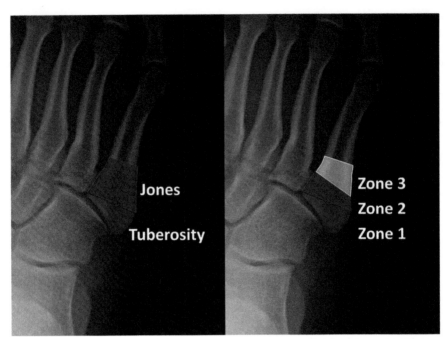

Fig. 3. Classification of fifth proximal metatarsal fractures. (*Left*) Stewart classification. (*Right*) Lawrence and Botte classification. (*Data from* Stewart IM. Jones's fracture: fracture of base of fifth metatarsal. Clin Orthop. 1960;(16):190-198 and Lawrence SJ, Botte MJ. Jones' fractures and related fractures of the proximal fifth metatarsal. Foot Ankle. 1993;14(6):358-365.)

specimens and determined that Jones fractures occur 5 mm distal to the peroneus brevis insertion and adjacent or just distal to the fourth to fifth intermetatarsal joint. Importantly, they reported a high rate of delayed union overall (67%). Kavanaugh and coworkers were also the first group to describe intramedullary screw fixation in this injury.

In 1984, Torg and colleagues[20] reported a case series of 46 proximal fifth metatarsal fractures, all distal to the tuberosity. These authors considered a Jones fracture to be anything other than a fracture of the styloid (still in line with the binary classification proposed by Stewart). However, Torg and colleagues proposed that these fractures should be further classified as an acute fracture, delayed union, or nonunion. They recommended that acute fractures be treated nonoperatively, whereas delayed unions or nonunions should be treated operatively. Importantly, their description of acute fractures allowed for "previous pain or discomfort" and also allowed for "minimal cortical hypertrophy or evidence of periosteal reaction to chronic stress." Thus, this description of acute, delayed union, and nonunion fractures was actually referencing stress fractures, although a few nonstress fractures may have been included in the case series (**Table 1**).

In 1993, Lawrence and Botte[4] proposed that three fracture types occur in the proximal fifth metatarsal (see **Fig. 3**, **Table 1**). Tuberosity avulsion fractures (zone 1) were described as a fracture of the styloid process sustained because of an acute hindfoot inversion force that caused avulsion of the tuberosity from the firm attachment of the lateral band of the plantar aponeurosis.[1] The bony avulsion may be extra-articular, or it

Table 1		
Types of proximal fifth metatarsal fractures		
Classification	**Chronicity**	**Radiographic Location/Features**
Zone 1: tuberosity avulsion	Acute	Tuberosity Extra-articular or extending into the cuboid-5th metatarsal articulation
Zone 2	Acute	Junction of metaphysis-diaphysis Extending into the 4th–5th intermetatarsal articulation
Zone 3: diaphyseal stress	Chronic	Proximal diaphysis Chronic stress reaction with acute or chronic superimposed fracture Categorized by Torg type (below)
Torg 1: early		Narrow fracture line with sharp margins Minimal cortical hypertrophy or periosteal reaction No intramedullary sclerosis
Torg 2: delayed union		Widened fracture line with adjacent radiolucency related to bone resorption Intramedullary sclerosis
Torg 3: nonunion		Complete obliteration of the medullary canal at the fracture site by sclerotic bone

Data from Torg JS, Balduini FC, Zelko RR, et al. Fractures of the base of the fifth metatarsal distal to the tuberosity: classification and guidelines for non-surgical and surgical management. J Bone Joint Surg Am. 1984;66(2):209-214 and Lawrence SJ, Botte MJ. Jones' fractures and related fractures of the proximal fifth metatarsal. Foot Ankle. 1993;14(6):358-365.

may involve the cuboid-fifth metatarsal articulation. These fractures may occasionally be multifragmentary.

Lawrence and Botte described zone 2 (Jones fractures) as acute fractures extending into the fourth to fifth intermetatarsal articulation along the metaphyseal-diaphyseal junction between the insertions of the peroneus brevis and peroneus tertius tendons.[4] These fractures are typically short oblique or transverse fractures, and medial comminution is common. These fractures are thought to occur because of forceful adduction of the foot with a plantarflexed ankle.

Lawrence and Botte[4] described diaphyseal stress fractures (zone 3) as pathologic fractures of the proximal shaft caused by repetitive forces that cause fatigue of the bone microarchitecture. These fractures are most appropriately further characterized using the Torg and colleagues[20] classification.

WHAT ARE THE INDICATIONS FOR OPERATIVE TREATMENT OF ZONE 1 TUBEROSITY FRACTURES?

Nonoperative treatment of zone 1 tuberosity fractures is typically recommended,[21–25] because these fractures have excellent healing potential.[4,19] Numerous high-quality studies show near 100% clinical union rates and high patient-reported outcome scores (PROs) with nonoperative treatment.[26] Patients are typically allowed to weight-bear as tolerated. PROs may be better when removable support is used (eg, walking boot, hard-sole shoe, or compressive dressing) rather than a cast.[26] When comparing different types of removable support, one study demonstrated a significantly faster rate of radiographic healing with use of a removable boot compared with a hard-sole shoe (7.2 weeks vs 8.6 weeks).[27] Asymptomatic nonunions may occur rarely and are typically treated with observation.

In the nonathlete, there is no evidence to support operative treatment of zone 1 fractures. There were no differences in visual analog scale score or American Orthopedic Foot and Ankle Society score at final follow-up in the only randomized controlled trial that has compared open reduction internal fixation with nonoperative treatment in displaced zone 1 fractures (displacement >2 mm).[28] In fact, tuberosity avulsion fractures have been found to have excellent outcomes with nonoperative treatment regardless of fracture displacement and extension into the cuboid-fifth metatarsal articulation in multiple studies.[28–33]

Anecdotally, many surgeons report that athletes with widely displaced zone 1 fractures have worse clinical outcomes with nonoperative treatment. Symptomatic nonunions of zone 1 fractures have been reported in athletes requiring operative treatment with fragment excision, internal fixation, and/or bone grafting.[34,35]

WHAT IS THE EVIDENCE FOR OPTIMAL TREATMENT OF ACUTE ZONE 2 FRACTURES?

The natural history of zone 2 fractures has been misunderstood in the past because of the grouping of multiple types of proximal fifth metatarsal fractures in historical and more recent studies.

Table 2 reports the results of studies that clearly described the treatment and outcomes for acute zone 2 fractures without mixing the results with zone 1 or zone 3 fractures. Five retrospective studies reported nonoperative treatment of zone 2 fractures. In one study, patients were treated nonweightbearing for 4 to 6 weeks, resulting in a union rate of 82.4%.[36] In four studies, patients were treated weightbearing as tolerated in a boot or hard-sole shoe. These studies demonstrated high clinical union rates of 96% to 100%.[30,31,33,37] No refractures were reported in any of these studies. In two studies, PROs were found to be similar to those for patients treated for zone 1 fractures.[30,31] One study found no difference in outcomes based on displacement.[31]

Three studies reported operative treatment of acute zone 2 fractures. Two of these studies included only fractures displaced greater than 2 mm,[30,36] and the other study included only elite athletes from the NFL.[38] All patients were treated with intramedullary screw fixation. Union rates were 89% to 100%. The study in NFL players reported a 22% refracture rate.

Two studies compared nonoperative treatment with operative treatment.[30,36] In both studies, less displaced fractures were treated nonoperatively, and displaced fractures were treated operatively. There were no statistically significant differences in union rates, time to union, or PROs. One study demonstrated a significantly faster return to sports (15 vs 30 weeks) for patients treated operatively.[36]

IS THERE ANY ROLE FOR NONOPERATIVE TREATMENT OF ZONE 3 PROXIMAL DIAPHYSEAL STRESS FRACTURES?

Historical case series of Jones fractures have reported high rates of delayed union/nonunion of 25% to 67%[7,19,39] and refracture rates of up to 50%.[7,39] These studies brought early attention to the importance of evaluating radiographs for evidence of stress phenomena in the bone, and many authors began to advocate for operative treatment of stress fractures.

Only one paper reported the outcomes for zone 3 fractures treated nonoperatively, without mixing the results with zone 1 or zone 2 fractures (**Table 3**). Chuckpaiwong and colleagues[36] reported the results of eight zone 3 fractures (all Torg I) treated nonweightbearing in a cast or boot for 4 to 6 weeks. The union rate was 88% and the time to return to sports was 26.3 weeks.

Table 2
Treatment and outcomes for zone 2 fractures

Study (Country)	Zone 2 Fractures	Treatment[a] (Follow-Up)	Union Rate	Refracture Rate
Nonoperative treatment				
Chuckpaiwong et al,[36] 2008 (United States)	17 displaced <2–3 mm	NWB in cast or boot 4–6 wk (40 mo)	82% (3 delayed unions)	NR
Baumbach et al,[31] 2017 (Germany)	16 (mixed displacement)	WBAT in HSS (22 mo)	100%	0%
Monteban et al,[30] 2018 (Belgium)[b]	49 displaced <2 mm	WBAT (37.5 mo)	100%	NR
Marecek et al,[37] 2016 (United States)	27 (displacement not specified)	WBAT in boot (short-term follow-up)	96% (1 nonunion)	NR
Biz et al,[33] 2017 (Italy, Spain, France)	42 displaced <2 mm	WBAT in cast or HSS (15 mo)	100%	0%
Operative treatment				
Chuckpaiwong et al,[36] 2008 (United States)	18 Displaced >2 mm or athlete	Screw fixation (40 mo)	89% (2 ASX nonunions)	NR
Lareau et al,[38] 2016 (United States)	18 athletes (mixed displacement)	Screw fixation, DBM, BMAC, and bone stimulator (minimum 6 mo)	100%	22%
Monteban et al,[30] 2018 (Belgium)	10 Displaced ≥2 mm	Screw fixation (38 mo)	100%	NR

Abbreviations: ASX, asymptomatic; BMAC, bone marrow aspirate concentrate; DBM, demineralized bone matrix; HSS, hard-sole shoe; NR, not reported/not specifically mentioned in the article; NWB, nonweightbearing; WBAT, weightbearing as tolerated.
[a] All studies included were retrospective studies.
[b] Study author was contacted to confirm union rate.
Data from Refs.[30,31,33,36–38]

Nine studies reported the results of operatively treated zone 3 stress fractures. Three studies did not specify the Torg classification of the included fractures, but all three reported 100% union with axial screw fixation in athletes.[38,40,41] The remaining studies specified their subsets of Torg fractures. Union rates were 76% to 100% with screw fixation.[36,42–44] Union rates were 86% to 100% with plantar plating[45] and 83% to 94% with tension band fixation.[46] Four studies reported a 0% refracture rate after operative treatment.[38,40–42] Three studies reported refracture rates between 3% and 11%.[44–46] Return to sport ranged from 8 to 15 weeks in six studies.[36,38,40–42,44] Miller and colleagues[44] reported the highest rate of delayed union in professional soccer players who returned to play at 8 weeks or less postoperatively. Lee and colleagues[47] reported a longer time to union in patients with stress fractures and a preoperative plantar fracture gap greater than 1 mm.

One study of operative versus nonoperative treatment of zone 3 fractures found a faster return to sports (15 weeks vs 26 weeks) with operative treatment, but no difference in time to radiographic union or overall union rate.[36] In that study, however, all

Table 3
Treatment and outcomes for zone 3 fractures

Study (Country)	Zone 3[a] Fractures	Treatment[b] (Follow-Up)	Union Rate	Refracture Rate
Nonoperative treatment				
Chuckpaiwong et al,[36] 2008 (United States)	8 Torg I	NWB in cast or boot 4–6 wk (Torg I only) (40 mo)	88% (1 delayed union)	NR
Operative treatment				
DeLee et al,[40] 1983 (United States)	10 athletes	Screw fixation (15 mo)	100%	0%
Fernandez Fairen et al,[41] 1999 (Spain)	9 athletes	Screw fixation (19 mo)	100%	0%
Portland et al,[43] 2003 (United States)	7 Torg II	Screw fixation (21 mo)	100%	NR
Porter et al,[42] 2005 (United States)	21 athletes 10 Torg II 11 Torg III	Screw fixation (22 mo)	100%	0%
Chuckpaiwong et al,[36] 2008 (United States)	22 Torg II and III	Screw fixation (40 mo)	91% (2 ASX nonunions)	NR
Lee et al,[46] 2013 (Korea)	86 athletes 23 Torg I 47 Torg II 16 Torg III	Tension band fixation Torg III also had bone grafting (unclear follow-up)	100% Torg I 83% Torg II 94% Torg III	9%
Lareau et al,[38] 2016 (United States)	7 athletes	Screw fixation, DBM, BMAC, and bone stimulator (minimum 6 mo)	100%	0%
Miller et al,[44] 2019 (United Kingdom)	37 athletes Torg II and III	Screw fixation, bone grafting, BMAC, and bone stimulator (61 mo)	76% (8 delayed union, 1 nonunion)	3%
Young et al,[45] 2020 (Korea)	38 athletes 20 Torg I 14 Torg II 4 Torg III	Plantar plating 12 with bone grafting (23 mo)	90% Torg I 86% Torg II 100% Torg III	11% All 10% Torg I 14% Torg II 0% Torg III

Abbreviations: ASX, asymptomatic; BMAC, bone marrow aspirate concentrate; DBM, demineralized bone matrix; HSS, hard-sole shoe; NR, not reported/not specifically mentioned in the article; NWB, nonweightbearing; WBAT, weightbearing as tolerated.

[a] In cases where zones were not specified, patients with radiographic signs of stress fracture were included.

[b] All studies included were retrospective studies.

Data from Refs.[36,38,40–46]

patients treated nonoperatively were Torg I, whereas all patients treated operatively were Torg II or III.

WHEN PERFORMING AXIAL SCREW FIXATION, WHAT TYPE OF SCREW SHOULD BE USED?

The canal of the fifth metatarsal is elliptical, with the narrowest width seen on the anteroposterior view and the narrowest width seen on the lateral view.[48,49] In computed tomography studies of fifth metatarsal morphology, the average canal diameter was found to be 5.0 mm at the isthmus[49] and 4.0 mm at the apex of the curvature.[48] The average distance from the apex to the base was 42.6 mm in the anteroposterior view in one study[48] and the average length of the straight segment was 52 mm in another study.[49]

The appropriate screw size and design is controversial. In terms of screw length, most authors suggest using the greatest length screw that will remain in the straight segment of the bone, because extension into the curved portion of the metatarsal may lead to distraction or displacement.[48]

Most authors also suggest that the largest diameter screw possible should be used for each patient. In one systematic review of proximal fifth metatarsal fractures, the most commonly used screw size was 4.5 mm, with a range from 4.0 to 6.5 mm.[50] Porter and colleagues[51] retrospectively compared clinical outcomes in 43 patients who underwent fixation with either 4.5-mm or 5.0-mm diameter cannulated screws. All fractures healed, and there were no refractures in either group. However, there were 3 out of 20 bent screws in the 4.5-mm group versus 0 out of 23 bent screws in the 5.5-mm group. Carreira and Sandilands[52] reported a series of 56 athletes treated operatively with intramedullary screw fixation with multiple types of screws. Screw size did not correlate with nonunion. Biomechanically, larger screw sizes have better fatigue bending strength[53] and greater pull-out strength.[54]

Another major controversy has been whether to use cannulated or solid screws for fixation. Cannulated screws offer the theoretic advantage of technical ease and precision when placed over a guidewire. However, some authors have cautioned against use of cannulated screws because of decreased strength. When comparing screws from the same implant company (with the same design and diameter), solid screws have been shown to have higher fatigue bending strength compared with cannulated screws.[53] The bending strength of a screw is proportional to the radius of the screw to the fourth power. Cannulation decreases the cross-sectional moment of inertia, but the effect of cannulation is typically small because of the small diameter of the central defect.[53] In a cadaver model of simulated proximal fifth metatarsal fractures fixed with either 4.5-mm cannulated or 4.5-mm solid malleolar screws, there was no significant difference between the force at initial fracture displacement and the force at complete displacement.[55] Despite the biomechanical differences between cannulated and solid screws, no clinical studies have provided convincing evidence of difference in failures or clinical outcomes. Porter and colleagues[42] reported no refractures and a 100% clinic union rate in 24 proximal fifth metatarsal fractures in athletes treated with 4.5-mm cannulated screws. Carreira and Sandilands[52] reported a series of 56 athletes treated operatively with intramedullary screw fixation. Screws used were 59% cannulated, 30% solid, and 11% tapered. Screw design did not correlate with the nonunion rate.

Some authors have questioned whether stainless steel or titanium implants are superior for fixation of proximal fifth metatarsal fractures. DeVries and colleagues[56] found no statistically significant difference in time radiographic union, overall union, or refracture when comparing patients who underwent screw fixation with cannulated titanium or stainless-steel screws.

Some surgeons have advocated fixing Jones fractures with variable pitch headless compression screws. One study reported excellent clinical outcomes using these variable pitch screws in 60 patients, resulting in a 97% union rate and 0% refracture rate.[57] However, biomechanical testing has demonstrated that variable pitch headless compression screws generate significantly less (30% less) compression at the fracture site than partially threaded constant pitch screws throughout physiologic cyclic loading.[58] Variable pitch headless compression screws also have inferior fatigue strength compared with partially threaded constant pitch screws.[53,59]

Finally, there has been discussion about whether there is any difference in outcome when using traditional screws versus indication-specific screws. These screws have been found to have improved fatigue bending strength compared with traditional malleolar screws,[59] cannulated partially threaded screws,[59] and variable pitch screws.[53,59] In a comparison between indication-specific and traditional screws, Metzl and colleagues[60] found no adverse events in a group of 26 patients treated with an indication-specific screw. There was a significantly higher adverse event rate in the group of 21 patients treated with traditional screws (two implant failures, one intraoperative fracture, one symptomatic hardware). There were no differences in union rate, activity limitations, footwear modifications, recovery time, satisfaction, willingness to repeat the surgery, or visual analog scale scores between the groups.

WHEN ARE BONE GRAFTING OR BONE MARROW ASPIRATE CONCENTRATE INJECTION RECOMMENDED?

There are an increasing number of retrospective reports of adjunctive treatment with bone grafting or bone marrow aspirate concentrate (BMAC) injection during internal fixation of zone 2 and 3 fractures of the proximal fifth metatarsal. These studies include acute and chronic fractures and previous nonunions or refractures.

Eight studies have described internal fixation with bone grafting for zone 2 and 3 fractures.[13,45,46,60–64] When combined, these studies contain 61 patients, with an overall union rate of 93%. Four of these studies included only elite athletes. Sources of bone autograft were the calcaneus and the iliac crest. Sample indications for bone grafting in these studies included acute fractures,[61] Torg II and Torg III stress fractures,[60] Torg III stress fractures only,[46] refractures,[61,62] previous nonunions,[62] and stress fractures with a remaining gap at the fracture site after fracture reduction.[45]

Four studies have described internal fixation with iliac crest BMAC injection in zone 2 and 3 fractures.[13,60,62,64] When combined, these studies contain 21 patients, with an overall union rate of 95%. Two studies included only elite athletes.

One study reported the combination of bone grafting and BMAC injection during screw fixation of 37 stress fractures in professional soccer players.[44] In this study, there were eight delayed unions (21.6%), although these all healed to complete union by 23 weeks. At final follow-up, there was one nonunion (3%).

We were unable to identify any published studies specifically designed to compare outcomes after internal fixation with and without bone grafting or BMAC. Hunt and Anderson reported their study of 21 athletes with refractures or previous nonunions of zone 2 and 3 fractures.[62] One patient received screw fixation, 12 patients received screw fixation plus bone grafting, and eight patients received screw fixation plus BMAC and demineralized bone matrix injection. The authors found that the time to return to sport was not affected by the use of bone graft versus BMAC and demineralized bone matrix.

None of these studies specifically reported increased risk of complications with the addition of a bone grafting or BMAC injection compared with screw fixation alone. However, donor site morbidity must be considered.

SUMMARY AND FUTURE DIRECTIONS

Based on this review of the history and nomenclature of proximal fifth metatarsal fractures, we advocate the use of a hybrid combination of the Lawrence and Botte and Torg classifications moving forward to allow for greater clarity in the literature.

In terms of treatment recommendations, the literature supports nonoperative treatment of zone 1 fractures in nonathletes. Studies demonstrate excellent outcomes in the treatment of zone 2 fractures either operatively or nonoperatively, suggesting that further research is needed in this area. The literature supports operative treatment of zone 3 stress fractures in nonathletes.

Excellent results have been found with internal fixation of zone 2 and 3 fractures with axial screws, plantar plating, and tension banding. When performing screw fixation, no single screw type has been found to be superior clinically. In additional to internal fixation, bone grafting and BMAC injection have been described with successful results; however, the optimal indications for their use remains unclear.

Although additional research is indicated in all of these areas, the answer to one important clinical question remains unclear: What is the optimal treatment of acute zone 2 fractures? A randomized controlled trial comparing nonoperative treatment protocols would be helpful in further answering this question. It is suspected that allowing patients to be weightbearing as tolerated as soon as their pain allows (typically 1–2 weeks) would allow for excellent results comparable with a more traditional protocol of nonweightbearing for 4 to 6 weeks. Based on the existing literature, we suspect that operative treatment may be avoided in many acute zone 2 fractures, particularly in nonathletes.

CLINICS CARE POINTS

What is a Jones fracture?
- A Jones fracture represents many fracture types depending on the article using this term.
- To promote clarity in the reporting of research results, a proximal fifth metatarsal fracture should be described by its anatomic zone (Lawrence and Botte classification).
- Zone 3 stress fractures should also be subclassified according to the Torg classification.
- The Torg classification should not be used to describe zone 1 or zone 2 proximal fifth metatarsal fractures, even in cases of nonunion (see **Table 1**).

Operative indications for operative treatment of zone 1 tuberosity fractures
- In the nonathlete, strong evidence supports nonoperative treatment of zone 1 fractures, regardless of fracture displacement, comminution, or intra-articular extension.
- Nonoperative treatment should consist of a period of weightbearing as tolerated in a removable support (eg, a walking boot, hard-sole shoe, or compressive dressing) rather than a cast.

Optimal treatment of acute zone 2 fractures
- There are few studies of true acute zone 2 fractures, and therefore there is insufficient evidence to support operative versus nonoperative treatment.

- Previously reported high rates of nonunion and refracture with nonoperative treatment of Jones fractures are not substantiated in studies where true acute zone 2 fractures are isolated.
- The existing data support operative treatment in cases where the patient requires faster return to sport or vigorous activities (eg, competitive athletes).
- When treating a patient nonoperatively, the need for nonweightbearing is unclear because the data demonstrate excellent rates of union with nonoperative treatment with a weightbearing as tolerated protocol (see **Table 2**).

Any role for nonoperative treatment of zone 3 fractures?

- Excellent union rates nearing 100% and low refracture rates have been found in multiple studies of surgical treatment of zone 3 fractures.
- The literature supports operative fixation of zone 3 fractures to decrease the risk for nonunion and refracture. However, the literature is of low quality (mostly retrospective case series) (see **Table 3**).

Screw fixation

- The largest diameter screw possible should be used for each patient when performing intramedullary screw fixation.
- There is considerable biomechanical evidence against the use of variable pitch headless compression screws, and there is no demonstrable clinical advantage to their use.
- Although biomechanical properties vary among screw types, clinical studies have not shown any definitive link between these parameters and clinical outcomes.

Bone graft and BMAC

- There are no high-quality studies demonstrating superior results with adjunctive use of bone grafting or BMAC during internal fixation of proximal fifth metatarsal fractures.
- Excellent overall union rates have been reported with bone graft and BMAC use in athletes, stress fractures, and revision cases.

DISCLOSURE

The authors declare no conflict of interest associated with this article.

REFERENCES

1. Richli WR, Rosenthal DI. Avulsion fracture of the fifth metatarsal: experimental study of pathomechanics. Am J Roentgenol 1984;143:889–91.
2. Smith JW, Arnoczky SP, Hersh A. The intraosseous blood supply of the fifth metatarsal: implications for proximal fracture healing. Foot Ankle 1992;13(3):143–52.
3. Shereff MJ, Yang QM, Kummer FJ, et al. Vascular anatomy of the fifth metatarsal. Foot Ankle Int 1991;11(6):350–3.
4. Lawrence SJ, Botte MJ. Jones' fractures and related fractures of the proximal fifth metatarsal. Foot Ankle Int 1993;14(6):358–65.
5. Petrisor BA, Ekrol I, Court-Brown C. The epidemiology of metatarsal fractures. Foot Ankle Int 2006;27(3):172–4.
6. Kane JM, Sandrowski K, Saffel H, et al. The epidemiology of fifth metatarsal fracture. Foot Ankle Spec 2015;8(5):354–9.
7. Kavanaugh JH, Brower TD, Mann RV. The Jones fracture revisited. J Bone Joint Surg Am 1978;60-A(6):776–82.
8. Porter DA. Fifth metatarsal Jones fractures in the athlete. Foot Ankle Int 2018; 39(2):250–8.

9. Le M, Anderson R. Zone II and III fifth metatarsal fractures in athletes. Curr Rev Musculoskelet Med 2017;10:86–93.
10. Pugliese M, De Meo D, Sinno E, et al. Can body mass index influence the fracture zone in the fifth metatarsal base? A retrospective review. J Foot Ankle Res 2020; 13(9):1–4.
11. Karnovsky SC, Rosenbaum AJ, DeSandis B, et al. Radiographic analysis of National Football League players' fifth metatarsal morphology relationship to proximal fifth metatarsal fracture risk. Foot Ankle Int 2019;40(3):318–22.
12. Yoho RM, Vardaxis V, Dikis J. A retrospective review of the effect of metatarsus adductus on healing time in the fifth metatarsal Jones fracture. Foot 2015;(25): 215–9.
13. O'Malley M, Desandis B, Allen A, et al. Operative treatment of fifth metatarsal Jones fractures (zones II and III) in the NBA. Foot Ankle Int 2016;37(5):488–500.
14. Raikin SM, Slenker N, Ratigan B. The association of a varus hindfoot and fracture of the fifth metatarsal metaphyseal-diaphyseal junction: the Jones fracture. Am J Sports Med 2008;36(7):1367–72.
15. Hetsroni I, Nyska M, Ben-Sira D, et al. Analysis of foot structure in athletes sustaining proximal fifth metatarsal stress fracture. Foot Ankle Int 2010;31(3):203–11.
16. Fujitaka K, Tanaka Y, Taniguchi A, et al. Pathoanatomy of the Jones fracture in male university soccer players. Am J Sports Med 2020;48(2):424–31.
17. Jones RI. Fracture of the base of the fifth metatarsal bone by indirect violence. Ann Surg 1902;35(6):697–700.
18. Stewart IM. Jones's fracture: fracture of base of fifth metatarsal. Clin Orthop 1960; 16:190–8.
19. Dameron TB. Fractures and anatomical variations of the proximal portion of the fifth metatarsal. J Bone Joint Surg Am 1975;57-A(6):788–92.
20. Torg JS, Balduini FC, Zelko RR, et al. Fractures of the base of the fifth metatarsal distal to the tuberosity. Classification and guidelines for non-surgical and surgical management. J Bone Joint Surg Am 1984;66-A(2):209–14.
21. Polzer H, Polzer S, Mutschler W, et al. Acute fractures to the proximal fifth metatarsal bone: development of classification and treatment recommendations based on the current evidence. Injury 2012;43:1626–32.
22. Nunley JA. Fractures of the base of the fifth metatarsal: the Jones fracture. Orthop Clin North Am 2001;32(1):171–80.
23. Rosenberg GA, Sferra JJ. Treatment strategies for acute fractures and nonunions of the proximal fifth metatarsal. J Am Acad Orthop Surg 2000;8(1):332–8.
24. Dameron TB. Fractures of the proximal fifth metatarsal: selecting the best treatment option. J Am Acad Orthop Surg 1995;3(2):110–4.
25. Quill GE. Fractures of the proximal fifth metatarsal. Orthop Clin North Am 1995; 26(2):353–61.
26. Pituckanotai K, Arirachakaran A, Piyapittayanun P, et al. Comparative outcomes of cast and removable support in fracture fifth metatarsal bone: systematic review and meta-analysis. J Foot Ankle Surg 2018;57(1):982–6.
27. Nishikawa DRC, Aires Duarte F, Saito GH, et al. Treatment of zone 1 fractures of the proximal fifth metatarsal with CAM-walker boot vs hard-soled shoes. Foot Ankle Int 2020;1–5. https://doi.org/10.1177/1071100720903259.
28. Lee TH, Lee JH, Chay SW, et al. Comparison of clinical and radiologic outcomes between non-operative and operative treatment in 5th metatarsal base fractures (zone 1). Injury 2016;47(1):1789–93.
29. Egol K, Walsh M, Rosenblatt K, et al. Avulsion fractures of the fifth metatarsal base: a prospective outcome study. Foot Ankle Int 2007;28(5):581–3.

30. Monteban P, van den Berg J, van Hees J, et al. The outcome of proximal fifth metatarsal fractures: redefining treatment strategies. Eur J Trauma Emerg Surg 2018;44(1):727–34.

31. Baumbach SF, Prall WC, Kramer M, et al. Functional treatment for fractures to the base of the 5th metatarsal: influence of fracture location and fracture characteristics. BMC Musculoskelet Disord 2017;18(1):534.

32. Baumbach SF, Urresti-Gundlach M, Böcker W, et al. Results of functional treatment of epi-metaphyseal fractures of the base of the fifth metatarsal. Foot Ankle Int 2020;41(6):666–73.

33. Biz C, Zamperetti M, Gasparella A, et al. Early radiographic and clinical outcomes of minimally displaced proximal fifth metatarsal fractures: cast vs functional bandage. Muscles Ligaments Tendons J 2017;7(3):532–40.

34. Rettig AC, Shelbourne KD, Wilckens J. The surgical treatment of symptomatic nonunions of the proximal (metaphyseal) fifth metatarsal in athletes. Am J Sports Med 1992;20(1):50–4.

35. Ritchie JD, Shaver JC, Anderson RB, et al. Excision of symptomatic nonunions of proximal fifth metatarsal avulsion fractures in elite athletes. Am J Sports Med 2011;39(11):2466–9.

36. Chuckpaiwong B, Queen RM, Easley ME, et al. Distinguishing Jones and proximal diaphyseal fractures of the fifth metatarsal. Clin Orthop Relat Res 2008; 466:1966–70.

37. Marecek GS, Earhart JS, Croom WP, et al. Treatment of acute Jones fractures without weightbearing restriction. J Foot Ankle Surg 2016;55:961–4.

38. Lareau CR, Hsu AR, Anderson RB. Return to play in National Football League players after operative Jones fracture treatment. Foot Ankle Int 2016;37(1):8–16.

39. Zelko RR, Torg JS, Rachun A. Proximal diaphyseal fractures of the fifth metatarsal: treatment of the fractures and their complications in athletes. Am J Sports Med 1979;7(2):95–101.

40. Delee JC, Evans JP, Julian J. Stress fracture of the fifth metatarsal. Am J Sports Med 1983;11(5):349–53.

41. Fernández Fairen M, Guillen J, Busto JM, et al. Fractures of the fifth metatarsal in basketball players. Knee Surg Sports Traumatol Arthrosc 1999;7:373–7.

42. Porter DA, Duncan M, Meyer SJF. Fifth metatarsal Jones fracture fixation with a 4.5-mm cannulated stainless steel screw in the competitive and recreational athlete: a clinical and radiographic evaluation. Am J Sports Med 2005;33(5): 726–33.

43. Portland G, Kelikian A, Kodros S. Acute surgical management of Jones' fractures. Foot Ankle Int 2003;24(11):829–33.

44. Miller D, Marsland D, Jones M, et al. Early return to playing professional football following fixation of 5th metatarsal stress fractures may lead to delayed union but does not increase the risk of long-term non-union. Knee Surg Sports Traumatol Arthrosc 2019;27:2796–801.

45. Young KW, Kim JS, Lee HS, et al. Operative results of plantar plating for fifth metatarsal stress fracture. Foot Ankle Int 2020;1–9. https://doi.org/10.1177/1071100719895273.

46. Lee KT, Park YU, Jegal H, et al. Prognostic classification of fifth metatarsal stress fracture using plantar gap. Foot Ankle Int 2013;34(5):691–6.

47. Lee KT, Park YU, Young KW, et al. The plantar gap: another prognostic factor for fifth metatarsal stress fracture. Am J Sports Med 2011;39(10):2206–11.

48. DeSandis B, Murphy C, Rosenbaum A, et al. Multiplanar CT analysis of fifth meta-tarsal morphology: implications for operative management of zone II fractures. Foot Ankle Int 2016;37(5):528–36.

49. Ochenjele G, Ho B, Switaj PJ, et al. Radiographic study of the fifth metatarsal for optimal intramedullary screw fixation of Jones fracture. Foot Ankle Int 2015;36(3): 293–301.

50. Roche AJ, Calder JDF. Treatment and return to sport following a Jones fracture of the fifth metatarsal: a systematic review. Knee Surg Sports Traumatol Arthrosc 2013;21:1307–15.

51. Porter DA, Dobslaw R, Duncan M. Comparison of 4.5- and 5.5-mm cannulated stainless steel screws for fifth metatarsal Jones fracture fixation. Foot Ankle Int 2009;30(1):27–33.

52. Carreira DS, Sandilands SM. Radiographic factors and effect of fifth metatarsal Jones and diaphyseal stress fractures on participation in the NFL. Foot Ankle Int 2013;34(4):518–22.

53. Jastifer J, McCullough KA. Fatigue bending strength of Jones fracture specific screw fixation. Foot Ankle Int 2018;39(4):493–9.

54. Kelly IP, Glisson RR, Fink C, et al. Intramedullary screw fixation of Jones fractures. Foot Ankle Int 2001;22(7):585–9.

55. Pietropaoli MP, Wnorowski DC, Werner FW, et al. Intramedullary screw fixation of Jones fractures: a biomechanical study. Foot Ankle Int 1999;20(9):560–3.

56. DeVries JG, Cuttica DJ, Hyer CF. Cannulated screw fixation of Jones fifth meta-tarsal fractures: a comparison of titanium and stainless steel screw fixation. J Foot Ankle Surg 2011;50:207–12.

57. Nagao M, Saita Y, Kameda S, et al. Headless compression screw fixation of Jones fractures: an outcomes study in Japanese athletes. Am J Sports Med 2012;40(11):2578–82.

58. Orr JD, Glisson RR, Nunley JA. Jones fracture fixation: a biomechanical compar-ison of partially threaded screws versus tapered variable pitch screws. Am J Sports Med 2012;40(3):691–8.

59. Nunley JA, Glisson RR. A new option for intramedullary fixation of Jones fractures: the Charlotte™ Carolina™ Jones fracture system. Foot Ankle Int 2008;29(12): 1216–21.

60. Metzl J, Olson K, Davis WH, et al. A clinical and radiographic comparison of two hardware systems used to treat Jones fracture of the fifth metatarsal. Foot Ankle Int 2013;34(7):956–61.

61. Bernstein DT, Mitchell RJ, McCulloch PC, et al. Treatment of proximal fifth meta-tarsal fractures and refractures with plantar plating in elite athletes. Foot Ankle Int 2018;39(12):1410–5.

62. Hunt KJ, Anderson RB. Treatment of Jones fracture nonunions and refractures in the elite athlete. Am J Sports Med 2011;39(9):1948–54.

63. Seidenstricker CL, Blahous EG, Bouché RT, et al. Plate fixation with autogenous calcaneal dowel grafting proximal fourth and fifth metatarsal fractures: technique and case series. J Foot Ankle Surg 2017;56:975–81.

64. Larson CM, Almekinders LC, Taft TN, et al. Intramedullary screw fixation of Jones fractures: analysis of failure. Am J Sports Med 2002;30(1):55–60.

UNITED STATES POSTAL SERVICE®

Statement of Ownership, Management, and Circulation
(All Periodicals Publications Except Requester Publications)

1. Publication Title: FOOT AND ANKLE CLINICS OF NORTH AMERICA

2. Publication Number: 016 - 368

3. Filing Date: 9/18/2020

4. Issue Frequency: MAR, JUN, SEP, DEC

5. Number of Issues Published Annually: 4

6. Annual Subscription Price: $340.00

7. Complete Mailing Address of Known Office of Publication (Not printer) (Street, city, county, state, and ZIP+4®)
ELSEVIER INC.
230 Park Avenue, Suite 800
New York, NY 10169

Contact Person: Malathi Samayan
Telephone (Include area code): 91-44-4299-4507

8. Complete Mailing Address of Headquarters or General Business Office of Publisher (Not printer)
ELSEVIER INC.
230 Park Avenue, Suite 800
New York, NY 10169

9. Full Names and Complete Mailing Addresses of Publisher, Editor, and Managing Editor (Do not leave blank)

Publisher (Name and complete mailing address)
DOLORES MELONI, ELSEVIER INC.
1600 JOHN F KENNEDY BLVD. SUITE 1800
PHILADELPHIA, PA 19103-2899

Editor (Name and complete mailing address)
LAUREN BOYLE, ELSEVIER INC.
1600 JOHN F KENNEDY BLVD. SUITE 1800
PHILADELPHIA, PA 19103-2899

Managing Editor (Name and complete mailing address)
PATRICK MANLEY, ELSEVIER INC.
1600 JOHN F KENNEDY BLVD. SUITE 1800
PHILADELPHIA, PA 19103-2899

10. Owner (Do not leave blank. If the publication is owned by a corporation, give the name and address of the corporation immediately followed by the names and addresses of all stockholders owning or holding 1 percent or more of the total amount of stock. If not owned by a corporation, give the names and addresses of the individual owners. If owned by a partnership or other unincorporated firm, give its name and address as well as those of each individual owner. If the publication is published by a nonprofit organization, give its name and address.)

Full Name	Complete Mailing Address
WHOLLY OWNED SUBSIDIARY OF REED/ELSEVIER, US HOLDINGS	1600 JOHN F KENNEDY BLVD. SUITE 1800 PHILADELPHIA, PA 19103-2899

11. Known Bondholders, Mortgagees, and Other Security Holders Owning or Holding 1 Percent or More of Total Amount of Bonds, Mortgages, or Other Securities. If none, check box ▶ ☐ None

Full Name	Complete Mailing Address
N/A	

12. Tax Status (For completion by nonprofit organizations authorized to mail at nonprofit rates) (Check one)
The purpose, function, and nonprofit status of this organization and the exempt status for federal income tax purposes:
☒ Has Not Changed During Preceding 12 Months
☐ Has Changed During Preceding 12 Months (Publisher must submit explanation of change with this statement)

PS Form **3526**, July 2014 [Page 1 of 4 (see instructions page 4)] PSN 7530-01-000-9931   PRIVACY NOTICE: See our privacy policy on www.usps.com.

---

13. Publication Title: FOOT AND ANKLE CLINICS OF NORTH AMERICA

14. Issue Date for Circulation Data Below: JUNE 2020

15. Extent and Nature of Circulation

		Average No. Copies Each Issue During Preceding 12 Months	No. Copies of Single Issue Published Nearest to Filing Date
a. Total Number of Copies (Net press run)		266	232
b. Paid Circulation (By Mail and Outside the Mail)	(1) Mailed Outside-County Paid Subscriptions Stated on PS Form 3541 (Include paid distribution above nominal rate, advertiser's proof copies, and exchange copies)	160	150
	(2) Mailed In-County Paid Subscriptions Stated on PS Form 3541 (Include paid distribution above nominal rate, advertiser's proof copies, and exchange copies)	0	0
	(3) Paid Distribution Outside the Mails Including Sales Through Dealers and Carriers, Street Vendors, Counter Sales, and Other Paid Distribution Outside USPS®	78	65
	(4) Paid Distribution by Other Classes of Mail Through the USPS (e.g., First-Class Mail®)	0	0
c. Total Paid Distribution [Sum of 15b (1), (2), (3), and (4)]	▶	238	215
d. Free or Nominal Rate Distribution (By Mail and Outside the Mail)	(1) Free or Nominal Rate Outside-County Copies included on PS Form 3541	13	3
	(2) Free or Nominal Rate In-County Copies Included on PS Form 3541	0	0
	(3) Free or Nominal Rate Copies Mailed at Other Classes Through the USPS (e.g., First-Class Mail)	0	0
	(4) Free or Nominal Rate Distribution Outside the Mail (Carriers or other means)	0	0
e. Total Free or Nominal Rate Distribution (Sum of 15d (1), (2), (3) and (4))	▶	13	3
f. Total Distribution (Sum of 15c and 15e)	▶	251	218
g. Copies not Distributed (See Instructions to Publishers #4 (page 83))	▶	15	14
h. Total (Sum of 15f and g)	▶	266	232
i. Percent Paid (15c divided by 15f times 100)		94.82%	98.62%

* If you are claiming electronic copies, go to line 16 on page 3. If you are not claiming electronic copies, skip to line 17 on page 3.

16. Electronic Copy Circulation

		Average No. Copies Each Issue During Preceding 12 Months	No. Copies of Single Issue Published Nearest to Filing Date
a. Paid Electronic Copies	▶		
b. Total Paid Print Copies (Line 15c) + Paid Electronic Copies (Line 16a)	▶		
c. Total Print Distribution (Line 15f) + Paid Electronic Copies (Line 16a)	▶		
d. Percent Paid (Both Print & Electronic Copies) (16b divided by 16c × 100)	▶		

☒ I certify that 50% of all my distributed copies (electronic and print) are paid above a nominal price.

17. Publication of Statement of Ownership
☒ If the publication is a general publication, publication of this statement is required. Will be printed in the DECEMBER 2020 issue of this publication.
☐ Publication not required.

18. Signature and Title of Editor, Publisher, Business Manager, or Owner
Malathi Samayan   **Date** 9/18/2020

Malathi Samayan - Distribution Controller

I certify that all information furnished on this form is true and complete. I understand that anyone who furnishes false or misleading information on this form or who omits material or information requested on the form may be subject to criminal sanctions (including fines and imprisonment) and/or civil sanctions (including civil penalties).

PS Form **3526**, July 2014 (Page 3 of 4)   PRIVACY NOTICE: See our privacy policy on www.usps.com

Moving?

Make sure your subscription moves with you!

To notify us of your new address, find your **Clinics Account Number** (located on your mailing label above your name), and contact customer service at:

Email: journalscustomerservice-usa@elsevier.com

800-654-2452 (subscribers in the U.S. & Canada)
314-447-8871 (subscribers outside of the U.S. & Canada)

Fax number: 314-447-8029

Elsevier Health Sciences Division
Subscription Customer Service
3251 Riverport Lane
Maryland Heights, MO 63043

ELSEVIER